J. P. Marques de Sá

Pattern Recognition

Springer-Verlag Berlin Heidelberg GmbH

J. P. Marques de Sá

Pattern Recognition

Concepts, Methods and Applications

With 197 Figures

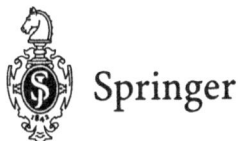 Springer

Prof. Joaquim P. Marques de Sá
Universidade do Porto
Faculdade de Engenharia
Rua Dr. Roberto Frias
4200-465 Porto
Portugal
e-mail: jmsa@fe.up.pt

Additional material to this book can be downloaded from http://extras.springer.com

ISBN 978-3-642-62677-7

Cip data applied for

Die Deutsche Bibliothek - Cip-Einheitsaufnahme
Sa, Joaquim P. Marques de:
Pattern recognition : concepts, methods and applications / J. P. Marques de Sa.
- Berlin ; Heidelberg ; New York ; Barcelona; Hong Kong ; London ; Milan ;
Paris ; Singapore ; Tokyo : Springer, 2001
  ISBN 978-3-642-62677-7   ISBN 978-3-642-56651-6 (eBook)
  DOI 10.1007/978-3-642-56651-6

http://www.springer.de
© Springer-Verlag Berlin Heidelberg 2001
Originally published by Springer-Verlag Berlin Heidelberg New York in 2001

Typesetting: data delivered by author
Cover design: de'blik, Berlin
Printed on acid free paper   SPIN: 10844202   62/3020/M – 5 4 3 2 1 0

To
my wife Wiesje
and our son Carlos,
lovingly.

Preface

Pattern recognition currently comprises a vast body of methods supporting the development of numerous applications in many different areas of activity. The generally recognized relevance of pattern recognition methods and techniques lies, for the most part, in the general trend of "intelligent" task emulation, which has definitely pervaded our daily life. Robot assisted manufacture, medical diagnostic systems, forecast of economic variables, exploration of Earth's resources, and analysis of satellite data are just a few examples of activity fields where this trend applies. The pervasiveness of pattern recognition has boosted the number of task-specific methodologies and enriched the number of links with other disciplines. As counterbalance to this dispersive tendency there have been, more recently, new theoretical developments that are bridging together many of the classical pattern recognition methods and presenting a new perspective of their links and inner workings.

This book has its origin in an introductory course on pattern recognition taught at the Electrical and Computer Engineering Department, Oporto University. From the initial core of this course, the book grew with the intent of presenting a comprehensive and articulated view of pattern recognition methods combined with the intent of clarifying practical issues with the aid of examples and applications to real-life data. The book is primarily addressed to undergraduate and graduate students attending pattern recognition courses of engineering and computer science curricula. In addition to engineers or applied mathematicians, it is also common for professionals and researchers from other areas of activity to apply pattern recognition methods, e.g. physicians, biologists, geologists and economists. The book includes real-life applications and presents matters in a way that reflects a concern for making them interesting to a large audience, namely to non-engineers who need to apply pattern recognition techniques in their own work, or who happen to be involved in interdisciplinary projects employing such techniques.

Pattern recognition involves mathematical models of objects described by their features or attributes. It also involves operations on abstract representations of what is meant by our common sense idea of similarity or proximity among objects. The mathematical formalisms, models and operations used, depend on the type of problem we need to solve. In this sense, pattern recognition is "mathematics put into action". Teaching pattern recognition without getting the feedback and insight provided by practical examples and applications is a quite limited experience, to say the least. We have, therefore, provided a CD with the book, including real-life data that the reader can use to practice the taught methods or simply to follow the explained examples. The software tools used in the book are quite popular, in the academic environment and elsewhere, so closely following the examples and checking the presented results should not constitute a major difficulty. The CD also includes a set of complementary software tools for those topics where the availability of such tools is definitely a problem. Therefore, from the beginning of the book, the reader should be able to follow the taught methods with the guidance of practical applications, without having to do any programming, and concentrate solely on the correct application of the learned concepts.

The main organization of the book is quite classical. Chapter 1 presents the basic notions of pattern recognition, including the three main approaches (statistical, neural networks and structural) and important practical issues. Chapter 2 discusses the discrimination of patterns with decision functions and representation issues in the feature space. Chapter 3 describes data clustering and dimensional reduction techniques. Chapter 4 explains the statistical-based methods, either using distribution models or not. The feature selection and classifier evaluation topics are also explained. Chapter 5 describes the neural network approach and presents its main paradigms. The network evaluation and complexity issues deserve special attention, both in classification and in regression tasks. Chapter 6 explains the structural analysis methods, including both syntactic and non-syntactic approaches. Description of the datasets and the software tools included in the CD are presented in Appendices A and B.

Links among the several topics inside each chapter, as well as across chapters, are clarified whenever appropriate, and more recent topics, such as support vector machines, data mining and the use of neural networks in structural matching, are included. Also, topics with great practical importance, such as the dimensionality ratio issue, are presented in detail and with reference to recent findings.

All pattern recognition methods described in the book start with a presentation of the concepts involved. These are clarified with simple examples and adequate illustrations. The mathematics involved in the concepts and the description of the methods is explained with a concern for keeping the notation cluttering to a minimum and using a consistent symbology. When the methods have been sufficiently explained, they are applied to real-life data in order to obtain the needed grasp of the important practical issues.

Starting with chapter 2, every chapter includes a set of exercises at the end. A large proportion of these exercises use the datasets supplied with the book, and constitute computer experiments typical of a pattern recognition design task. Other exercises are intended to broaden the understanding of the presented examples, testing the level of the reader's comprehension.

Some background in probability and statistics, linear algebra and discrete mathematics is needed for full understanding of the taught matters. In particular, concerning statistics, it is assumed that the reader is conversant with the main concepts and methods involved in statistical inference tests.

All chapters include a list of bibliographic references that support all explanations presented and constitute, in some cases, pointers for further reading. References to background subjects are also included, namely in the area of statistics.

The CD datasets and tools are for the Microsoft Windows system (95 and beyond). Many of these datasets and tools are developed in Microsoft Excel and it should not be a problem to run them in any of the Microsoft Windows versions.

The other tools require an installation following the standard Microsoft Windows procedure. The description of these tools is given in Appendix B. With these descriptions and the examples included in the text, the reader should not have, in principle, any particular difficulty in using them.

Acknowledgements

In the preparation of this book I have received support and encouragement from several persons. My foremost acknowledgement of deep gratitude goes to Professor Willem van Meurs, researcher at the Biomedical Engineering Research Center and Professor at the Applied Mathematics Department, both of the Oporto University, who gave me invaluable support by reviewing the text and offering many stimulating comments. The datasets used in the book include contributions from several people: Professor C. Abreu Lima, Professor Aurélio Campilho, Professor João Bernardes, Professor Joaquim Góis, Professor Jorge Barbosa, Dr. Jacques Jossinet, Dr. Diogo A. Campos, Dr. Ana Matos and João Ribeiro. The software tools included in the CD have contributions from Eng. A. Garrido, Dr. Carlos Felgueiras, Eng. F. Sousa, Nuno André and Paulo Sousa. All these contributions of datasets and software tools are acknowledged in Appendices A and B, respectively. Professor Pimenta Monteiro helped me review the structural pattern recognition topics. Eng. Fernando Sereno helped me with the support vector machine experiments and with the review of the neural networks chapter. João Ribeiro helped me with the collection and interpretation of economics data. My deepest thanks to all of them. Finally, my thanks also to Jacqueline Wilson, who performed a thorough review of the formal aspects of the book.

Joaquim P. Marques de Sá
May, 2001
Oporto University, Portugal

Contents

Symbols and Abbreviations

Global Symbols

d	number of features or primitives
c	number of classes or clusters
n	number of patterns
w	number of weights
ω_i	class or cluster i, $i=1, \dots, c$
n_i	number of patterns of class or cluster ω_i
w_i	weight i
w_0	bias
E	approximation error
X	pattern set
Ω	class set

Mathematical Symbols

x	variable
$x^{(r)}$	value of x at iteration r
x_i	i-th component of vector or string $\mathbf{x}$
$x_{k,i}$	i-th component of vector $\mathbf{x}_k$
$\mathbf{x}$	vector (column) or string
$\mathbf{x}'$	transpose vector (row)
$\Delta\mathbf{x}$	vector $\mathbf{x}$ increment
$\mathbf{x}'\mathbf{y}$	inner product of $\mathbf{x}$ and $\mathbf{y}$
a_{ij}	i-th row, j-th column element of matrix $\mathbf{A}$
$\mathbf{A}$	matrix
$\mathbf{A}'$	transpose of matrix $\mathbf{A}$
$\mathbf{A}^{-1}$	inverse of matrix $\mathbf{A}$
$|\mathbf{A}|$	determinant of matrix $\mathbf{A}$
$\mathbf{A}^*$	pseudo inverse of matrix $\mathbf{A}$
$\mathbf{I}$	identity matrix
$k!$	factorial of k, $k!= k(k-1)(k-2)...2.1$
$C(n, k)$	combinations of n elements taken k at a time
$\left.\dfrac{\partial E}{\partial \mathbf{w}}\right|_{\mathbf{w}^*}$	derivative of E relative to $\mathbf{w}$ evaluated at $\mathbf{w}^*$

$g(x)$	function g evaluated at x
erf	error function
ln	natural logarithm function
$\log_2$	logarithm in base 2 function
sgn	sign function
$\Re$	real numbers set
η	learning rate
λ_i	eigenvalue i
λ	null string
$|x|$	absolute value of x
$\|\ \|$	norm
$\Rightarrow$	implies
$\rightarrow$	converges to
$\mapsto$	produces

Statistical Symbols

m	sample mean
s	sample standard deviation
$\mathbf{m}$	sample mean vector
$\mathbf{C}$	sample covariance matrix
$\boldsymbol{\mu}$	mean vector
$\boldsymbol{\Sigma}$	covariance matrix
$E[\mathbf{x}]$	expected value of $\mathbf{x}$
$E[\mathbf{x} \mid \mathbf{y}]$	expected value of $\mathbf{x}$ given $\mathbf{y}$ (conditional expectation)
$N(m,s)$	normal distribution with mean m and standard deviation s
$P(\mathbf{x})$	discrete probability of random vector $\mathbf{x}$
$P(\omega_i|\mathbf{x})$	discrete conditional probability of ω_i given $\mathbf{x}$
$p(\mathbf{x})$	probability density function p evaluated at $\mathbf{x}$
$p(\mathbf{x}|\omega_i)$	conditional probability density function p evaluated at $\mathbf{x}$ given ω_i
Pe	probability of misclassification (error)
$\hat{Pe}$	estimate of Pe
Pc	probability of correct classification

Abbreviations

CAM	Content Addressed Memory
CART	Classification And Regression Trees
ECG	Electrocardiogram
ERM	Empirical Risk Minimization

ERM   Empirical Risk Minimization
FHR   Foetal Heart Rate
IPS   Intelligent Problem Solver (*Statistica*)
KFM   Kohonen's Feature Map
k-NN   k - Nearest Neighbours
ISODATA   Iterative Self-Organizing Data Analysis Technique
LMS   Least Mean Square
MLP   Multi-layer perceptron
PAC   Probably Approximately Correct
pdf   Probability Density Function
PDL   Picture Description Language
PR   Pattern Recognition
RBF   Radial Basis Functions
RMS   Root Mean Square
ROC   Receiver Operating Characteristic
SRM   Structural Risk Minimization
SVM   Support Vector Machine
UPGMA   Un-weighted Pair-Group Method using arithmetic Averages
UWGMA   Un-weighted Within-Group Method using arithmetic Averages
VC   Vapnik-Chervonenkis (dimension)
XOR   Exclusive OR

Tradenames

Matlab   The MathWorks, Inc.
Excel   Microsoft Corporation
SPSS   SPSS, Inc.
Statistica   Statsoft, Inc.
Windows   Microsoft Corporation

1 Basic Notions

1.1 Object Recognition

Object recognition is a task performed daily by living beings and is inherent to their ability and necessity to deal with the environment. It is performed in the most varied circumstances – navigation towards food sources, migration, identification of predators, identification of mates, etc. - with remarkable efficiency. Recognizing objects is considered here in a broad cognitive sense and may consist of a very simple task, like when a micro-organism flees from an environment with inadequate pH, or refer to tasks demanding non-trivial qualities of inference, description and interpretation, for instance when a human has to fetch a pair of scissors from the second drawer of a cupboard, counting from below.

The development of methods capable of emulating the most varied forms of object recognition has evolved along with the need for building "intelligent" automated systems, the main trend of today's technology in industry and in other fields of activity as well. In these systems objects are represented in a suitable way for the type of processing they are subject to. Such representations are called *patterns*. In what follows we use the words object and pattern interchangeably with similar meaning.

Pattern Recognition (PR) is the scientific discipline dealing with methods for object description and classification. Since the early times of computing the design and implementation of algorithms emulating the human ability to describe and classify objects has been found a most intriguing and challenging task. Pattern recognition is therefore a fertile area of research, with multiple links to many other disciplines, involving professionals from several areas.

Applications of pattern recognition systems and techniques are numerous and cover a broad scope of activities. We enumerate only a few examples referring to several professional activities:

Agriculture:
> **Crop analysis**
> **Soil evaluation**

Astronomy:
> **Analysis of telescopic images**
> **Automated spectroscopy**

Biology:
> **Automated cytology**
> **Properties of chromosomes**
> **Genetic studies**

Civil administration:

> **Traffic analysis and control**
> **Assessment of urban growth**

Economy:

> **Stocks exchange forecast**
> **Analysis of entrepreneurial performance**

Engineering:

> **Fault detection in manufactured products**
> **Character recognition**
> **Speech recognition**
> **Automatic navigation systems**
> **Pollution analysis**

Geology:

> **Classification of rocks**
> **Estimation of mining resources**
> **Analysis of geo-resources using satellite images**
> **Seismic analysis**

Medicine:

> **Analysis of electrocardiograms**
> **Analysis of electroencephalograms**
> **Analysis of medical images**

Military:

> **Analysis of aerial photography**
> **Detection and classification of radar and sonar signals**
> **Automatic target recognition**

Security:

> **Identification of fingerprints**
> **Surveillance and alarm systems**

As can be inferred from the above examples the patterns to be analysed and recognized can be signals (e.g. electrocardiographic signals), images (e.g. aerial photos) or plain tables of values (e.g. stock exchange rates).

1.2 Pattern Similarity and PR Tasks

A fundamental notion in pattern recognition, independent of whatever approach we may follow, is the notion of *similarity*. We recognize two objects as being similar because they have similarly valued common attributes. Often the similarity is stated in a more abstract sense, not among objects but between an object and a target *concept*. For instance, we recognise an object as being an apple because it corresponds, in its features, to the idealized image, concept or *prototype*, we may have of an apple, i.e., the object is similar to that concept and dissimilar from others, for instance from an orange.

Assessing the similarity of patterns is strongly related to the proposed pattern recognition task as described in the following.

1.2.1 Classification Tasks

When evaluating the similarity among objects we resort to *features* or *attributes* that are of distinctive nature. Imagine that we wanted to design a system for discriminating green apples from oranges. Figure 1.1 illustrates possible representations of the prototypes "green apple" and "orange". In this discrimination task we may use as obvious distinctive features the colour and the shape, represented in an adequate way.

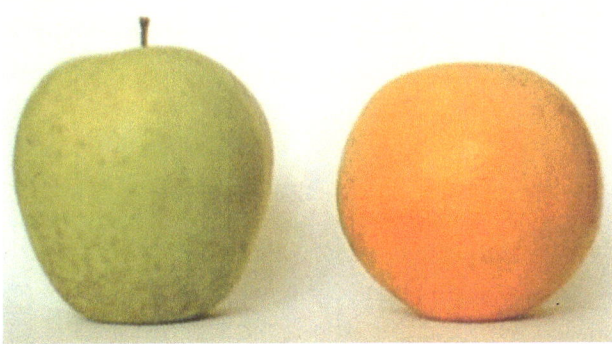

Figure 1.1. Possible representations of the prototypes "green apple" and "orange".

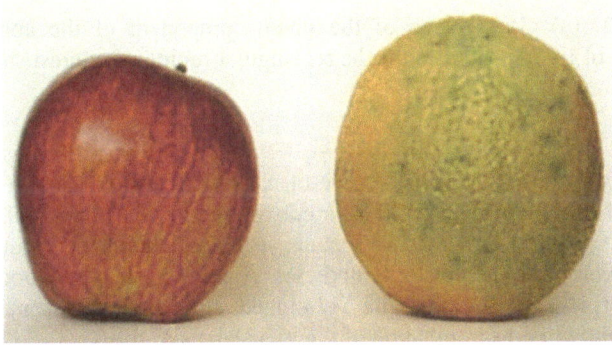

Figure 1.2. Examples of "red apple" and "greenish orange" to be characterized by shape and colour features.

In order to obtain a numeric representation of the *colour* feature we may start by splitting the image of the objects into the red-green-blue components. Next we may, for instance, select a central region of interest in the image and compute, for that region, the ratio of the maximum histogram locations for the red and green components in the respective ranges (usually [0, 255]; 0=no colour, 255=full colour). Figure 1.3 shows the grey image corresponding to the green component of the apple and the light intensity histogram for a rectangular region of interest. The maximum of the histogram corresponds to 186. This means that the green intensity value occurring most often is 186. For the red component we would obtain the value 150. The ratio of these values is 1.24 revealing the predominance of the green colour vs. the red colour.

In order to obtain a numeric representation of the *shape* feature we may, for instance, measure the distance, away from the top, of the maximum width of the object and normalize this distance by the height, i.e., computing x/h, with x, h shown in Figure 1.3a. In this case, x/h=0.37. Note that we are assuming that the objects are in a standard upright position.

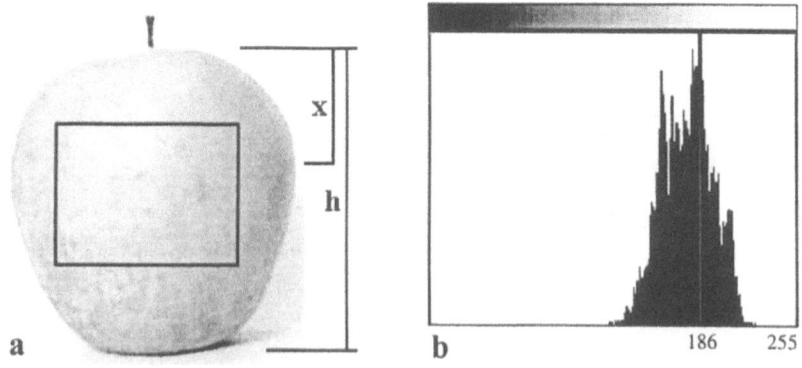

Figure 1.3. (a) Grey image of the green component of the apple image; (b) Histogram of light intensities for the rectangular region of interest shown in (a).

If we have made a sensible choice of prototypes we expect that representative samples of green apples and oranges correspond to clusters of points around the prototypes in the 2-dimensional feature space, as shown in Figure 1.4a by the curves representing the cluster boundaries. Also, if we made a good choice of the features, it is expected that the mentioned clusters are reasonably separated, therefore allowing discrimination of the two classes of fruits.

The PR task of assigning an object to a class is said to be a *classification task*. From a mathematical point of view it is convenient in classification tasks to represent a pattern by a vector, which is 2-dimensional in the present case:

$$\mathbf{x} = \begin{bmatrix} x_1 \\ x_2 \end{bmatrix} \equiv \begin{bmatrix} colour \\ shape \end{bmatrix}.$$

For the green apple prototype we have therefore:

$$\mathbf{x}_{green\ apple} = \begin{bmatrix} 1.24 \\ 0.37 \end{bmatrix}.$$

The points corresponding to the feature vectors of the prototypes are represented by a square and a circle, respectively for the green apple and the orange, in Figure 1.4.

Let us consider a machine designed to separate green apples from oranges using the described features. A piece of fruit is presented to the machine, its features are computed and correspond to the point $\mathbf{x}$ (Figure 1.4a) in the colour-shape plane. The machine, using the feature values as inputs, then has to decide if it is a green apple or an orange. A reasonable decision is based on the Euclidian distance of the point $\mathbf{x}$ from the prototypes, i.e., for the machine the similarity is a *distance* and in this case it would decide "green apple". The output of the machine is in this case any two-valued variable, e.g., 0 corresponding to green apples and 1 corresponding to oranges. Such a machine is called a *classifier*.

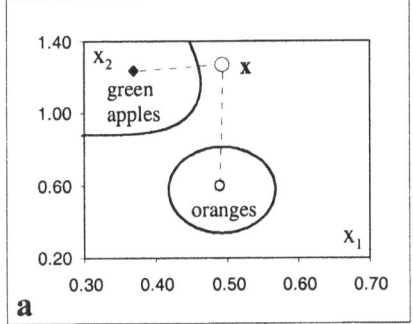 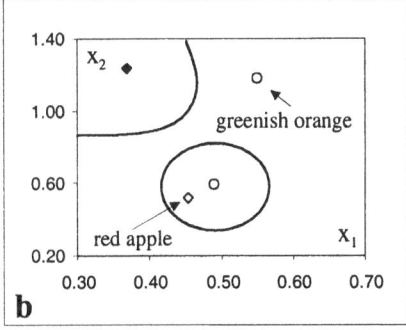

Figure 1.4. (a) Green apples and oranges in the feature space; (b) A red apple "resembling" an orange and a problematic greenish orange.

Imagine that our classifier receives as inputs the features of the red apple and the greenish orange presented in Figure 1.2. The feature vectors correspond to the points shown in Figure 1.4b. The red apple is wrongly classified as an orange since it is much closer to the orange prototype than to the green apple prototype. This is not a surprise since, after all, the classifier is being used for an object clearly outside its scope. As for the greenish orange its feature vector is nearly at equal distance from both prototypes and its classification is problematic. If we use, instead of the Euclidian distance, another distance measure that weighs more heavily vertical deviations than horizontal deviations, the greenish orange would also be wrongly classified.

In general practice pattern classification systems are not flawless and we may expect errors due to several causes:

− The features used are inadequate or insufficient. For instance, the classification of the problematic greenish orange would probably improve by using an additional texture feature measuring the degree of surface roughness.
− The pattern samples used to design the classifier are not sufficiently representative. For instance, if our intention is to discriminate apples from oranges we should have to include in the apples sample a representative variety of apples, including the red ones as well.
− The classifier is not efficient enough in separating the classes. For instance, an inefficient distance measure or inadequate prototypes are being used.
− There is an intrinsic overlap of the classes that no classifier can resolve.

In this book we will focus our attention on the aspects that relate to the selection of adequate features and to the design of efficient classifiers. Concerning the initial choice of features it is worth noting that this is more an art than a science and, as with any art, it is improved by experimentation and practice. Besides the appropriate choice of features and similarity measures, there are also other aspects responsible for the high degree of classifying accuracy in humans. Aspects such as the use of contextual information and advanced knowledge structures fall mainly in the domain of an artificial intelligence course and will be not dealt with in this book. Even the human recognition of objects is not always flawless and contextual information risks classifying a greenish orange as a lemon if it lies in a basket with lemons.

1.2.2 Regression Tasks

We consider now another type of task, directly related to the cognitive inference process. We observe such a process when animals start a migration based on climate changes and physiological changes of their internal biological cycles. In daily life, inference is an important tool since it guides decision optimisation. Well-known examples are, for instance, keeping the right distance from the vehicle driving ahead in a road, forecasting weather conditions, predicting firm revenue of investment and assessing loan granting based on economic variables.

Let us consider an example consisting of forecasting firm A share value in the stock exchange market, based on past information about: the share values of firm A and of other firms; the currency exchange rates; the interest rate. In this situation we want to predict the value of a variable based on a sequence of past values of the same and other variables, which in the one-day forecast situation of Figure 1.5 are: r_A, r_B, r_C, Euro-USD rate, Interest rate for 6 months.

As can be appreciated this time-series prediction task is an example of a broader class of tasks known in mathematics as function approximation or *regression task*. A system providing the regression solution will usually make forecasts (black circles in Figure 1.5) somewhat deviated from the true value (curve, idem). The difference between the predicted value and the true value, also known as *target value*, constitutes a *prediction error*. Our aim is a solution yielding predicted values *similar* to the targets, i.e., with small errors.

As a matter of fact regression tasks can also be cast under the form of classification tasks. We can divide the dependent variable domain (r_A) into sufficiently small intervals and interpret the regression solution as a classification solution, where a correct classification corresponds to a predicted value falling inside the correct interval ≡ class. In this sense we can view the sequence of values as a feature vector, $[r_A \quad r_B \quad r_C$ Euro-USD-rate   Interest-rate-6-months]' and again, we express the similarity in terms of a distance, now referred to the predicted and target values (classifications). Note that a coarse regression could be: predict whether or not $r_a(t)$ is larger than the previous value, $r_a(t\text{-}1)$. This is equivalent to a 2-class classification problem with the class labelling function $\text{sgn}(r_a(t)\text{-} r_a(t\text{-}1))$.

Sometimes regression tasks are also performed as part of a classification. For instance, in the recognition of living tissue a merit factor is often used by physicians, depending on several features such as colour, texture, light reflectance and density of blood vessels. An automatic tissue recognition system attempts then to regress the merit factor evaluated by the human expert, prior to establishing a tissue classification.

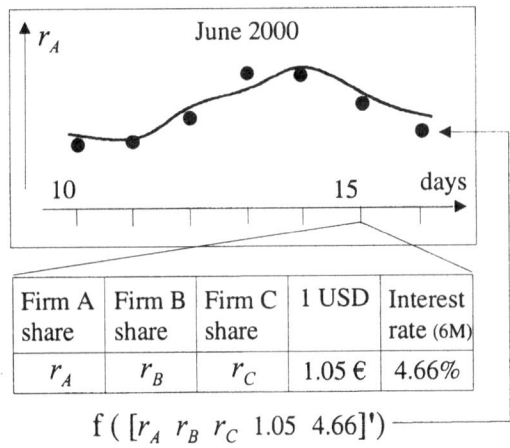

Figure 1.5. Share value forecast one-day ahead. r_A, r_B, r_C are share values of three firms. Functional approximation (black circles) of the true value of r_A (solid curve), is shown for June 16 depending on the values of the shares, euro-dollar exchange rate and interest rate for June 15.

1.2.3 Description Tasks

In both classification and regression tasks similarity is a distance and therefore evaluated as a numeric quantity. Another type of similarity is related to the feature structure of the objects. Let us assume that we are presented with tracings of foetal heart rate during some period of time. These tracings register the instantaneous frequency of the foetus' heart beat (between 50 and 200 b.p.m.) and are used by obstetricians to assess foetal well-being. One such tracing is shown in Figure 1.6.

These tracings show ups and downs relative to a certain baseline corresponding to the foetus' basal rhythm of the heart (around 150 b.p.m. in Figure 1.6a). Some of these ups and downs are idiosyncrasies of the heart rate to be interpreted by the obstetrician. Others, such as the vertical downward strokes in Figure 1.6, are artefacts introduced by the measuring equipment. These artefacts or spikes are to be removed. The question is: when is an up or a down wave a spike?

In order to answer this question we may start by describing each tracing as a sequence of segments connecting successive heart beats as shown in Figure 1.6b. These segments could then be classified in the tracing elements or *primitives* listed in Table 1.1.

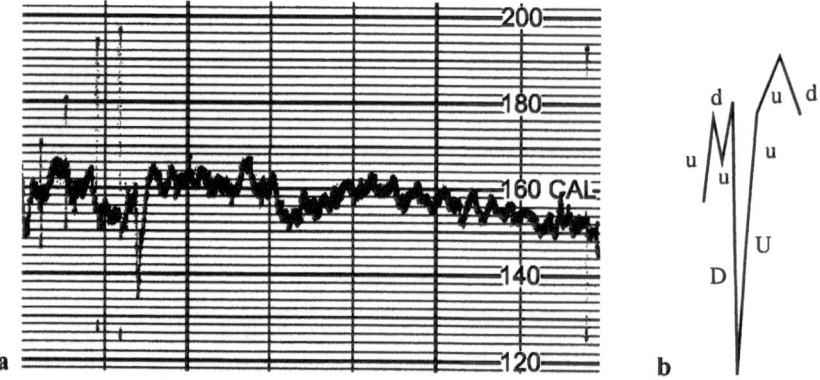

Figure 1.6. (a) Foetal heart rate tracing with the vertical scale in b.p.m. (b) A detail of the first prominent downward wave is shown with its primitives.

Table 1.1 Primitives of foetal heart rate tracings.

Primitive Name	Symbol	Description
Horizontal	h	A segment of constant value
Up slope	u	An upward segment with slope $< \Delta$
Down slope	d	A downward segment with slope $> -\Delta$
Strong up slope	U	An upward segment with slope $\geq \Delta$
Strong down slope	D	A downward segment with slope $\leq -\Delta$

Δ is a minimum slope value specified beforehand.

Based on these elements we can describe a spike as any sequence consisting of a subsequence of U primitives followed by a subsequence of D primitives or vice-versa, with at least one U and one D and no other primitives between. Figures 1.7a and 1.7b show examples of spikes and non-spikes according to this rule.

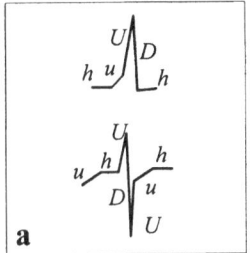
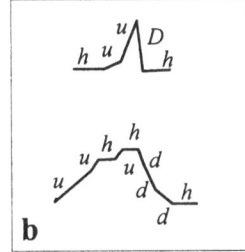
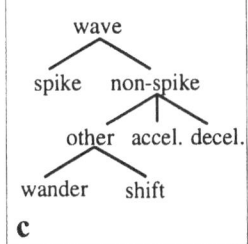

Figure 1.7 Wave primitives for FHR signal: (a) Spikes; (b) Non-spikes; (c) Wave hierarchy.

The non-spikes could afterwards be classified as accelerations, decelerations or other wave types. The rule for acceleration could be: any up wave sequence starting with at least one u primitive with no d's in between, terminating with at least one d primitive with no u's in between. An example is shown at the bottom of Figure 1.7b. With these rules we could therefore establish a hierarchy of wave descriptions as shown in Figure 1.7c.

In this *description task* the similarity of the objects (spikes, accelerations, decelerations, etc., in this example) is assessed by means of a *structural rule*. Two objects are similar if they obey the same rule. Therefore all spikes are similar, all accelerations are similar, and so on. Note in particular that the bottom spike of Figure 1.7a is, in this sense, more similar to the top spike than the top wave of Figure 1.7b, although applying a distance measure to the values of the signal amplitudes, using the first peak as time alignment reference, would certainly lead to a different result!

The structural rule is applied here to the encoded sequence of the primitives, in the form of a *string of primitives*, in order to see if the rule applies. For instance, a machine designed to describe foetal heart rate tracings would encode the segment shown in Figure 1.6b as "*uduDUuud*", thereby recognizing the presence of a spike.

1.3 Classes, Patterns and Features

In the pattern recognition examples presented so far a quite straightforward correspondence existed between patterns and classes. Often the situation is not that simple. Let us consider a cardiologist intending to diagnose a heart condition based on the interpretation of electrocardiographic signals (ECG). These are electric signals acquired by placing electrodes on the patient's chest. Figure 1.8 presents four ECGs, each one corresponding to a distinct physiological condition: N – normal; LVH – left ventricle hypertrophy; RVH – right ventricle hypertrophy; MI – myocardial infarction.

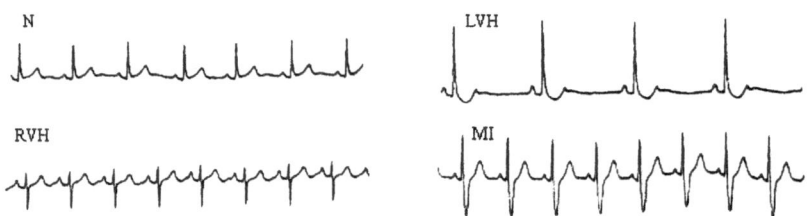

Figure 1.8. ECGs of 4 diagnostic classes: (N) Normal; (LVH) Left ventricular hypertrophy; (RVH) Right ventricular hypertrophy; (MI) Myocardial infarction.

Each ECG tracing exhibits a "wave packet" that repeats itself in a more or less regular way over time. Figure 1.9 shows an example of such a "wave packet", whose components are sequentially named P, Q, R, S and T. These waves reflect the electrical activity of distinct parts of the heart. A P wave reflects the atrial activity of the heart. The Q, R, S and T waves reflect the subsequent ventricular activity.

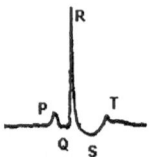

Figure 1.9. ECG wave packet with sequentially named waveforms P, Q, R, S, T.

Cardiologists learn to interpret the morphology of these waves in correspondence with the physiological state of the heart. The situation can be summarized as follows:

– There is a set of *classes* (states) in which can be found a certain studied entity. In the case of the heart we are considering the mentioned four classes.
– Corresponding to each class (state) is a certain set of representations (signals, images, etc.), the *patterns*. In the present case the ECGs are the patterns.

– From each pattern we can extract information characterizing it, the *features*. In the ECG case the features are related to wave measurements of amplitudes and durations. A feature can be, for instance, the ratio between the amplitudes of the Q and R waves, Q/R ratio.

In order to solve a PR problem we must have clear definitions of the class, pattern and feature spaces. In the present case these spaces are represented in Figure 1.10.

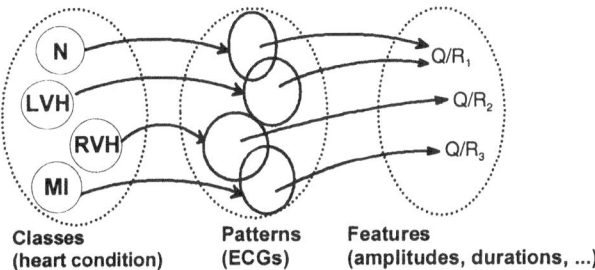

Classes	Patterns	Features
(heart condition)	(ECGs)	(amplitudes, durations, ...)

Figure 1.10. PR spaces for the heart condition classification using ECG features.

A PR system emulating the cardiologist abilities, when presented with a feature vector, would have to infer the heart condition (diagnostic class) from the feature vector. The problem is that, as we see from Figure 1.10, there are annoying overlaps: the same Q/R ratio can be obtained from ECGs corresponding to classes N and LVH; the same ECG can be obtained from classes MI and RVH. The first type of overlap can be remedied using additional features; the second type of overlap is intrinsic to the method and, as a matter of fact, the best experts in electrocardiography have an upper limit to their performance (about 23% overall classification error when using the standard "12-lead ECG system" composed of 12 ECG signals). Therefore, a PR system frequently has a non-zero performance error, independent of whatever approach is used, and usually one is satisfied if it compares equally or favourably with what human experts can achieve.

Summarizing some notions:

Classes

Classes are *states* of "nature" or *categories* of objects associated with *concepts* or *prototypes*.

In what follows we assume c classes denoted $\omega_i \in \Omega$, $(i = 1, \ldots, c)$, where Ω is the set of all classes, known as the *interpretation space*. The interpretation space has *concept-driven* properties such as unions, intersections and hierarchical trees of classes.

Patterns

Patterns are "physical" representations of the objects. Usually signals, images or simple tables of values. Often we will refer to patterns as *objects*, *cases* or *samples*.

In what follows we will use the letter n to indicate the total number of available patterns for the purpose of designing a PR system, the so-called *training* or *design set*.

Features

Features are *measurements*, *attributes* or *primitives* derived from the patterns, that may be useful for their characterization.

We mentioned previously that an initial choice of adequate features is often more an art than a science. By simplicity reasons (and for other compelling reasons to be discussed later) we would like to use only a limited number of features. Frequently there is previous knowledge guiding this choice. In the case of the ECGs a 10s tracing sampled at a convenient 500 Hz would result in 5000 signal samples. However it would be a disastrous choice to use these 5000 signal samples as features! Fortunately there is previous medical knowledge guiding us in the choice of a quite reduced set of features. The same type of problem arises when we want to classify images in digitised form. For a greyscale 256x256 pixels image we have a set of 65536 values (light intensities). To use these values as features in a PR system is unthinkable! However, frequently a quite reduced set of image measurements is sufficient as feature vector.

Table 1.2 presents a list of common types of features used for signal and image recognition. These can be obtained by signal and image processing techniques described in many textbooks (see e.g. Duda and Hart, 1973 and Schalkoff, 1992).

Table 1.2. Common types of signal and image features.

Signal Features	Image Features
Wave amplitudes, durations	Region size
Histogram measurements	Region colour components
Wave moments (e.g. standard deviation)	Region average light intensity
	Image moments
Wave morphology (e.g. symmetry)	Histogram measurements
Zero crossings	Spectral peaks (Fourier transform)
Autocorrelation peaks	Topological features (e.g. region connectivity)
Spectral peaks (Fourier transform)	Mathematical morphology features

In what follows we assume a set of d features or primitives. In classification or regression problems we consider features represented by real numbers; a pattern is, therefore, represented by a *feature vector*:

$$\mathbf{x} = \begin{bmatrix} x_1 \\ x_2 \\ \vdots \\ x_d \end{bmatrix} \in X \subset \Re^d ,$$

where X is the d-dimensional domain of the feature vectors.

For description problems a pattern is often represented by a *string* of symbolic primitives x_i:

$$\mathbf{x} = x_1 x_2 ... x_d \in S ,$$

where S is the set of all possible strings built with the primitives. We will see in Chapter 6 other representational alternatives to strings.

The feature space is also called the *representation space*. The representation space has *data-driven* properties according to the defined similarity measure.

1.4 PR Approaches

There is a multiplicity of PR approaches and no definite consensus on how to categorize them. The objective of a PR system is to perform a mapping between the representation space and the interpretation space. Such mapping, be it a classification, a regression or a description solution, is also called a *hypothesis*.

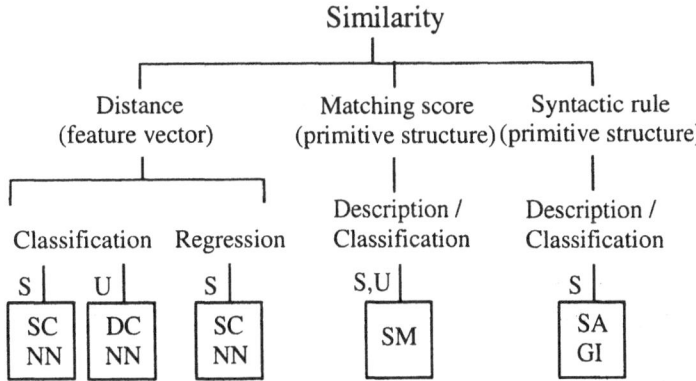

Figure 1.11. PR approaches: S - supervised; U - unsupervised; SC – statistical classification; NN – neural networks; DC – data clustering; SM – structural matching; SA – syntactic analysis; GI – grammatical inference.

There are two distinct ways such hypotheses can be obtained:

- *Supervised, concept driven or inductive hypotheses*: find in the representation space a hypothesis corresponding to the structure of the interpretation space. This is the approach of the previous examples, where given a set of patterns we hypothesise a solution. In order to be useful, any hypothesis found to approximate the target values in the training set must also approximate unobserved patterns in a similar way.
- *Unsupervised, data-driven or deductive hypotheses*: find a structure in the interpretation space corresponding to the structure in the representation space. The unsupervised approach attempts to find a useful hypothesis based only on the similarity relations in the representation space.

The hypothesis is derived using learning methods which can be of statistical, approximation (error minimization) or structural nature.

Taking into account how the hypothesis is derived and pattern similarity is measured, we can establish the hierarchical categorization shown in Figure1.11.

We proceed to briefly describe the main characteristics and application scope of these approaches, to be explained in detail in the following chapters.

1.4.1 Data Clustering

The objective of *data clustering* is to organize data (patterns) into meaningful or useful groups using some type of similarity measure. Data clustering does not use any *prior* class information. It is therefore an unsupervised classification method, in the sense that the solutions arrived at are data-driven, i.e., do not rely on any supervisor or teacher.

Data clustering is useful when one wants to extract some meaning from a pile of unclassified information or in an exploratory phase of pattern recognition research for assessing internal data similarities. In section 5.9 we will also present a neural network approach that relies on a well-known data clustering algorithm as a first processing stage.

Example of data clustering: Given a table containing crop yields per hectare for several soil lots the objective is to cluster these lots into meaningful groups.

1.4.2 Statistical Classification

Statistical classification is a long-established and classic approach of pattern recognition whose mathematics dwell on a solid body of methods and formulas. It is essentially based on the use of probabilistic models for the feature vector distributions in the classes in order to derive classifying functions. Estimation of these distributions is based on a training set of patterns whose classification is known beforehand (e.g. assigned by human experts). It is therefore a supervised method of pattern recognition, in the sense that the classifier is concept-driven, taught from labelled patterns how to perform the classification. If the classifier is efficiently designed it will be able to perform well on new patterns.

There are variants of the statistical classification approach, which depend on whether a known, parametrizable, distribution model is being used or not. There are also important by-products of statistical classification such as decision trees and tables.

The statistical classification approach is adequate when the patterns are distributed in the features space, among the several classes, according to simple topologies and preferably with known probabilistic distributions.

Example of statistical classification system: A machine is given the task of separating cork stoppers into several categories according to the type of defects they present. For that purpose defects are characterized by several features, which can be well modelled by the normal distribution. The machine uses a statistical classifier based on these features in order to achieve the separation.

1.4.3 Neural Networks

Neural networks (or neural nets) are inspired by physiological knowledge of the organization of the brain. They are structured as a set of interconnected identical units known as *neurons*. The interconnections are used to send signals from one neuron to the others, in either an enhanced or inhibited way. This enhancement or inhibition is obtained by adjusting connection *weights*.

Neural nets can perform classification and regression tasks in either a supervised or non-supervised way. They accomplish this by appropriate methods of *weight adjustment*, whereby the outputs of the net hopefully converge to the right target values.

Contrary to statistical classification, neural nets have the advantage of being model free machines, behaving as universal approximators, capable of adjusting to any desired output or topology of classes in the feature space. One disadvantage of neural nets compared with statistical classification is that its mathematics are more intricate and, as we will see later on, for some important decisions the designer has often little theoretically based guidance, and has to rely on trial-and-error heuristics. Another disadvantage, which can be important in some circumstances, is that practically no semantic information is available from a neural net. In order to appreciate this last point, imagine that a physician performs a diagnostic task aided by a neural net and by a statistical classifier, both fed with the same input values (symptoms) and providing the correct answer, maybe contrary to the physician's knowledge or intuition. In the case of the statistical classifier the physician is probably capable of perceiving how the output was arrived at, given the distribution models. In the case of the neural net this perception is usually impossible.

Neural nets are preferable to classic statistical model-free approaches, especially when the training set size is small compared with the dimensionality of the problem to be solved. Model-free approaches, either based on classic statistical classification or on neural nets, have a common body of analysis provided by the *Statistical Learning Theory* (see e.g. Cherkassky and Mulier, 1998).

Example of a neural net application: Foetal weight estimation is important for assessing antepartum delivery risk. For that purpose a set of echographic measurements of the foetus are obtained and a neural net is trained in order to provide a useful estimate of the foetal weight.

1.4.4 Structural PR

Structural pattern recognition is the approach followed whenever one needs to take into consideration the set of relations applying to the parts of the object to be recognized. Sometimes the recognition assumes the form of *structural matching*, when one needs to assess how well an unknown object or part of it relates to some prototype. A *matching score* is then computed for this purpose, which does not necessarily have the usual properties of a distance measure.

A particular type of structural PR, known as *syntactic* PR, may be followed when one succeeds in formalizing rules for describing the relations among the object's parts. The goal of the recognizing machine is then to verify whether a sequence of pattern primitives obeys a certain set of rules, known as syntactic rules or *grammar*. For that purpose a syntactic analyser or *parser* is built and the sequence of primitives inputted to it.

Structural analysis is quite distinctive from the other approaches. It operates with symbolic information, often in the form of strings, therefore using appropriate non-numeric operators. It is sometimes used at a higher level than the other methods, for instance in image interpretation, after segmenting an image into primitives using a statistical or a neural net approach, the structure or relation linking these primitives can be elucidated using a structural approach.

Some structural approaches can be implemented using neural nets. We will see an example of this in Chapter 6.

Example of structural analysis: Given the foetal heart rate tracings mentioned in section 1.2.3 design a parser that will correctly describe these tracings as sequences of wave events such as spikes, accelerations and decelerations.

1.5 PR Project

1.5.1 Project Tasks

PR systems, independent of the approach followed to design them, have specific functional units as shown in Figure 1.12. Some systems do not have pre-processing and/or post-processing units.

The PR system units and corresponding project tasks are:

1. *Pattern acquisition*, which can take several forms: signal or image acquisition, data collection.
2. *Feature extraction*, in the form of measurements, extraction of primitives, etc.

3. *Pre-processing*. In some cases the features values are not directly fed into the classifier or descriptor. For instance in neural net applications it is usual to standardize the features in some way (e.g. imposing a [0, 1] range).

4. The *classification*, *regression* or *description* unit is the kernel unit of the PR system.

5. *Post-processing*. Sometimes the output obtained from the PR kernel unit cannot be directly used. It may need, for instance, some decoding operation. This, along with other operations that will be needed eventually, is called post-processing.

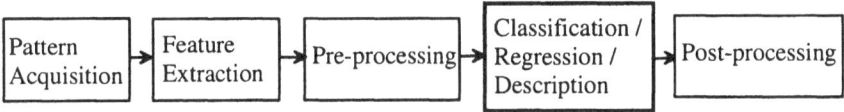

Figure 1.12. PR system with its main functional units. Some systems do not have pre-processing and/or post-processing units.

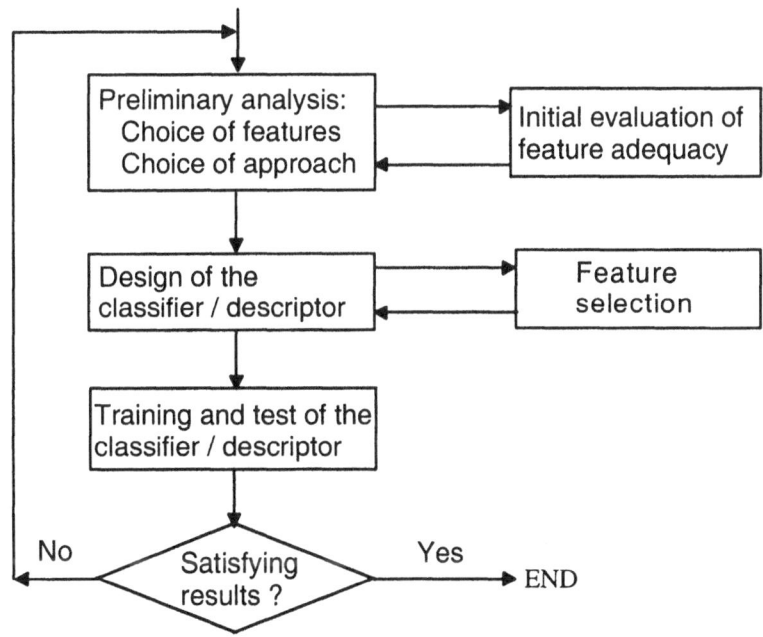

Figure 1.13. PR project phases. Note the feature assessment at two distinct phases.

Although these tasks are mainly organised sequentially, as shown in Figure 1.12, some feedback loops may be present, at least during the design phase, since there is interdependence of the solutions adopted at each unit level. For instance, the type of pattern acquisition used may influence the choice of features, and therefore the other units as well. Other influences are more subtle: for instance, the type of pre-processing performed on the features inputted to a neural net may influence the overall performance in a way that is difficult to foresee.

A PR project has to consider all the mentioned tasks and evolves in a schematic way through the phases shown in Figure 1.13.

1.5.2 Training and Testing

As mentioned in the previous section the development of a PR application starts with the evaluation of the type of features to be used and the adequate PR approach for the problem at hand. For this purpose an initial set of patterns is usually available. In the supervised approaches this initial set, represented by n d-dimensional feature vectors or n strings built with d primitives, is used for developing the PR kernel. It constitutes the *training set*.

The performance of a PR system is usually evaluated in terms of error rates for all classes and an overall error rate. When this performance evaluation is based on the patterns of the training set we obtain, on average, optimistic figures. This somewhat intuitive result will be further clarified in later chapters. In order to obtain better estimates of a PR system performance it is indispensable to evaluate it using an independent set of patterns, i.e., patterns not used in its design. This independent set of patterns is called a *test set*. Test set estimates of a PR system performance give us an idea of how well the system is capable of generalizing its recognition abilities to new patterns.

For classification and regression systems the degree of confidence we may have on estimates of a PR system performance, as well as in its capability of generalization, depends strongly on the n/d ratio, the *dimensionality ratio*.

1.5.3 PR Software

There are many software products for developing PR applications, which can guide the design of a PR system from the early stages of the specifications until the final evaluation. A mere search through the Internet will disclose many of these products and tools, either freeware, shareware or commercial. Many of these are method-specific, for instance in the neural networks area. Generally speaking, the following types of software products can be found:

1. Tool libraries (e.g. in C) for use in the development of applicative software.
2. Tools running under other software products (e.g. *Microsoft Excel* or *The MathWorks Matlab*).
3. Didactic purpose products.
4. Products for the design of PR applications using a specific method.
5. Products for the design of PR applications using a panoply of different methods.

Concerning the flexibility of PR design software, there is a broad spectrum of possibilities. At one end we find "closed" products where the user can only perform menu operations. At the other end we find "open" products allowing the user to program any arbitrarily complex PR algorithm. A popular example of such a product is *Matlab* from *The MathWorks, Inc.*, a mathematical software product. Designing a PR application in *Matlab* gives the user the complete freedom to implement specific algorithms and perform complex operations, namely using the routines available in the *Matlab* Toolboxes. For instance, one can couple routines from the Neural Networks Toolbox with routines from the Image Processing Toolbox in order to develop image classification applications. The penalty to be paid for this flexibility is that the user must learn to program in the Matlab language, with non-trivial language learning and algorithm development times.

Some statistical software packages incorporate relevant tools for PR design. Given their importance and wide popularisation two of these products are worth mentioning: *SPSS* from *SPSS Inc.* and *Statistica* from *StatSoft Inc.* Both products require minimal time for familiarization and allow the user to easily perform classification and regression tasks using a scroll-sheet based philosophy for operating with the data. Figure 1.14 illustrates the *Statistica* scroll-sheet for a cork stoppers classification problem with column C filled in with numeric codes of the supervised class labels and the other columns (ART to PRT) filled in with feature values. Concerning flexibility, both *SPSS* and *Statistica* provide macro constructions. As a matter of fact *Statistica* is somewhere between a "closed" type product and *Matlab*, since it provides programming facilities such as the use of external code (DLLs) and application programming interfaces (API). In this book we will extensively use the *Statistica* (kernel release 5.5A for *Windows*), with a few exceptions, for illustrating PR methods with appropriate examples and real data.

NUME VALU	1 C	2 ART	3 N	4 PRT	5 ARM	6 PRM	7 ARTG	8 NG	9 PRT
48	1	187	76	492	2.46	6.47	33.0	3.0	40
49	1	125	52	348	2.40	6.69	0.0	0.0	0
50	1	179	89	520	2.01	5.84	21.8	2.8	29
51	2	240	76	596	3.16	7.84	9.0	1.0	12
52	2	224	77	576	2.91	7.48	12.0	1.0	14
53	2	265	81	624	3.27	7.70	33.0	2.0	34

Figure 1.14. *Statistica* scroll-sheet for the cork stoppers data. Each row corresponds to a pattern. C is the class label column. The other columns correspond to the features.

Concerning software for specific PR methodologies it is worth mentioning the impressive number of software products and tools in the Neural Network and Data Mining areas. In chapter 5 we will use one such tool, namely the *Support Vector Machine Toolbox* for *Matlab*, developed by S.R. Gunn at the University of Southampton.

Unfortunately there are practically no software tools for structural PR, except for a few non user-friendly parsers. There is also a lack of tools for guiding important project decisions such as the choice of a reasonable dimensionality ratio. The CD offered with this book is intended to fill in the gaps of available software, supplying the necessary tools in those topics where none exist (or are not readily available).

All the main PR approaches and techniques described in the book are illustrated with applications to real-life problems. The corresponding datasets, described in Appendix A, are also supplied in the CD. At the end of the following chapters several exercises are proposed, many involving computer experiments with the supplied datasets.

With *Statistica*, *Matlab*, *SPSS* or any other equivalent product and the complementary tools of the included CD the reader is encouraged to follow the next chapters in a hands-on fashion, trying the presented examples and freeing his/her imagination.

Bibliography

Bishop CM (1995) Neural Networks for Pattern Recognition. Clarendon Press, Oxford.

Cherkassky V, Mulier F (1998) Learning from Data. John Wiley & Sons, Inc.

Duda RO, Hart PE (1973) Pattern Classification and Scene Analysis. Wiley, New York.

Friedman M, Kandel A (1999) Introduction to Pattern Recognition. World Scientific, Imperial College Press.

Fu KS (1977) Introduction to Syntactic Pattern Recognition. In: Fu KS (ed) Syntactic Pattern Recognition, Applications. Springer-Verlag, Berlin, Heidelberg.

Hartigan, JA (1975) Clustering algorithms. Wiley, New York.

Jain AK, Duin RPW, Mao J (2000). Statistical Pattern Recognition: A Review. IEEE Tr Patt An Mach Intel 1:4-37.

Mitchell TM (1997) Machine Learning. McGraw Hill Book Co., Singapore.

Schalkoff R (1992) Pattern Recognition. Wiley.

Schürmann J (1996) Pattern Classification. A Unified View of Statistical and Neural Approaches. John Wiley & Sons, Inc.

Simon JC, Backer E, Sallentin J (1982) A Unifying Viewpoint on Pattern Recognition. In: Krishnaiah PR and Kanal LN (eds) Handbook of Statistics vol.2, North Holland Pub. Co., 451-477.

2 Pattern Discrimination

2.1 Decision Regions and Functions

We saw in the previous chapter that in classification or regression tasks, patterns are represented by feature vectors in an $\Re^d$ feature space. In the particular case of a classifier, the main goal is to divide the feature space into regions assigned to the classification classes. These regions are called *decision regions*. If a feature vector falls into a certain decision region the associated pattern is assigned to the corresponding class.

Let us assume two classes ω_1 e ω_2 of patterns described by two-dimensional feature vectors (coordinates x_1 and x_2) as shown in Figure 2.1.

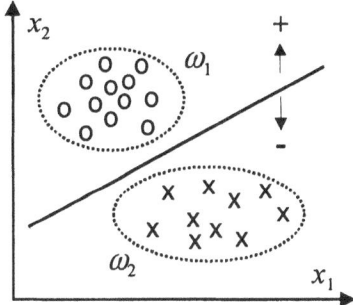

Figure 2.1. Two classes of patterns described by two-dimensional feature vectors (features x_1 and x_2).

Each pattern is represented by a vector $\mathbf{x} = [x_1 \quad x_2]' \in \Re^2$. In Figure 2.1 we used "o" to denote class ω_1 patterns and "x" to denote class ω_2 patterns. In general, the patterns of each class will be characterized by random distributions of the corresponding feature vectors, as illustrated in Figure 2.1 where the ellipses represent "boundaries" of the distributions, also called *class limits*.

Figure 2.1 also shows a straight line separating the two classes. We can easily write the equation of the straight line in terms of the coordinates (features) x_1, x_2

using coefficients or *weights* w_1 and w_2 and a *bias* term w_0 as shown in equation (2-1). The weights determine the slope of the straight line; the bias determines the deviation from the origin of the straight line intersects with the coordinates.

$$d(\mathbf{x}) = w_1 x_1 + w_2 x_2 + w_0 = 0. \tag{2-1}$$

Equation (2-1) also allows interpretation of the straight line as the roots set of a linear function $d(\mathbf{x})$. We say that $d(\mathbf{x})$ is a *linear decision function* that divides (categorizes) $\mathfrak{R}^2$ into two decision regions: the upper half plane corresponding to $d(\mathbf{x}) > 0$ where each feature vector is assigned to ω_1; the lower half plane corresponding to $d(\mathbf{x}) < 0$ where each feature vector is assigned to ω_2. The classification is arbitrary for $d(\mathbf{x}) = 0$. Note that class limits do not have to coincide with decision region boundaries.

The generalization of the linear decision function for a d-dimensional feature space in $\mathfrak{R}^d$ is straightforward:

$$d(\mathbf{x}) = \mathbf{w}^{*\prime} \mathbf{x}^* = \mathbf{w}' \mathbf{x} + \mathbf{w}_0, \tag{2-2}$$

where

$\mathbf{w} = [w_1 \ \dots \ w_d]'$ is the weight vector; $\tag{2-2a}$

$\mathbf{w}^* = [w_0 \ w_1 \ \dots \ w_d]'$ is the augmented weight vector with the bias term; $\tag{2-2b}$

$\mathbf{x}^* = [1 \ x_1 \ \dots \ x_d]$ is the augmented feature vector. $\tag{2-2c}$

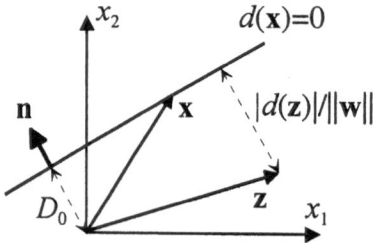

Figure 2.2. Two-dimensional linear decision function with normal vector **n** and at a distance D_0 from the origin.

The roots set of $d(\mathbf{x})$, the *decision surface*, or *discriminant*, is now a linear d-dimensional surface called a *hyperplane* that can be characterized (see Figure 2.2) by its distance D_0 from the coordinates origin and its unitary normal vector **n** in the positive direction ($d(\mathbf{x}) > 0$) as follows (see e.g. Friedman and Kandel, 1999):

$$D_0 = \frac{|w_0|}{\|\mathbf{w}\|}; \qquad \mathbf{n} = \frac{\mathbf{w}}{\|\mathbf{w}\|}, \qquad\qquad (2\text{-}2d)$$

where $\|\mathbf{w}\|$ represents the vector $\mathbf{w}$ length.

Notice also that $|d(\mathbf{z})|/\|\mathbf{w}\|$ is precisely the distance of any point $\mathbf{z}$ to the hyperplane.

2.1.1 Generalized Decision Functions

In pattern classification we are not confined to using linear decision functions. As long as the classes do not overlap one can always find a *generalized decision function* defined in $\Re^d$ that separates a class ω_i from a total of c classes, so that the following decision rule applies:

$$d_i(\mathbf{x}) > 0 \quad \text{if } \mathbf{x} \in \omega_i; \quad d_i(\mathbf{x}) < 0 \quad \text{if } \mathbf{x} \in \omega_j \text{ with } j \neq i. \qquad (2\text{-}3)$$

For some generalized decision functions we will establish a certain threshold Δ for class discrimination:

$$d_i(\mathbf{x}) > \Delta \quad \text{if } \mathbf{x} \in \omega_i; \quad d_i(\mathbf{x}) < \Delta \quad \text{if } \mathbf{x} \in \omega_j \text{ with } j \neq i. \qquad (2\text{-}3a)$$

For instance, in a two-class one-dimensional classification problem with a quadratic decision function $d(x) = x^2$, one would design the classifier by selecting an adequate threshold Δ so that the following decision rule would apply:

$$\text{If} \quad d(x) = x^2 \geq \Delta \quad \text{then } x \in \omega_1 \quad \text{else} \quad x \in \omega_2. \qquad (2\text{-}3b)$$

In this decision rule we chose to assign the equality case to class ω_1. Figure 2.3a shows a two-class discrimination using a quadratic decision function with a threshold $\Delta=49$, which will discriminate between the class $\omega_1 = \{x; \ x \in [-7, 7]\}$ and $\omega_2 = \{x; \ x \in \,]-7, 7[\,\}$.

It is important to note that as far as class discrimination is concerned, any functional composition of $d(\mathbf{x})$ by a monotonic function will obviously separate the classes in exactly the same way. For the quadratic classifier (2-3b) we may, for instance, use a monotonic logarithmic composition:

$$\text{If} \quad \ln(d(x)) \geq \ln(\Delta) \quad \text{then } x \in \omega_1 \quad \text{else} \quad x \in \omega_2. \qquad (2\text{-}3c)$$

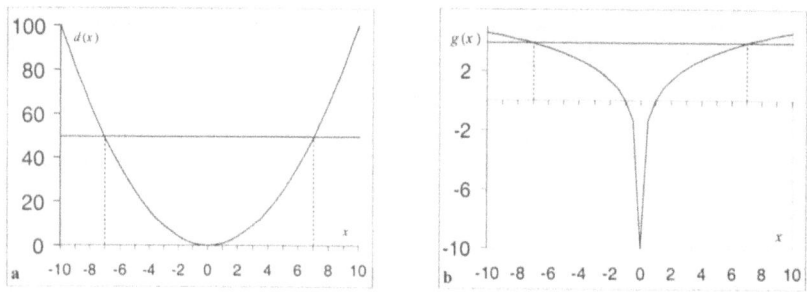

Figure 2.3. (a) Quadratic decision function, $d(x) = x^2$; (b) Logarithmic decision function, $g(x) = \ln(d(x))$.

Figure 2.3b illustrates this logarithmic decision function for the quadratic classifier example using the new threshold value $\ln(49) = 3.89$. The resulting class discrimination is exactly the same as before the logarithmic transformation. The benefit that can be derived from the use of a monotonic transformation will become clear in later chapters.

It is sometimes convenient to express a generalized decision function as a functional linear combination:

$$d(\mathbf{x}) = w_1 f_1(\mathbf{x}) + \ldots + w_k f_k(\mathbf{x}) + w_0 = \mathbf{w}^{*\prime} \mathbf{y}^*, \qquad (2\text{-}4)$$

$$\text{with} \quad \mathbf{y}^* = \begin{bmatrix} 1 & f_1(\mathbf{x}) & f_2(\mathbf{x}) \ldots f_k(\mathbf{x}) \end{bmatrix}^\prime . \qquad (2\text{-}4a)$$

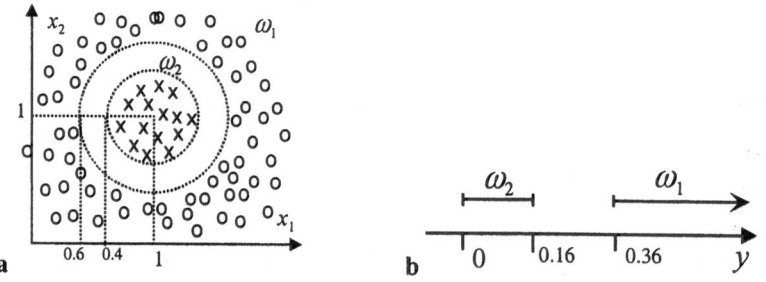

Figure 2.4. A two-class discrimination problem in the original feature space (a) and in a transformed one-dimensional feature space (b).

In this way, an arbitrarily complex decision function is expressed linearly in the space of the feature vectors **y**. Imagine, for instance, that we had two classes with circular limits as shown in Figure 2.4a. A quadratic decision function capable of separating the classes is:

$$d(\mathbf{x}) = (x_1 - 1)^2 + (x_2 - 1)^2 + 0.25 .$$ (2-5a)

Instead of working with a quadratic decision function in the original two-dimensional feature space, we may decide to work in a transformed one-dimensional feature space:

$$\mathbf{y}^* = \begin{bmatrix} 1 & y \end{bmatrix}' \quad \text{with} \quad y = f(\mathbf{x}) = (x_1 - 1)^2 + (x_2 - 1)^2 .$$ (2-5b)

In this one-dimensional space we rewrite the decision function simply as a linear decision function:

$$g(\mathbf{y}) = \begin{bmatrix} 0.25 & 1 \end{bmatrix}' \mathbf{y}^* = y + 0.25 .$$ (2-5c)

Figure 2.4b illustrates the class discrimination problem in this transformed one-dimensional feature space. Note that if there are small scaling differences in the original features x_1 and x_2, as well as deviations from the class centres, it would be, in principle, easier to perform the discrimination in the $\mathbf{y}$ space than in the $\mathbf{x}$ space.

A particular case of interest is the polynomial expression of a decision function $d(\mathbf{x})$. For instance, the decision function (2-5a) can be expressed as a degree 2 polynomial in x_1 and x_2. Figure 2.5 illustrates an example of 2-dimensional classes separated by a decision boundary obtained with a polynomial decision function of degree four:

$$\begin{aligned} d(\mathbf{x}) = & w_{14}x_1^4 + w_{13}x_2^4 + w_{12}x_1^2 x_2^2 + w_{11}x_1^3 x_2 + w_{10}x_1 x_2^3 + w_9 x_1^3 + w_8 x_2^3 + \\ & w_7 x_1^2 x_2 + w_6 x_1 x_2^2 + w_5 x_1^2 + w_4 x_2^2 + w_3 x_1 x_2 + w_2 x_1 + w_1 x_2 + w_0 . \end{aligned}$$ (2-6)

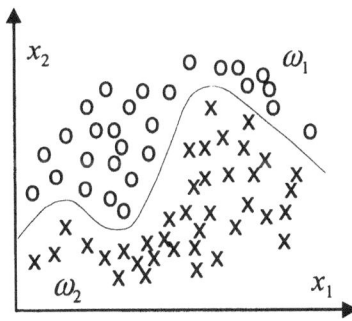

Figure 2.5. Decision regions and boundary for a degree 4 polynomial decision function.

In the original feature space we are dealing with 2 features and will have to compute (adjust) 15 weights. We may choose instead to operate in a *transformed feature space*, the space of the monomial functions $x_1^p x_2^q$ (x_1^4, x_2^4, $x_1^2 x_2^2$, x_1^3, etc.). We will then have to compute in a straightforward way 14 features plus a bias term (w_0). The eventual benefit derived from working in this higher dimensionality space is that it may be possible to determine a linear decision function involving easier computations and weight adjustments (see Exercises 2.3 and 2.4). However, working in high dimensional spaces raises a number of difficulties as explained later.

For a PR problem originally stated in a d features space, it can be shown that in order to determine a polynomial decision function of degree k one has to compute:

$$C(d+k,k) = \frac{(d+k)!}{d!k!} \text{ polynomial coefficients,} \tag{2-7}$$

with $C(n, k)$ denoting the number of combinations of n elements taken k at a time.

For $d=2$ and $k=4$ expression (2-7) yields 15 polynomial coefficients. For quadratic decision functions one would need to compute:

$$C(d+2,2) = \frac{(d+2)!}{d!2!} = \frac{(d+2)(d+1)}{2} \text{ polynomial coefficients.} \tag{2-7a}$$

Linear decision functions are quite popular, as they are easier to compute and have simpler mathematics. This is why in the following we lend more attention to linear separability.

2.1.2 Hyperplane Separability

Let us consider again the situation depicted in Figure 2.1. The decision "surface" divides the feature space into two decision regions: the half plane above the straight line containing class ω_1, and the half plane below the straight line containing class ω_2.

In a multiple class problem, with several decision surfaces, arbitrarily complex decision regions can be expected and the separation of the classes can be achieved in essentially two ways: each class can be separated from all the others (*absolute separation*); the classes can only be separated into pairs (*pairwise separation*). In the following we analyse these two types of class discrimination assuming linear separability by hyperplanes.

Absolute separation

Absolute separation corresponds strictly to definition (2-3): any class is separable from all the others. Figure 2.6 illustrates the absolute separation for $d=2$ and $c=3$.

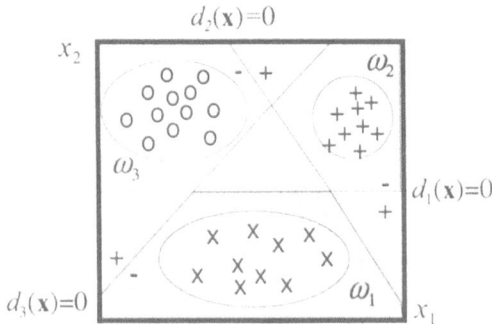

Figure 2.6. Example of absolute separation of three classes in a two-dimensional space.

Figure 2.6 also shows linear decision "surfaces". The decision regions (shaded areas) are defined as:

$$R_i = \{\mathbf{x};\ d_i(\mathbf{x}) > 0,\ d_j(\mathbf{x}) < 0,\ i, j = 1, \ldots, c,\ j \neq i\}. \tag{2-8}$$

Absolute separation lends itself to a hierarchical classification approach as shown in Figure 2.7. At each level of the hierarchical tree a decision is made regarding the discrimination of a disjointed group of classes. Each feature vector (right side of Figure 2.7) is accordingly passed through a decision function. For the ω_2 vs. ω_3 discrimination we may use $d_{23}(\mathbf{x}) = d_2(\mathbf{x}) - d_3(\mathbf{x})$.

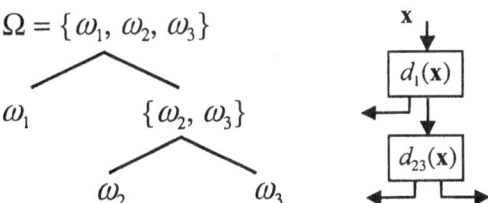

Figure 2.7. Hierarchical classification of a feature vector into one of the classes exemplified in Figure 2.6.

In this example a dichotomic tree, also known as a *binary tree*, is illustrated. Although this is a popular type of hierarchical tree, other types of multi-group discrimination at each level can of course be considered.

In a multi-class PR problem complying, at least approximately, with an absolute separation structure, design criteria derived for a two-class setting can be easily generalized. We will have the opportunity to apply such generalization when discussing the dimensionality ratio issue in section 4.2.4.

Pairwise separation

Sometimes absolute separation is not achievable, however, the classes may be separated into pairs as shown in Figure 2.8.

In this case one can establish c decision surfaces separating pairs of classes, using decision functions defined as follows:

$$d_{ij}(\mathbf{x}) > 0 \quad \forall \mathbf{x} \in \omega_i \quad \text{and} \quad d_{ij}(\mathbf{x}) < 0 \quad \forall \mathbf{x} \in \omega_j \qquad (d_{ij}(\mathbf{x}) = -d_{ji}(\mathbf{x})). \quad (2\text{-}9)$$

The decision regions are now defined in the following way:

$$R_i = \{\, \mathbf{x}; \quad d_{ij}(\mathbf{x}) > 0, \quad i, j = 1, \ldots, c, \quad j \neq i \,\}. \qquad (2\text{-}9\text{a})$$

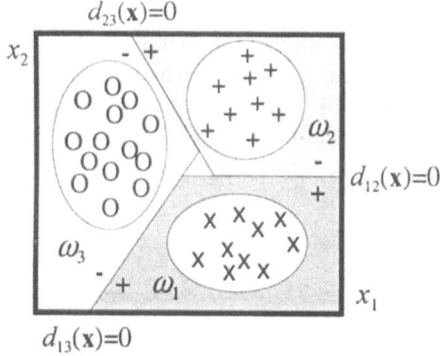

Figure 2.8. Pairwise separation of three classes in a two-dimensional space.

Notice that pairwise separability may not lend itself to hierarchical implementation, since decision surfaces at each level may cut through the classes. Also, in this case, the hyperplanes separating the classes work in a coupled way, which makes it risky to generalize for this situation design criteria established for a two-class setting.

2.2 Feature Space Metrics

In the previous chapter we used a distance measure for assessing pattern similarity in the feature space. A measuring rule $d(\mathbf{x},\mathbf{y})$ for the distance between two vectors $\mathbf{x}$ and $\mathbf{y}$ is considered a *metric* if it satisfies the following properties:

$$d(\mathbf{x},\mathbf{y}) \geq d_0 \; ; \qquad\qquad\qquad\qquad\qquad\qquad\qquad (2\text{-}10a)$$

$$d(\mathbf{x},\mathbf{y}) = d_0 \quad \text{if and only if} \quad \mathbf{x} = \mathbf{y} \, ; \qquad\qquad (2\text{-}10b)$$

$$d(\mathbf{x},\mathbf{y}) = d(\mathbf{y},\mathbf{x}) \, ; \qquad\qquad\qquad\qquad\qquad\qquad (2\text{-}10c)$$

$$d(\mathbf{x},\mathbf{y}) \leq d(\mathbf{x},\mathbf{z}) + d(\mathbf{z},\mathbf{y}) \, . \qquad\qquad\qquad\qquad (2\text{-}10d)$$

If the metric has the property

$$d(a\mathbf{x}, a\mathbf{y}) = |a| \, d(\mathbf{x},\mathbf{y}) \quad \text{with } a \in \Re \, , \qquad\qquad (2\text{-}10e)$$

it is called a norm and denoted $d(\mathbf{x},\mathbf{y}) = \|\mathbf{x} - \mathbf{y}\|$.

The most "natural" metric is the Euclidian norm when an adequate system of coordinates is used. For some classification problems it may be convenient to evaluate pattern similarity using norms other than the Euclidian. The four most popular norms for evaluating the distance of a feature vector $\mathbf{x}$ from a prototype $\mathbf{m}$, all with $d_0 = 0$, are:

Euclidian norm:
$$\|\mathbf{x} - \mathbf{m}\|_e = \left(\sum_{i=1}^{d} (x_i - m_i)^2 \right)^{1/2} \qquad (2\text{-}11a)$$

Squared Euclidian norm[1]:
$$\|\mathbf{x} - \mathbf{m}\|_s = \sum_{i=1}^{d} (x_i - m_i)^2 \qquad (2\text{-}11b)$$

City-block norm:
$$\|\mathbf{x} - \mathbf{m}\|_c = \sum_{i=1}^{d} |x_i - m_i| \qquad (2\text{-}11c)$$

Chebychev norm:
$$\|\mathbf{x} - \mathbf{m}\|_C = \max_i (|x_i - m_i|) \qquad (2\text{-}11d)$$

Compared with the usual Euclidian norm the squared Euclidian norm grows faster with patterns that are further apart. The city-block norm dampens the effect of single large differences in one dimension since they are not squared. The Chebychev norm uses the biggest deviation in any of the dimensions to evaluate the distance. It can be shown that all these norms are particular cases of the *power norm*[1]:

---

[1] Note that for $\|\mathbf{x} - \mathbf{m}\|_s$ and $\|\mathbf{x} - \mathbf{m}\|_{p/r}$ we will have to relax the norm definition, allowing a scale factor for $|a|$.

$$\|\mathbf{x} - \mathbf{m}\|_{p/r} = \left(\sum_{i=1}^{d} |x_i - m_i|^p \right)^{1/r} \tag{2-11e}$$

Parameter p controls the weight placed on any dimension dissimilarity. Parameter r controls the distance growth of patterns that are further apart. The special case $r=p$ is called the *Minkowsky norm*. For $r=p=2$, one obtains the Euclidian norm; for $r=p=1$, the city-block norm; for $r=p \to \infty$, the Chebychev norm.

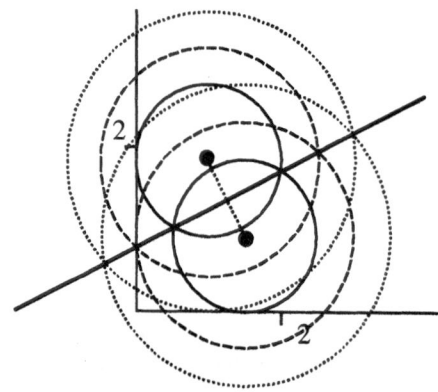

Figure 2.9. Equidistant "surfaces" for Euclidian metric. The straight line is the set of equidistant points from the means.

Notice that strictly speaking a *similarity* measure $s(\mathbf{x}, \mathbf{y})$ should respect the inequality $s(\mathbf{x}, \mathbf{y}) \le s_0$ instead of (2-10a). A distance is, therefore, a *dissimilarity* measure.

For the Euclidian metric the equidistant surfaces are *hyperspheres*. Figure 2.9 illustrates this situation for $d=2$ and $c=2$ classes represented by the class means [1 2]' and [1.5 1]'. The circles in this case represent distances of 1, 1.5 and 2.

Note that by using the Euclidian (or squared Euclidian) metric, the set of equidistant points from the class means, i.e., the decision surface, is just one hyperplane perpendicular to the straight-line segment between the class means and passing through the middle point of this line segment.

With the city-block or Chebychev metric this excellent property is not always verified as illustrated in Figure 2.10.

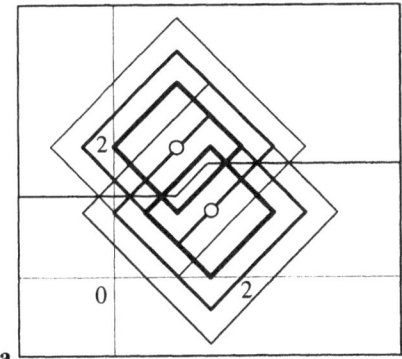 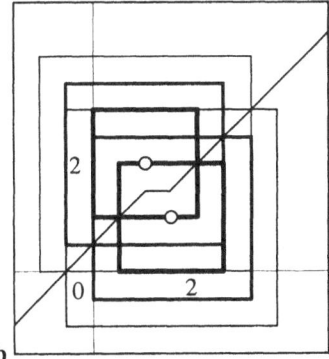

Figure 2.10. Equidistant "surfaces" for city-block (a) and Chebychev (b) metrics.

In both cases the decision surfaces are stepwise linear. In the city-block case the surfaces are parallel to the coordinate axis with smaller distance of the class means (horizontal axis in Figure 2.10a); in the Chebychev case the surfaces bisect the axes. Therefore, as we will see next chapter, the city-block metric is well suited for separating flattened clusters aligned along the axes; the Chebychev metric is adequate when the clusters are aligned along the quadrant bisectors.

The choice of one type of metric must take into account the particular shape of the pattern clusters around the class means. This common sense rule will be further explored in the following chapters. Let us present now a more sophisticated type of metric, which can be finely adjusted to many cluster shapes. For that purpose consider the following linear transformation in the feature space:

$\mathbf{y} = \mathbf{Ax}$, with symmetric matrix $\mathbf{A}$.   (2-12)

Let us assume a cluster of 2-dimensional patterns around the class mean $[1\ 1]'$ with a circular structure, i.e., the patterns whose corresponding vectors fall on the same circle are equally similar. Figure 2.11 shows one of these circles and illustrates the influence of a linear transformation on the circular equidistant surface, using the following matrix $\mathbf{A}$:

$$\mathbf{A} = \begin{bmatrix} 2 & 1 \\ 1 & 1 \end{bmatrix}.$$ (2-12a)

Therefore:

$$y_1 = 2x_1 + x_2 \quad ; \quad y_2 = x_1 + x_2.$$ (2-12b)

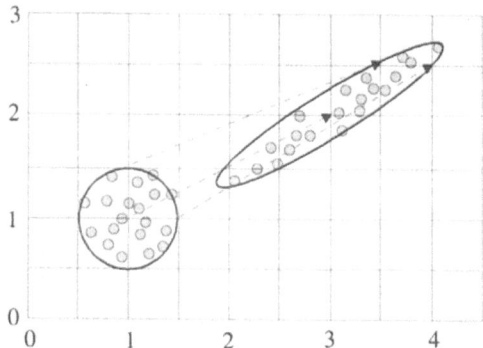

Figure 2.11. Linear transformation of a circular pattern cluster into an elliptic one. The dots represent feature vectors.

We see that this linear transformation amounts to a *scaling operation* (e.g. x_1 is stretched by a factor of 2) concomitant with a *translation effect* of the mean due to a_{11} and a_{22}, plus a *mirroring effect* due to a_{12} and a_{21}. If the matrix A is anti-symmetric with $a_{12} = -a_{21}$, a *rotation effect* is observed instead (see Exercise 2.7).

The transformed mean is:
$$\begin{bmatrix} 2x_1+x_2 \\ x_1+x_2 \end{bmatrix} = \begin{bmatrix} 3 \\ 2 \end{bmatrix}. \qquad (2\text{-}12c)$$

We see that the cluster structure changed from circular to ellipsoidal equidistant surfaces, whose shape is dependent on the particular matrix **A**, i.e., in the transformed space similar patterns have feature vectors lying on the same ellipsis. The generalization to any *d*-dimensional space is straightforward: the equidistant surfaces in the transformed space for the **y** vectors are *hyperellipsoids*, whose distance from the prototype is given by the *Mahalanobis metric* (in a broad sense):

$$p(\mathbf{y}) = \|\mathbf{y} - \mathbf{m}\|_m = ((\mathbf{y} - \mathbf{m})' \mathbf{A}(\mathbf{y} - \mathbf{m}))^{\frac{1}{2}}. \qquad (2\text{-}13)$$

Notice that for **A=I**, unity matrix, one obtains the Euclidian metric as a particular case of the Mahalanobis metric. In order for formula (2-13) to represent a distance, matrix **A** must be such that $p(\mathbf{y}) > 0$ for all $\mathbf{y} \neq 0$. **A** is then called a *positive definite* matrix and $p(\mathbf{y})$ a *positive definite form* of matrix **A**, known as a *quadratic form*. For *d*=2 the quadratic form is:

$$p(\mathbf{y}) = a_{11}y_1^2 + 2a_{12}y_1y_2 + a_{22}y_2^2. \qquad (2\text{-}13a)$$

Notice that with hyperellipsoidal equidistant surfaces one can obtain decision surfaces that are either linear or quadratic as shown in Figure 2.12.

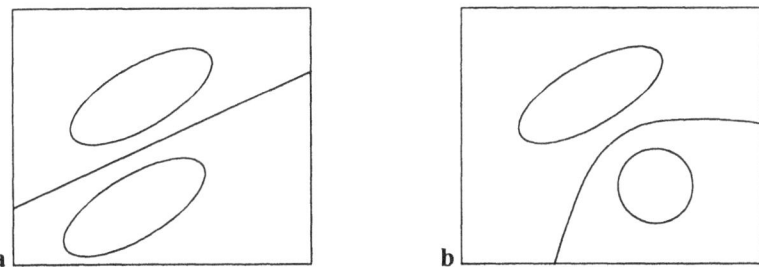

Figure 2.12. Examples of two-class discriminants with pattern similarity measured according to a Mahalanobis metric: (a) Linear; (b) Quadratic.

2.3 The Covariance Matrix

Consider the first two classes of cork stoppers from the dataset described in Appendix A (*Cork Stoppers.xls*). Figure 2.13 shows the scatter plot of these two classes, ω_1 and ω_2, using features N (number of defects) and PRT10=PRT/10 (total perimeter of the defects in tens of pixels).

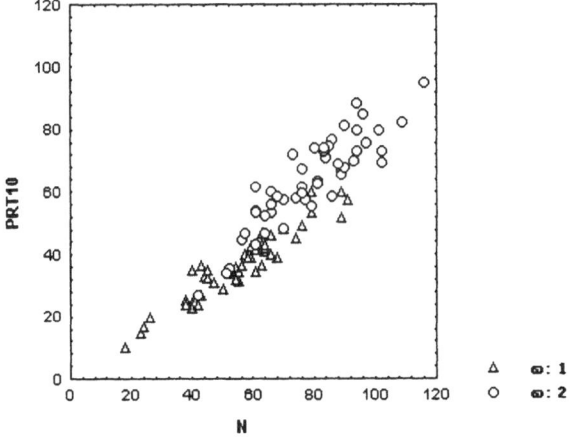

Figure 2.13. Scatter plot for two classes of cork stoppers with features N, PRT10.

The scatter plot shown in Figure 2.13 uses the same scale for the coordinate axes. This allows the evaluation under equal conditions of the features' contributions to the Euclidian distance measures, the ones that we are accustomed to appreciating visually. As can be seen in Figure 2.13 there is a certain amount of correlation between the features. One might wonder what would happen if the features were not measured in approximately the same ranges, if for instance we used the original PRT feature. We can do this by increasing the PRT10 scale ten times as shown in Figure 2.14, where we also changed the axes orientation in order to reasonably fit the plot in the book sheet.

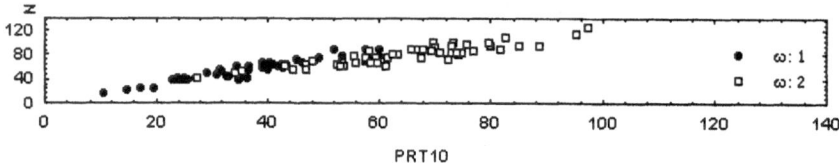

Figure 2.14. Scatter plot for two classes of cork stoppers with PRT10 scale increased ten times.

It is now evident that the measurement unit has a profound influence on the Euclidian distance measures, and in the visual clustering of the patterns as well. Namely, in Figure 2.14, the contribution of N to class discrimination is, in the Euclidian distance sense, negligible.

The usual form of equalizing the features contributions consists of performing some scaling operation. A well-known scaling method consists of subtracting the mean and dividing by the standard deviation:

$$y_i = (x_i - m_i)/s_i \quad , \tag{2-14}$$

where m_i is the sample mean and s_i is the sample standard deviation of feature x_i.

Using this common scaling method (yielding features with zero mean and unit variance), the squared Euclidian distance of the scaled feature vector $\mathbf{y}$ relative to the origin is expressed as:

$$\|\mathbf{y}\|_s = \sum_{i=1}^{d} (x_i - m_i)^2 / s_i^2 . \tag{2-14a}$$

Thus, the original squared Euclidian distance $(x_i - m_i)^2$ has been scaled by $1/s_i^2$, shrinking large variance features with $s_i > 1$ and stretching low variance features with $s_i < 1$, therefore balancing the feature contribution to the squared Euclidian distance. We can obtain some insight into this scaling operation by imagining what it would do to an elliptical cluster with axes aligned with the coordinate axes. The simple scaling operation of (2-14a) would transform equidistant ellipses into equidistant circles. As a matter of fact, any linear transformation of $\mathbf{x}$ with a diagonal matrix, amounting to a multiplication of each feature x_i by some quantity a_i, would now be scaled by a new variance $a_i^2 s_i^2$, therefore preserving $\|\mathbf{y}\|_s$. However, this simple scaling method would fail to preserve distances for the general linear transformation, such as the one illustrated in Figure 2.11.

In order to have a distance measure that will be invariant to linear transformations we need to first consider the notion of *covariance*, an extension of the more popular variance notion, measuring the tendency of two features x_i and x_j varying in the same direction. The covariance between features x_i and x_j is estimated as follows for n patterns:

$$c_{ij} = \frac{1}{n-1} \sum_{k=1}^{n} (x_{k,i} - m_i)(x_{k,j} - m_j) .$$ (2-15)

Notice that covariances are symmetric, $c_{ij} = c_{ji}$, and that c_{ii} is in fact the usual estimation of the variance of x_i.

The covariance is related to the well-known Pearson correlation, estimated as:

$$r_{ij} = \frac{\sum_{k=1}^{n}(x_{k,i} - m_i)(x_{k,j} - m_j)}{(n-1)s_i s_j} = \frac{c_{ij}}{s_i s_j}, \quad \text{with} \quad r_{ij} \in [-1,1].$$ (2-16)

Therefore, the correlation can be interpreted as a standardized covariance.

Looking at Figure 2.9, one may rightly guess that circular clusters have no privileged direction of variance, i.e., they have equal variance along any direction. Consider now the products $v_{ij} = (x_{k,i} - m_i)(x_{k,j} - m_j)$. For any feature vector yielding a given v_{ij} value, it is a simple matter for a sufficiently large population to find another, orthogonal, feature vector yielding $-v_{ij}$. The v_{ij} products therefore cancel out (the variation along one direction is uncorrelated with the variation in any other direction), resulting in a covariance that apart from a scale factor is the unit matrix, $\mathbf{C}=\mathbf{I}$.

Let us now turn to the elliptic clusters shown in Figure 2.11. For such ellipses, with the major axis subtending a positive angle measured in an anti-clockwise direction from the abscissas, one will find more and higher positive v_{ij} values along directions around the major axis than negative v_{ij} values along directions around the minor axis, therefore resulting in a positive cross covariance $c_{12} = c_{21}$. If the major axis subtends a negative angle the covariance is negative. The higher the covariance, the "thinner" the ellipsis (feature vectors concentrated around the major axis). In the cork stoppers example of Figure 2.13, the correlation (and therefore also the covariance) between N and PRT10 is high: 0.94.

Given a set of n patterns we can compute all the covariances using formula (2-15), and then establish a symmetric covariance matrix:

$$
\mathbf{C} = \begin{bmatrix} c_{11} & c_{12} & \cdots & c_{1d} \\ c_{21} & c_{22} & \cdots & c_{2d} \\ \cdots & \cdots & \cdots & \cdots \\ c_{d1} & c_{d2} & \cdots & c_{dd} \end{bmatrix}.
\tag{2-17}
$$

The covariance matrix $\mathbf{C}$ can be expressed compactly as the sum of the *direct products* of the difference vectors of $\mathbf{x}$ from the mean $\mathbf{m}$ by their transpose:

$$
\mathbf{C} = \frac{1}{n-1} \sum_{k=1}^{n} (\mathbf{x}_k - \mathbf{m})(\mathbf{x}_k - \mathbf{m})'.
\tag{2-17a}
$$

Suppose now that the feature vectors $\mathbf{x}$ undergo a linear transformation as in Figure 2.11. The transformed patterns will be characterized by a new mean vector and a new covariance matrix:

$$
\mathbf{m}_y = \mathbf{A}\mathbf{m}_x;
\tag{2-18a}
$$

$$
\mathbf{C}_y = \mathbf{A}\mathbf{C}_x\mathbf{A}'.
\tag{2-18b}
$$

Applying these formulas to the example shown in Figure 2.11 (matrix $\mathbf{A}$ presented in 2-12a), we obtain:

$$
\mathbf{m}_x = \begin{bmatrix} 1 \\ 1 \end{bmatrix} \quad \Rightarrow \quad \mathbf{m}_y = \begin{bmatrix} 2 & 1 \\ 1 & 1 \end{bmatrix}\begin{bmatrix} 1 \\ 1 \end{bmatrix} = \begin{bmatrix} 3 \\ 2 \end{bmatrix};
\tag{2-18c}
$$

$$
\mathbf{C}_x = \begin{bmatrix} 1 & 0 \\ 0 & 1 \end{bmatrix} \quad \Rightarrow \quad \mathbf{C}_y = \begin{bmatrix} 2 & 1 \\ 1 & 1 \end{bmatrix}\begin{bmatrix} 1 & 0 \\ 0 & 1 \end{bmatrix}\begin{bmatrix} 2 & 1 \\ 1 & 1 \end{bmatrix} = \begin{bmatrix} 5 & 3 \\ 3 & 2 \end{bmatrix}.
\tag{2-18d}
$$

The result (2-18c) was already obtained in (2-12c). The result (2-18d) shows that the transformed feature vectors have a variance of $\sqrt{5}$ along y_1 and $\sqrt{2}$ along y_2. It also shows that whereas in the original feature space the feature vectors were uncorrelated, there is now a substantial correlation in the transformed space.

In general, except for simple rotations or reflections, the Euclidian distances $\|\mathbf{x} - \mathbf{m}_x\|$ and $\|\mathbf{y} - \mathbf{m}_y\|$ will be different from each other. In order to maintain the distance relations before and after a linear transformation, we will have to generalize the idea of scaling presented at the beginning of this section, using the metric:

$$
\|\mathbf{x} - \mathbf{m}\|_m = (\mathbf{x} - \mathbf{m})'\mathbf{C}^{-1}(\mathbf{x} - \mathbf{m}).
\tag{2-19}
$$

This is a *Mahalanobis distance* already introduced in the preceding section. Notice that for the particular case of a diagonal matrix $\mathbf{C}$ one obtains the scaled distance formula (2-14a). The Mahalanobis distance is invariant to scaling operations, as can be illustrated for the preceding example, computing in the transformed space the distance corresponding to the feature vector $\begin{bmatrix} 1.5 & 1 \end{bmatrix}'$:

$$\mathbf{x} = \begin{bmatrix} 1.5 \\ 1 \end{bmatrix} \quad \Rightarrow \quad \mathbf{y} = \begin{bmatrix} 4 \\ 2.5 \end{bmatrix};$$

$$\mathbf{y} - \mathbf{m}_y = \begin{bmatrix} 1 \\ 0.5 \end{bmatrix} \quad \Rightarrow \quad (\mathbf{y} - \mathbf{m}_y)' \mathbf{C}_y^{-1} (\mathbf{y} - \mathbf{m}_y) = \begin{bmatrix} 1 & 0.5 \end{bmatrix} \begin{bmatrix} 2 & -3 \\ -3 & 5 \end{bmatrix} \begin{bmatrix} 1 \\ 0.5 \end{bmatrix} = 1.$$

Using the Mahalanobis metric with the appropriate covariance matrix we are able to adjust our classifiers to any particular hyperellipsoidal shape the pattern clusters might have.

We now present some important properties of the covariance matrix, to be used in following chapters.

Covariance estimation

Until now we have only used sample estimates of mean and covariance computed from a training set of n patterns per class. As already discussed in section 1.5.2, in order for a classifier to maintain an adequate performance when presented with new cases, our mean and covariance estimates must be sufficiently near the theoretical values, corresponding to $n \to \infty$.

Estimating $\mathbf{C}$ corresponds to estimating $d(d+1)/2$ terms c_{ij}. Looking at formula (2-17a), we see that $\mathbf{C}$ is the sum of $n-1$ independent $d{\times}d$ matrices of characteristic 1, therefore the computed matrix will be singular if $n \leq d$. The conclusion is that $n = d+1$ is the *minimum number of patterns per class* a training set must have in order for a classifier using the Mahalanobis distance to be designed. Near this minimum value numerical problems can arise in the computation of $\mathbf{C}^{-1}$.

Orthonormal transformation

The orthonormal transformation is a linear transformation which allows one to derive uncorrelated features from a set of correlated features. In order to see how this transformation is determined, let us consider the correlated features of Figure 2.11 (feature vector $\mathbf{y}$) and assume that we knew the linear transformation $\mathbf{y} = \mathbf{A}\mathbf{x}$, producing $\mathbf{y}$ based on the uncorrelated features corresponding to the feature vector $\mathbf{x}$, characterized by a simple unit covariance matrix $\mathbf{I}$ (circular cluster). Suppose now that we wished to find the uncorrelated feature vectors $\mathbf{z}$ that maintain the same direction after the transformation:

$$\mathbf{y} = \mathbf{A}\mathbf{z} = \lambda \mathbf{z} . \tag{2-20}$$

The determination of the scalars λ and the vectors $\mathbf{z}$ corresponds to solving the equation $(\lambda\mathbf{I}-\mathbf{A})\mathbf{z} = \mathbf{0}$, with $\mathbf{I}$ the unit $d{\times}d$ matrix, i.e. $|\lambda\mathbf{I}-\mathbf{A}| = 0$, in order to obtain non-trivial solutions. There are d scalar solutions λ called the *eigenvalues* of $\mathbf{A}$.

After solving the homogeneous system of equations for the different eigenvalues one obtains a family of *eigenvectors* **z**.

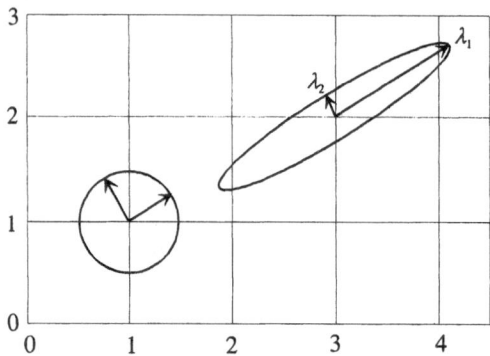

Figure 2.15. Eigenvectors of a linear transformation, maintaining the same direction before and after the transformation. The standard deviations along the eigenvectors are λ_1 and λ_2.

Let us compute the eigenvalues for the transformation of Figure 2.11:

$$\lambda \mathbf{I} - \mathbf{A} = \begin{bmatrix} \lambda - 2 & -1 \\ -1 & \lambda - 1 \end{bmatrix} = 0 \;\Rightarrow\; \lambda^2 - 3\lambda + 1 = 0 \;\Rightarrow\; \lambda_1 = 2.618, \; \lambda_2 = 0.382.$$

For λ_1 the homogeneous system of equations is:

$$\begin{bmatrix} -0.618 & -1 \\ -1 & 1.618 \end{bmatrix} \begin{bmatrix} z_1 \\ z_2 \end{bmatrix} = 0,$$

allowing us to choose the eigenvector: $\mathbf{z}_1 = \begin{bmatrix} 1 & 0.618 \end{bmatrix}'$. For λ_2 we can compute the following eigenvector orthogonal to $\mathbf{z}_1$: $\mathbf{z}_2 = \begin{bmatrix} -1 & 1.618 \end{bmatrix}'$.

For a real symmetric and non-singular matrix **A** one always obtains d distinct eigenvalues. Also, in this case, each pair of eigenvalues correspond to orthogonal eigenvectors. Figure 2.15 illustrates the eigenvectors for the example we have been solving. Using the eigenvectors one may obtain new features which are uncorrelated. As a matter of fact, consider the matrix **Z** of unitary eigenvectors:

$$\mathbf{Z} = \begin{bmatrix} \mathbf{z}_1 & \mathbf{z}_2 & \dots & \mathbf{z}_d \end{bmatrix}, \tag{2-21}$$

with $\mathbf{z}_i'\mathbf{z}_j = 0$ and $\mathbf{Z}'\mathbf{Z} = \mathbf{I}$ (i.e., **Z** is an *orthonormal matrix*). (2-21a)

Suppose that we apply a linear transformation with the transpose of $\mathbf{Z}$, $\mathbf{u} = \mathbf{Z'y}$, to the vectors $\mathbf{y}$ with covariance $\mathbf{C}$. Then, as shown in Appendix C, the new covariance matrix will be *diagonal* (uncorrelated features), having the squares of the eigenvalues as new variances and preserving the Mahalanobis distances. This *orthonormal transformation* is also called Karhunen-Loève transformation.

Notice that we have been using the eigenvectors computed from the original linear transformation matrix $\mathbf{A}$. Usually we do not know this matrix, and instead, we will compute the eigenvectors of $\mathbf{C}$ itself, which are the same. The corresponding eigenvalues of $\mathbf{C}$ are, however, the square of the ones computed from $\mathbf{A}$, and represent the variances along the eigenvectors or, equivalently, the eigenvectors of $\mathbf{A}$ represent the standard deviations, as indicated in Figure 2.15. It is customary to sort the eigenvectors by decreasing magnitude, the first one corresponding to the direction of maximum variance, as shown in Figure 2.15, the second one to the direction of the maximum remaining variance, and so on, until the last one (λ_2 in Figure 2.15) representing only a residual variance.

Appendix C also includes the demonstration of the positive definiteness of the covariance matrices and other equally interesting results.

2.4 Principal Components

As mentioned in the previous chapter the initial choice of features in PR problems is mostly guided by common sense ideas of pattern discrimination. Therefore, it is not unusual to have a large initial set constituted by features that may exhibit high correlations among them, and whose contribution to pattern discrimination may vary substantially. Large feature sets are inconvenient for a number of reasons, an obvious one being the computational burden. Less obvious and more compelling reasons will be explained later. A common task in PR problems is therefore to perform some type of feature selection. In the initial phase of a PR project, such selection aims to either discard features whose contribution is insignificant as will be described in section 2.5, or to perform some kind of dimensionality reduction by using an alternative and smaller set of features derived from the initial ones.

Principal components analysis is a method commonly used for data reduction purposes. It is based on the idea of performing an orthonormal transformation as described in the previous section, retaining only significant eigenvectors. As explained in the section on orthonormal transformation, each eigenvector is associated with a variance represented by the corresponding eigenvalue. Each eigenvector corresponding to an eigenvalue that represents a significant variance of the whole dataset is called a *principal component* of the data. For instance, in the example portrayed in Figure 2.15 the first eigenvector represents $\lambda_1^2 / (\lambda_1^2 + \lambda_2^2) =$ 98% of the total variance; in short, $\mathbf{z}_1$ alone contains practically all information about the data.

Let us see how this works in a real situation. Figure 2.16 shows the sorted list of the eigenvalues (classes ω_1, ω_2) of the cork stoppers data, computed with *Statistica*. The ninth eigenvalue, for instance, is responsible for about 0.01% of the total variance, certainly a negligible fraction. The first 3 eigenvalues, however, are responsible for more than 95% of the total variance, which suggests that it would probably be adequate to use the corresponding first 3 eigenvectors (computed as linear transformations of the original features) instead of the 10 original features.

FACTOR ANALYSIS	Extraction: Principal components			
Value	Eigenval	% total Variance	Cumul. Eigenval	Cumul. %
1	7.672	76.72	7.67	76.72
2	1.236	12.36	8.91	89.08
3	.726	7.26	9.63	96.34
4	.235	2.35	9.87	98.68
5	.086	.86	9.95	99.54
6	.029	.29	9.98	99.83
7	.009	.09	9.99	99.91
8	.006	.06	10.00	99.98
9	.001	.01	10.00	99.99
10	.001	.01	10.00	100.00

Figure 2.16. Sorted list of the eigenvalues for the cork stoppers data (two classes).

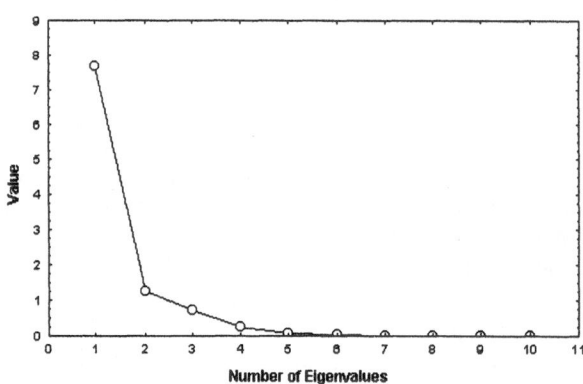

Figure 2.17. Plot of the eigenvalues for the cork stoppers data (two classes).

When using principal component analysis for dimensionality reduction, the decision one must make is how many eigenvectors (and corresponding eigenvalues) to retain. The *Kaiser criterion* discards eigenvalues below 1, which nearly corresponds to retaining the eigenvalues responsible for an amount of variance of one feature if the total variance was equally distributed. For the cork stoppers data this would correspond to retaining only the first 2 eigenvalues. It can also be useful to inspect a plot of the eigenvalues as illustrated in Figure 2.17. A criterion based on such a plot (called *scree test*) suggests discarding the eigenvalues starting where the plot levels off, which, in this case, would amount to retaining only the first 4 eigenvalues.

Principal components analysis as a dimensionality reduction method must be applied with caution, for the following reasons:

– Principal components are *linear transformations* of the original features, therefore, reduction to significant principal components may not appropriately reflect non-linearities that may be present in the data (see e.g. chapter eight of Bishop, 1995).
– Principal components with negligible contribution to the overall variance may nevertheless provide a crucial contribution to pattern discrimination. By discarding such components we may inadvertently impair the classification or regression performance (idem).
– It is usually difficult to attach any semantic meaning to principal components. Such semantic meaning, provided by the original features, is often useful when developing and applying classification or regression solutions.

Although principal components analysis suffers from these shortcomings there is still something to be gained from it since it provides the designer with desirable low dimensional representations of the original data, to be explored further in the next chapter. It also provides meaningful estimates of the intrinsic data dimensionality, which can somehow serve as reference for more sophisticated feature selection methods, to be explained in chapter four.

2.5 Feature Assessment

Assessing the discriminative capability of features is an important task either in the initial phase of a PR project or in a more advanced phase, for example, when choosing between alternative feature sets. This assessment is usually of great help in guiding subsequent project phases by giving some insight in what is going on in the feature space, e.g., concerning class separability.

The feature assessment task is usually conducted in the following sequence of subtasks:

1. Graphic inspection
2. Distribution model assessment
3. Statistic inference tests

We will illustrate now these subtasks using the cork stoppers data. We assume that the reader is familiar with the statistical techniques used, which are described in many textbooks on Statistics, namely Hoel (1975), and Siegel and Castellan (1998).

2.5.1 Graphic Inspection

Graphic inspection allows one to compare feature distributions for the several classes of the problem at hand, and therefore to obtain some insight into their usefulness for the class discrimination task. There are several types of graphic representations that can be used depending on the insight one wishes to obtain. Particularly useful in PR problems, besides histograms, are box plots and scatter plots.

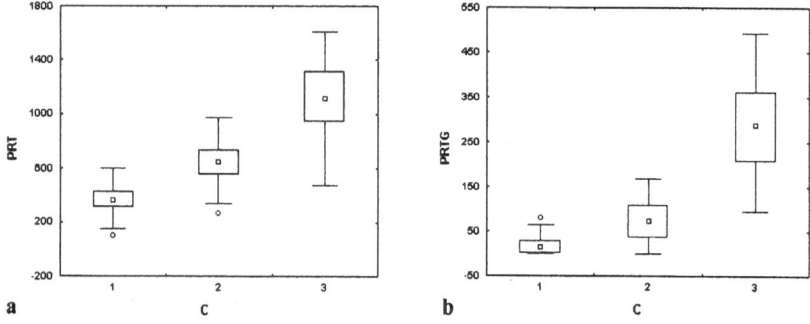

Figure 2.18. Box plots for the 3 classes of cork stoppers and features PRT (a) and PRTG (b): □ – median position; ⊥ - *extremes*, exceeding above or below the box 1.5 times the interquartile distance; o - *outliers*, exceeding above or below the box 3 times the interquartile distance.

A box plot depicts for each feature and each class a box representing the interquartile range of the distribution, i.e., covering 50% of the central feature values. Figure 2.18 shows box plots for features PRT and PRTG of the cork stoppers data. As shown in this figure, the box plot usually includes further information.

As can be appreciated from Figure 2.18, box plots give a clear indication of the discrimination capability of each feature and the amount of overlap of the several classes. In this example we see that feature PRT seems to discriminate the three classes well, meanwhile feature PRTG seems to be useful only in the discrimination of class ω_3 from classes ω_1 and ω_2.

Features with largely overlapped distributions are, of course, of little help for classification or regression purposes.

Scatter plots are useful for gaining some insight into the topology of the classes and clusters, especially for identifying features that are less correlated among them and have more discriminative capability.

Figure 2.19 shows the scatter plot for the three classes of cork stoppers using features ART and RAN, which, as we will see in a later section, are quite discriminative and less correlated than others.

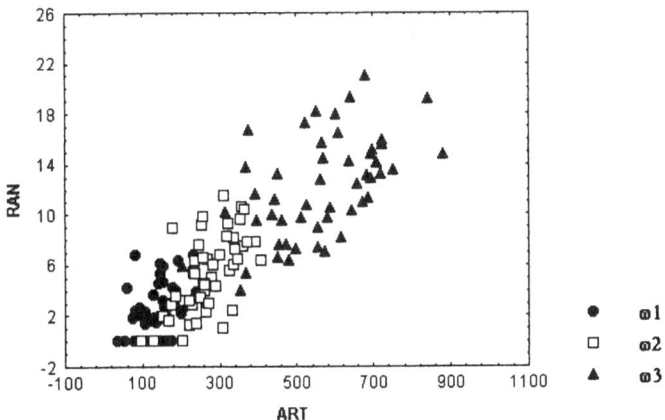

Figure 2.19. Scatter plot for the three classes of cork stoppers (features ART and RAN).

2.5.2 Distribution Model Assessment

Some pattern classification approaches assume a distribution model of the patterns. In these cases one has to assess whether the distributions of the feature vectors comply reasonably with the model used. Also, the statistical inference tests that are to be applied for assessing feature discriminative power may depend on whether the distributions obey a certain model or not. The distribution model that is by far the most popular is the Gaussian or normal model.

Statistical software products include tests on the acceptability of a given distribution model. On this subject *Statistica* offers results of the *Kolmogorov-Smirnov* (K-S) and the *Shapiro-Wilk* tests along with the representation of histograms.

Figure 2.20 shows the histograms of features PRT and ARTG for class ω_1, with overlaid normal curve (with same sample mean and variance) and results of normality tests on the top.

As can be appreciated, feature PRT is well modelled by a normal distribution (K-S $p > 0.2$), whereas for feature ARTG, the normality assumption has to be rejected (K-S $p < 0.01$). In all tests we are using a 95% confidence level. When using the *Komogorov-Smirnov* test one must take into account the *Lillefors* correction (use of sample mean and sample variance) as we did before. The *Shapiro-Wilk* test results should also be inspected, especially in the situation of small n ($n < 25$), where this test is more accurate.

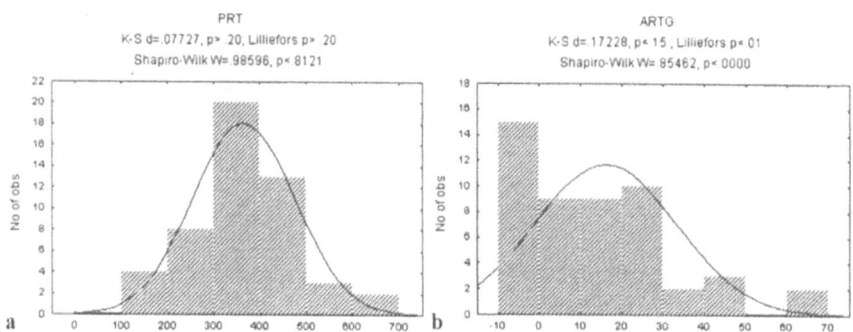

Figure 2.20. Histograms and normality tests for features PRT (a) and ARTG (b).

2.5.3 Statistical Inference Tests

Statistical inference tests provide a quantification of the features' discriminative powers. The well-known *t-Student* and *Anova* statistical tests can be applied to features complying to a normal distribution, for assessing the discrimination of two and more than two classes, respectively.

Frequently one has to deal with features showing appreciable departure from the normal model, at least for some classes. It is also not uncommon to have a reduced number of cases available at the beginning of a project, thereby decreasing the power of the normality tests. Therefore, it is reasonable, in many cases, to adopt a conservative attitude, avoiding the assumption of a distribution model when comparing features. We then resort to a non-parametric statistical test for independent samples, namely the *Kruskal-Wallis* test. Figure 2.21 shows the results of this test for the ART feature of the cork stoppers.

The Kruskal-Wallis test sorts the feature values and assigns ordinal ranks in corresponding order to the original values. The sums of these ranks for the classes are then used to compute the value of the governing statistic H, which reflects the difference of the ranks' sums. From Figure 2.21 we observe a significantly high ($p=0$) value of H, not attributable to chance. We therefore accept ART as a feature with definite discriminating capability.

NONPAR STATS	Independent variable: C H (2, N= 150) = 121.5896 p = .0000		
Depend.: ART	Code	Valid N	Sum of Ranks
Group 1	1	50	1409.0
Group 2	2	50	3717.5
Group 3	3	50	6198.5

Figure 2.21. Kruskal-Wallis test for feature ART of the cork stoppers data.

It is also useful, as we have seen in previous sections, to compute the correlations among the features in order to eventually discard features that are highly correlated with other ones. Figure 2.22 shows the correlation matrix for the cork stoppers features. All of them are significantly correlated. For instance, the total perimeter of the defects (PRT), not surprisingly, has a high correlation (0.98) with their total area (ART). The same happens for the big defects with a 0.99 correlation for the respective features (PRTG and ARTG). It is therefore reasonable to discard one of the PRT, ART features when the other one is used, and likewise for the PRTG, ARTG features.

Var.	N=150									
	ART	N	PRT	ARM	PRM	ARTG	NG	PRTG	RAAR	RAN
ART	1.00	.80	.98	.87	.88	.96	.94	.97	.86	.85
N	.80	1.00	.89	.45	.49	.68	.75	.72	.61	.55
PRT	.98	.89	1.00	.78	.81	.91	.92	.93	.82	.79
ARM	.87	.45	.78	1.00	.99	.88	.80	.87	.85	.89
PRM	.88	.49	.81	.99	1.00	.88	.81	.88	.86	.88
ARTG	.96	.68	.91	.88	.88	1.00	.91	.99	.92	.86
NG	.94	.75	.92	.80	.81	.91	1.00	.96	.85	.93
PRTG	.97	.72	.93	.87	.88	.99	.96	1.00	.91	.90
RAAR	.86	.61	.82	.85	.86	.92	.85	.91	1.00	.87
RAN	.85	.55	.79	.89	.88	.86	.93	.90	.87	1.00

Figure 2.22. Correlation matrix for the cork stoppers features. All correlations are significant at $p=0.05$ level.

Once all the inference tests have been performed it is convenient to summarize the results in a sorted table, as was done in Table 2.1 for the *Kruskal-Wallis* test results for all features. Sorting should be done for the p values and in case of ties for the H values. For the cork stopper features all p values are zero, therefore Table 2.1 lists only the H values from the most discriminative feature, ART, to the less discriminative, N.

Table 2.1. Cork stoppers features in descending order of Kruskal-Wallis' H (three classes).

Feature	H
ART	121.6
PRTM	117.6
PRT	115.7
ARTG	115.2
ARTM	113.5
PRTG	113.3
RA	105.2
NG	104.4
RN	94.3
N	74.5

2.6 The Dimensionality Ratio Problem

In section 2.1.1 we saw that a complex decision surface in a low dimensionality space can be made linear and therefore much simpler, in a higher dimensionality space. Let us take another look at formula (2-14a). It is obvious that by adding more features one can only increase the distance of a pattern to a class mean. Therefore, it seems that working in high dimensionality feature spaces, or equivalently, using arbitrarily complex decision surfaces (e.g. Figure 2.5), can only increase the classification or regression performance.

However, this expected performance increase is not verified in practice. The reason for this counterintuitive result, related to the reliable estimation of classifier or regressor parameters, is one of the forms of what is generally known as the *curse of dimensionality*.

In order to get some insight into what is happening, let us assume that we are confronted with a two-class classification problem whose data collection progresses slowly. Initially we only have available $n=6$ patterns for each class. The patterns are represented in a $d=2$ feature space as shown in Figure 2.23. The two classes seem linearly separable with 0% error. Fine!

Meanwhile, a few more cases were gathered and we now have available $n=10$ patterns. The corresponding scatter plot is shown in Figure 2.24. Hum! ... The situation is getting tougher. It seems that, after all, the classes were not so separable as we had imagined.... However, a quadratic decision function still seems to provide a solution...

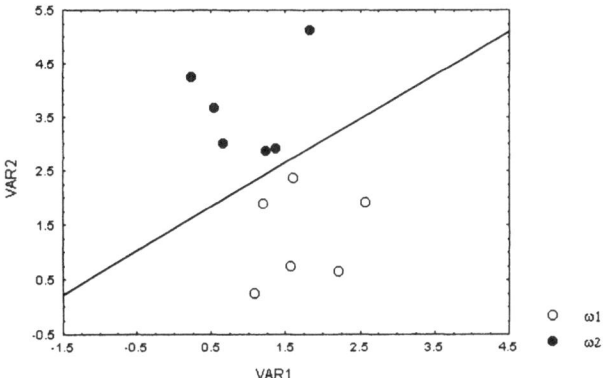

Figure 2.23. Two class linear discrimination with dimensionality ratio $n/d = 6$.

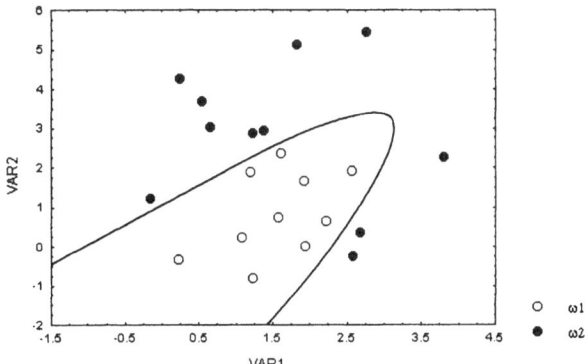

Figure 2.24. Two class quadratic discrimination with dimensionality ratio $n/d = 10$.

Later on, the data collection task has progressed considerably. We now have available 30 patterns of each class, distributed as shown in Figure 2.25.

What a disappointment! The classes are largely overlapped. As a matter of fact, all the data were generated with:

Class 1:	$Var1 = N(1.0, 1);$ [2]	$Var2 = N(1.0, 1)$
Class 2:	$Var1 = N(1.1, 1);$	$Var2 = N(1.2, 2)$

---

[2] $N(m, s)$ is the normal distribution with mean m and standard deviation s. In equally scaled scatter plots, class 1 is represented by a circular cluster and class 2 by an elliptic cluster with a vertical axis bigger than the horizontal axis.

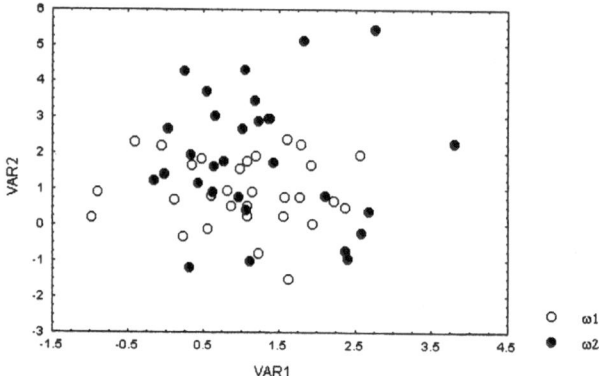

Figure 2.25. Two class scatter plot with dimensionality ratio $n/d = 30$.

This is a dramatic example of how the use of a reduced set of patterns compared to the number of features - i.e., the use of a low *dimensionality ratio, n/d* – can lead to totally wrong conclusions about a classifier (or regressor) performance evaluated in a training set. We can get more insight into this dimensionality problem by looking at it from the perspective of how many patterns one needs to have available in order to design a classifier, i.e., what is the minimum size of the training set. Consider that we would be able to train the classifier by deducing a rule based on the location of each pattern in the d-dimensional space. In a certain sense, this is in fact how the neural network approach works. In order to have a sufficient resolution we assume that the range of values for each feature is divided into m intervals; therefore we have to assess the location of each pattern in each of the m^d hypercubes. This number of hypercubes grows exponentially so that for a value of d that is not too low we have to find a mapping for a quite sparsely occupied space, i.e., with a poor representation of the mapping.

This phenomenon, generally called the *curse of dimensionality* phenomenon, also affects our common intuition about the concept of neighbourhood. In order to see this, imagine that we have a one-dimensional normal distribution. We know then that about 68% of the distributed values lie within one standard deviation around the mean. If we increase our representation to two independent dimensions, we now have only about 46% in a circle around the mean and for a d-dimensional representation we have $(0.68)^d \times 100\%$ samples in a hypersphere with a radius of one standard deviation, which means, as shown in Figure 2.26, that for $d=12$ less than 1% of the data is in the neighbourhood of the mean! For the well-known 95% neighbourhood, corresponding approximately to two standard deviations, we will find only about 54% of the patterns for $d=12$.

The dimensionality ratio issue is a central issue in PR with a deep influence on the quality of any PR project and, therefore, we will dedicate special attention to this issue at all opportune moments.

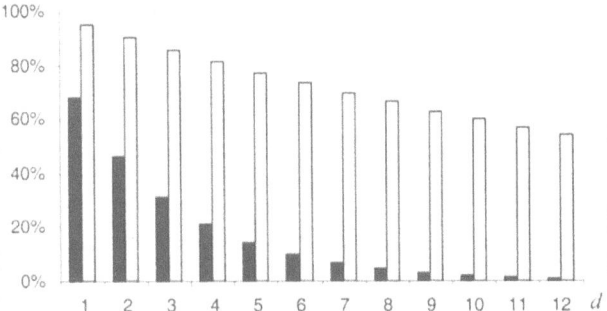

Figure 2.26. Percentage of normally distributed samples lying within one standard deviation neighbourhood (black bars) and two standard deviations neighbourhood (grey bars) for several values of d.

Bibliography

Andrews HC (1972) Introduction to Mathematical Techniques in Pattern Recognition, John Wiley & Sons, Inc.

Bishop CM (1995) Neural Networks for Pattern Recognition. Clarendon Press, Oxford.

Bronson R (1991) Matrix Methods. An Introduction. Academic Press, Inc.

Duda R, Hart P (1973) Pattern Classification and Scene Analysis. Wiley, New York.

Friedman M, Kandel A (1999) Introduction to Pattern Recognition. Statistical, Structural, Neural and Fuzzy Logic Approaches. World Scientific Co. Pte. Ltd., Singapore.

Fukunaga K (1990) Introduction to Statistical Pattern Recognition. Academic Press.

Hoel PG (1975) Elementary Statistics. John Wiley & Sons.

Looney CG (1997) Pattern Recognition Using Neural Networks. Theory and Algorithms for Engineers and Scientists. Oxford University Press.

Pipes LA, Hovanessian SA (1996) Matrix-Computer Methods in Engineering. Robert Krieger Pub. Co., Florida.

Schalkoff RJ (1992) Pattern Recognition. Statistical, Structural and Neural Approaches. John Wiley & Sons, Inc.

Siegel S, Castellan Jr NJ (1998) Nonparametric Statistics for the Behavioral Sciences. McGraw Hill Book Co., Sidney.

Späth H (1980) Cluster Analysis Algorithms. Ellis Horwood, Ltd., England.

Milton JS, McTeer PM, Corbet JJ (2000) Introduction to Statistics. McGraw Hill College Div.

Exercises

2.1 Consider the two-dimensional *Globular* data included in the *Cluster.xls* file. With the help of a scatter plot determine the linear decision function that separates the two visiually identifiable clusters, with slope minus one and at a minimum distance from the origin.

2.2 A classifier uses the following linear discriminant in a 3-dimensional space:

$$d(\mathbf{x}) = x_1 + 2x_2 + x_3 + 1.$$

  a) Compute the distance of the discriminant from the origin.
  b) Give an example of a pattern whose classification is borderline ($d(\mathbf{x})=0$).
  c) Compute the distance of the feature vector [1 -1 0]' from the discriminant.

2.3 A pattern classification problem has one feature x and two classes of points: $\omega_1=\{-2, 1, 1.5\}$; $\omega_2=\{-1, -0.5, 0\}$.
  a) Determine a linear discriminant of the two classes in a two-dimensional space, using features $y_1 = x$ and $y_2 = x^2$.
  b) Determine the quadratic classifier in the original feature space that corresponds to the previous linear classifier.

2.4 Consider a two-class one-dimensional problem with one feature x and classes $\omega_1=\{-1, 1\}$ and $\omega_2=\{0, 2\}$.
  a) Show that the classes are linearly separable in the two-dimensional feature space with feature vectors $\mathbf{y}=[x^2 \ x^3]'$ and write a linear decision rule.
  b) Using the previous linear decision rule write the corresponding rule in the original one-dimensional space.

2.5 Consider the equidistant surfaces relative to two prototype patterns, using the city-block and Chebychev metrics in a two-dimensional space, as shown in Figure 2.10. In which case do the decision functions correspond to simple straight lines?

2.6 Draw the scatter plot of the +Cross data (Cluster.xls) and consider it composed of two classes of points corresponding to the cross arms, with the same prototype, the cross center. Which metric must be used in order for a decision function, based on the distance to the prototypes, to achieve class separation?

2.7 Compute the linear transformation $\mathbf{y} = \mathbf{Ax}$ in a two-dimensional space using the sets of points $P=\{(0,0), (0.5,0), (0,1), (-1.5,0), (0,-2)\}$ and $Q=\{(1,1), (0,1), (1,0), (2,1), (1,2)\}$, observing:

- Simple scaling for $a_{21}=a_{12}=0$ with translation for set Q.
- Simple rotation for $a_{21}=-a_{12}=1$ and $a_{11}=a_{22}=0$.
- Simple mirroring for $a_{21}=a_{12}=1$ and $a_{11}=a_{22}=0$.

This analysis can be performed using Microsoft Excel. Combinations of scaling, translation with rotation or mirroring can also be observed.

2.8 Consider the linear transformation (2-12a) applied to pattern clusters with circular shape, as shown in Figure 2.11. Compute the correlation between the transformed features and explain which types of transformation matrices do not change the correlation values.

2.9 Which of the following matrices can be used in a 2-dimensional linear transformation preserving the Mahalanobis distance relations?

$$A = \begin{bmatrix} 2 & 1 \\ -1 & 1 \end{bmatrix}; \qquad B = \begin{bmatrix} 2 & 1 \\ 1 & 1 \end{bmatrix}; \qquad C = \begin{bmatrix} 1 & 0.5 \\ 0.5 & -1 \end{bmatrix}$$

Explain why.

2.10 Determine the orthonormal transformation for the data represented in Figure 2.11 in the y plane.

2.11 Consider the *Tissue* dataset. Determine, for each pattern class, which feature distributions can be reasonably described by the normal model.

2.12 Consider the *CTG* dataset. Perform Kruskal-Wallis tests for all the features and sort them by decreasing discriminative capacity (ten classes). Using the rank values of the tests and box plots determine the contributions for class discrimination of the best three features.

3 Data Clustering

3.1 Unsupervised Classification

In the previous chapters, when introducing the idea of similarity as a distance between feature vectors, we often computed this distance relative to a prototype pattern. We have also implicitly assumed that the shape of the class distributions in the feature space around a prototype was known, and based on this, we could choose a suitable distance metric. The knowledge of such class shapes and prototypes is obtained from a previously classified training set of patterns. The design of a PR system using this "teacher" information is called a *supervised* design. For the moment our interest is in classification systems and we will refer then to *supervised classification*.

We are often confronted with a more primitive situation where no previous knowledge about the patterns is available or obtainable (after all, we learn to classify a lot of things without being taught). Therefore our classifying system must "discover" the internal similarity structure of the patterns in a useful way. We then need to design our system using a so-called *unsupervised* approach. The present chapter is dedicated to the *unsupervised classification* of feature vectors, also called *data clustering*. This is essentially a *data-driven* approach, that attempts to discover structure within the data itself, grouping together the feature vectors in *clusters* of data.

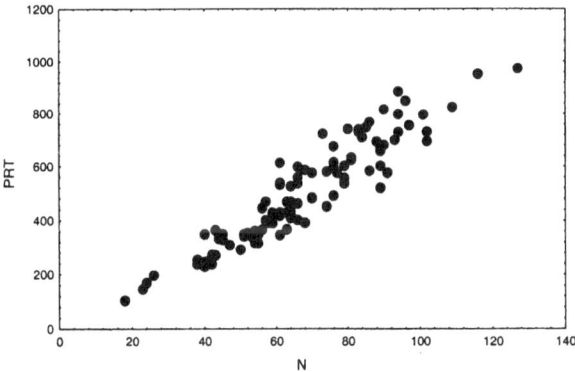

Figure 3.1. Scatter plot of the first 100 cork stoppers, using features N and PRT.

In order to show the basic difficulties of data clustering let us look to the scatter plot of the first two classes of the corker stoppers data, features N and PRT, without any pattern labelling, such as represented in Figure 3.1. Do we really see two clusters? If we were asked to delineate two clusters, where should we set the limits? Would such limits approximate the class limits?

From Figure 3.1 one readily gets the impression that data clustering is an ill-formulated problem with an arbitrary number of solutions, especially in the case where no cluster separation is visually identifiable. However, there are a number of reasons for applying clustering techniques, such as the following important ones:

- **In order to obtain a useful summary and interpretation of the problem data**. This is the classical purpose of clustering, applied to a wide variety of problems. A good review can be found in Hartigan (1975). Data is summarized by referring to the attributes of the clusters instead of the attributes of the individual patterns. Cluster interpretation can provide guidance on the development of scientific theories. Good examples of this last application are the clusters of stars, which inspired theories about the life of stars, and the clusters of animal species, which inspired evolutionary theories.
- **In order to initialise a supervised statistical classification approach**. This type of application is attractive when data collection is a very slow and costly process. Clustering is used then as an unsupervised classification method at a starting phase in order to obtain parametric estimates of the class distributions for a small initial set of patterns. These estimates will be updated, as more patterns become available. The reader can find a good description of this topic in Duda and Hart (1973).
- **In order to provide centroid estimates for neural network classifiers**. The *centroid* of a cluster is the average point in the multidimensional feature space. In a sense, it is the centre of gravity of the respective cluster. We will refer to this application in detail in chapter five, when discussing radial basis functions.

There are a large number of clustering algorithms, depending on the type of data, on the rules for pattern amalgamation in a cluster and on the approach followed for applying such rules. Regarding the type of amalgamation approach two categories of algorithms can be considered:

- **Hierarchical algorithms**

The hierarchical or tree clustering algorithms use linkage rules of the patterns in order to produce a hierarchical sequence of clustering solutions. Algorithms of this type are adequate for a reduced and meaningful set of patterns, i.e., the set must contain representative pattern exemplars.

- **Centroid adjustment algorithms**

Algorithms of this type use an iterative method in order to adjust prototypes, also called centroids, of the clusters, as a consequence of the patterns assignable to them. In section 3.3 a popular algorithm of this type will be explained.

An important aspect of data clustering is which patterns or cases to choose for deriving the cluster solution. Usually, in data clustering, one wants *typical cases* to be represented, i.e., cases that the designer suspects of typifying the structure of the data. If the clustering solution supports typical case, it is generally considered a good solution. A totally different perspective is followed in supervised classification, where no distinction is made between typical and atypical cases, since a classifier is expected to perform uniformly for all cases. Therefore, random data sampling, a requirement when designing supervised classifiers, is not usually needed. It is only when one is interested in generalizing the clustering results that the issue of random sampling should be considered.

3.2 The Standardization Issue

Data clustering explores the metric properties of the feature vectors in the feature space (described in 2.2) in order to join them into meaningful groups. As one has no previous knowledge concerning prototypes or cluster shape, there is an arbitrarily large number of data clustering solutions that can be radically different from each other. As an example, consider the +*Cross* data available in the *Cluster.xls* file, which is represented in Figure 3.2a.

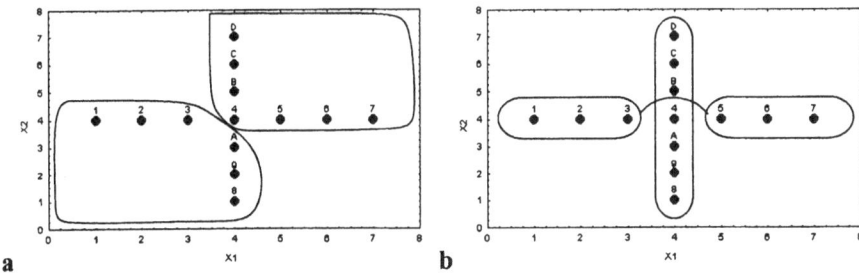

Figure 3.2. Cross data with: (a) Euclidian clustering; (b) City-block clustering.

Imagine that we are searching for a 2-cluster solution that minimizes the *within-cluster average error*:

$$E = \sum_{i=1}^{c} \frac{1}{n_i} \sum_{x,\, y \in \omega_i} \text{distance}(x, y),$$ (3-1)

with n_i different pairs of patterns x, y in cluster ω_i.

Therefore, minimizing E corresponds in a certain sense to minimizing the cluster volumes, which seems a sensible decision. If we use a Euclidian metric to evaluate the distance between the pairs of feature vectors, we obtain the cluster solution depicted in Figure 3.2a. This solution is quite distinct from the visual clustering solution, shown in Figure 3.2b, which is obtained using the city-block metric. If we had used the *xCross* data instead, it is easy to see that the only adequate metric to use in this case is the Chebychev metric.

As we see from the cross data example, clustering solutions may depend drastically on the metric used. There is, however, a subtle point concerning the measurement scale of the features that must be emphasized. Whereas in the following chapters we will design classifiers using supervised methods, which are in principle independent (or moderately dependent) of the measurement scale of the features, when performing data clustering, the solutions obtained may also vary drastically with the measurement scale or type of *standardization* of the features.

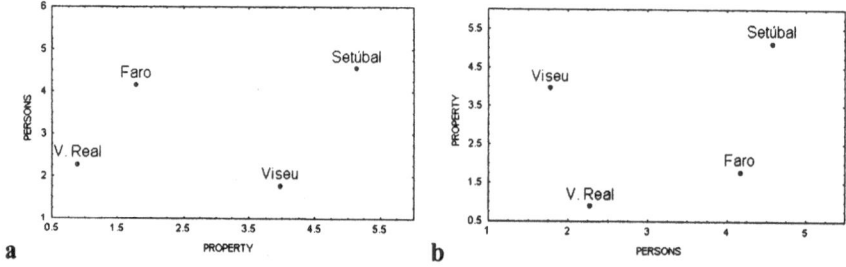

Figure 3.3. Visual clustering of crimes data with different coordinate axes. (a) {Faro, V. Real} {Setúbal, Viseu}; (b) {Viseu, V. Real} {Setúbal, Faro}.

An example of the influence of *feature standardization* can be seen in Figure 3.3, where the same patterns of the *Crimes* dataset are depicted changing the position and scale of the coordinate axes. In Figure 3.3a two clusters can be identified visually {Faro, V. Real} and {Setúbal, Viseu}; in Figure 3.3b the visual clustering is different: {Viseu, V. Real}, {Faro, Setúbal}. Notice that this contradictory result is a consequence of a different *representation scale* of the coordinate axes, which corresponds with situations of different *true scales*: in a) with a shrunken *persons* scale; in b) with a shrunken *property* scale. If the true scales were used then one would tend to choose only one cluster. The problem is aggravated when the features are of different nature, measured in different measurement units and occupying quite disparate value ranges. This scaling aspect was already referred to in section 2.3 (see Figure 2.14) when discussing features' contribution to pattern discrimination.

First of all, the need for any standardization must be questioned. If the interesting clusters are based on the original features, then any standardization method may distort or mask those clusters. It is only when there are grounds to search for clusters in a transformed space that some standardization rule should be used.

Several simple standardization methods have been proposed for achieving scale invariance or at least attempting a balanced contribution of all features to distance measurements:

$$y_i = (x_i - m)/s \quad \text{with } m, s \text{ resp. mean and standard deviation of } x_i; \qquad (3\text{-}2a)$$
$$y_i = (x_i - \min(x_i))/(\max(x_i)-\min(x_i)); \qquad (3\text{-}2b)$$
$$y_i = x_i /(\max(x_i)-\min(x_i)); \qquad (3\text{-}2c)$$
$$y_i = x_i /a . \qquad (3\text{-}2d)$$

There is also, of course, the more sophisticated orthonormal transformation, described in section 2.3, preserving the Mahalanobis distance. All these standardization methods have some pitfalls. Consider, for instance, the popular standardization method of obtaining scale invariance by using transformed features with zero mean and unit variance (3-2a). An evident pitfall is that semantic information from the features can be lost with this standardization. Another problem is that this unit variance standardization is only adequate if the differing feature variances are due only to random variation. However, if such variation is due to data partition in distinct clusters it may produce totally wrong results.

If we know beforehand the type of clusters we are dealing with, we can devise a suitable standardization method. This poses the following vicious circle:

1. In order to perform clustering we need an appropriate distance measure.
2. The appropriate distance measure depends on the feature standardization method.
3. In order to select the standardization method we need to know the type of clusters needed.

There is no methodological way out of this vicious circle except by a "trial and error" approach, experimenting with various alternatives and evaluating the corresponding solutions aided by visual inspection, data interpretation and utility considerations. An easy standardization method that we will often follow and frequently achieves good results is the division or multiplication by a simple scale factor (e.g. a power of 10), properly chosen so that all feature values occupy a suitable interval. This corresponds to method (3-2d). In this way we can balance the contribution of the features and still retain semantic information.

3.3 Tree Clustering

Hierarchical or tree clustering algorithms allow us to reveal the internal similarities of a given pattern set and to structure these similarities hierarchically. They are usually applied to a small set of typical patterns.

For n patterns these algorithms generate a sequence of 1 to n clusters. This sequence has the form of a binary tree (two branches for each tree node) and can be structured bottom up – *merging algorithm* –, starting with the individual patterns, or top down – *splitting algorithm* –, starting with a cluster composed of all patterns.

The merging algorithm consists of the following steps:

1. Given n patterns x_i consider initially $c = n$ singleton clusters $\omega_i = \{ x_i \}$
2. While $c \geq 1$ do
   2.1. Determine the two nearest clusters ω_i and ω_j using an appropriate similarity measure and rule.
   2.2. Merge ω_i and ω_j: $\omega_{ij}=\{\omega_i, \omega_j \}$, therefore obtaining a solution with c-1 clusters.
   2.3. Decrease c.

Notice that in step 2.1 the determination of the nearest clusters depends both on the similarity measure and the rule used to assess the similarity of pairs of clusters.

Let us consider the *Globular* data (*Cluster.xls*) shown in Figure 3.4a and assume that the similarity between two clusters is assessed by measuring the similarity of its furthest pair of patterns (each one from a distinct cluster). This is the so-called *complete linkage* rule. As the merging process evolves, the similarity measure of the merged clusters decreases or, putting it in another way, their dissimilarity increases. This is illustrated in the binary tree shown as a *vertical icicle plot* in Figure 3.5a, for the complete linkage merging process of the 18 patterns.

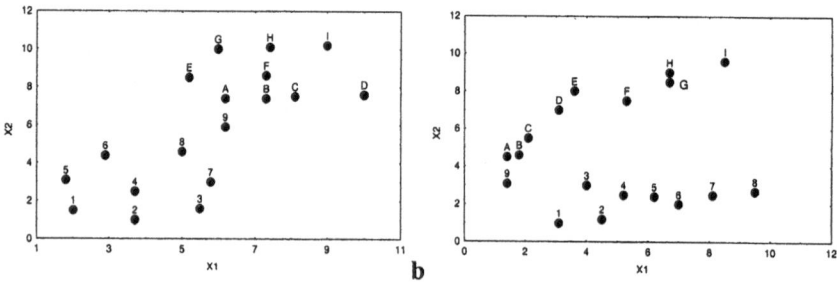

Figure 3.4. Globular (a) and filamentary (b) datasets for comparison of clustering methods.

The vertical icicle plot represents the hierarchical clustering tree and must be inspected bottom-up. Initially, as in step 1 of the merging algorithm, we have 18 clusters of singleton patterns. Next, patterns B and C are merged together as they are at the smallest Euclidian distance. Consider now that we are at a linkage distance of 4 with the following clusters: $\omega_1=\{I, D\}$, $\omega_2=\{A, B, C, E, F, G, H\}$, $\omega_3=\{8, 9\}$, $\omega_4=\{1, 2, 3, 4, 5, 6, 7\}$. In the next merging phase the distances of the furthest pair of patterns (each pattern from a distinct cluster) of $\{\omega_1, \omega_2\}$, $\{\omega_1, \omega_3\}$, $\{\omega_1, \omega_4\}$, $\{\omega_2, \omega_3\}$, $\{\omega_2, \omega_4\}$, $\{\omega_3, \omega_4\}$ are computed. The smallest of these distances corresponds to $\{\omega_1, \omega_2\}$, therefore these are clustered next. This process continues until finally all patterns are merged into one cluster.

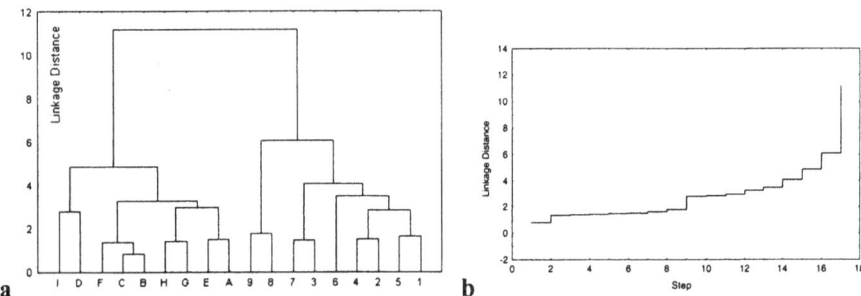

Figure 3.5. (a) Vertical icicle plot for the globular data; (b) Clustering schedule graph.

Figure 3.5b shows the clustering schedule graph, which may be of help for selecting the best cluster solutions. These usually correspond to a plateau before a high jump in the distance measure. In this case the best cluster solution has two clusters, corresponding to the somewhat globular clouds $\{1, 2, 3, 4, 5, 6, 7, 8, 9\}$ and $\{A, B, C, D, E, F, G, H, I\}$. Notice also that, usually, the more meaningful solutions have balanced clusters (in terms of the number of cases) or, to put it in another way, solutions with very small or even singleton clusters are rather suspicious.

Let us now consider the *crimes* data for the Portuguese towns represented by the scatter plot of Figure 3.6a. Using the complete linkage method the *dendrogram* of Figure 3.6b is obtained. A dendrogram is just like a horizontal icicle plot.

Dendrogram inspection shows that there is a substantial increase in the dissimilarity measure when passing from 3 to 2 clusters. It seems, therefore, that an interesting cluster solution from the point of view of summarizing the data is:

Cluster 1 = {Aveiro, Setúbal, V. Castelo}: High incidence of crimes against property; above average against persons.

Cluster 2 = {Beja, Braga, Bragança, Coimbra, Porto, Santarém, Viseu}: High incidence of crimes against property; below average against persons.

Cluster 3 = {C. Branco, Évora, Faro, Guarda, Leiria, Lisboa, Portalegre, V. Real}: Average incidence of crimes against property and persons.

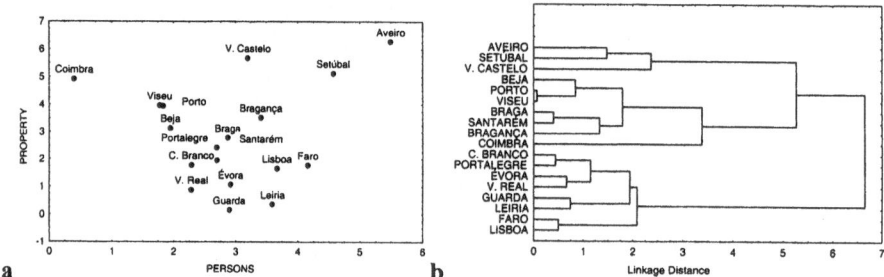

Figure 3.6. Crimes dataset: (a) Scatter plot; (b) Dendrogram using complete linkage clustering.

The splitting version of the hierarchical clustering algorithm, previously mentioned, operates in a top-down fashion, initially considering one cluster formed by all patterns. Afterwards, the algorithm proceeds to consider all possible partitions (2 in the first step, 3 in the second step, and so on until n in the last step), choosing at each step the partition that minimizes a dissimilarity measure. In this way a dendrogram with inverse structure, starting with one cluster and finishing with n clusters, is obtained.

As the merging algorithm is computationally easier and quicker than the splitting algorithm and produces similar solutions, it is the preferred approach.

3.3.1 Linkage Rules

In the examples presented so far we have made reference to two ways of evaluating the dissimilarity between clusters: the within-cluster average error and the complete linkage rule. Actually, there are several methods of evaluating the dissimilarity between clusters, the so-called *linkage rules*. The most used ones are now presented.

Single linkage

Also called *NN* (nearest neighbour) rule, the single linkage rule evaluates the dissimilarity between two clusters, $d(\omega_i, \omega_j)$, as the dissimilarity of the nearest patterns, one from each cluster:

$$d(\omega_i, \omega_j) = \min_{\mathbf{x} \in \omega_i, \mathbf{y} \in \omega_j} \|\mathbf{x} - \mathbf{y}\|. \tag{3-3a}$$

The norm $\|\mathbf{x} - \mathbf{y}\|$ is evaluated using any of the metrics described in section 2.2. Unless explicitly stated otherwise we will use the Euclidian norm.

The single linkage rule produces a chaining effect and is therefore adequate for clusters with filamentary shape.

Consider the globular data of Figure 3.4a. If we apply the single linkage rule no reasonable clustering solution is attained and the schedule graph increases smoothly to the uninteresting one cluster solution as shown in Figure 3.7. On the contrary, if we apply this rule to the filamentary data of Figure 3.4b, a clear two-cluster solution consistent with the visual clustering is obtained, as shown in Figure 3.8.

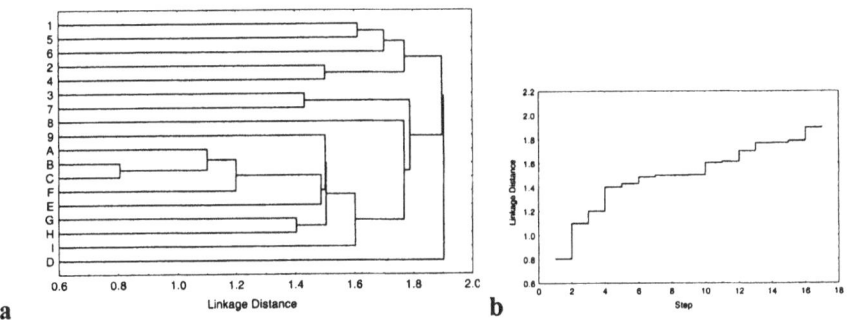

Figure 3.7. Single linkage clustering of globular data. (a) Dendrogram; (b) Clustering schedule graph.

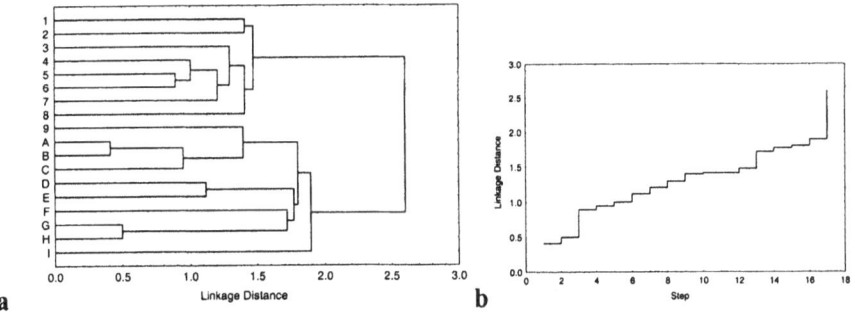

Figure 3.8. Single linkage clustering of filamentary data. (a) Dendrogram; (b) Clustering schedule graph.

Complete linkage

Also called *FN* (furthest neighbour) rule, this method (previously introduced) evaluates the dissimilarity between two clusters as the greatest distance between any two patterns, one from each cluster.

$$d(\omega_i, \omega_j) = \max_{x \in \omega_i, y \in \omega_j} \|x - y\|. \tag{3-3b}$$

This rule performs well when the clusters are compact, roughly globular and of equal size, as shown in the example of the globular data (Figure 3.5a). It is, however, inadequate for filamentary clusters. For instance, for the filamentary data of Figure 3.4b, the 2 and 3 cluster solutions obtained are of globular shape and therefore inadequate. The 2 cluster solution is: {*1, 2, 3, 4, 9, A, B, C*} and {*5, 6, 7, 8, D, E, F, G, H, I*}.

The single and complete linkage rules represent two extremes in dissimilarity assessment and tend to be sensitive to atypical patterns, since they depend only on nearest or furthest neighbours, thereby discarding a lot of information. The following rules use all available information in an averaging approach and are therefore less sensitive to atypical patterns.

Average linkage between groups

Also known as *UPGMA* (un-weighted pair-group method using arithmetic averages), this rule assesses the distance between two clusters as the average of the distances between all pairs of patterns, each pattern from a distinct cluster:

$$d(\omega_i, \omega_j) = \frac{1}{n_i n_j} \sum_{x \in \omega_i} \sum_{y \in \omega_j} \|x - y\|. \tag{3-3c}$$

This method is quite effective for several types of cluster shapes.

Average linkage within groups

This rule, known as *UWGMA* (un-weighted within-group method using arithmetic averages), is a variant of the previous one, where the distance between two clusters is taken to be the average of the distances of all possible pairs of patterns, as if they formed a single cluster:

$$d(\omega_i, \omega_j) = \frac{1}{C(n_i + n_j, 2)} \sum_{x, y \in \{\omega_i, \omega_j\}} \|x - y\|. \tag{3-3d}$$

Notice that this formula is equivalent to formula (3-1) when applied to all clusters.

This method is quite efficient when we intend to keep the "volume" of the resulting cluster as small as possible, minimizing the within-cluster average error of formula (3-1). The solution of the cross data (Figure 3.2b) was obtained with this rule (available in the *SPSS* software). Figure 3.9 shows the corresponding dendrogram.

Ward's method

In Ward's method the sum of the squared within-cluster distances, for the resulting merged cluster, is computed:

$$d\left(\omega_i, \omega_j\right) = \frac{1}{n_i + n_j} \sum_{x \in \omega_i, \omega_j} \|x - m\|^2, \tag{3-3e}$$

where **m** is the centroid of the merged clusters.

At each step the two clusters that merge are the ones that contribute to the smallest increase of the overall sum of the squared within-cluster distances. This method is reminiscent of the ANOVA statistical test, in the sense that it tries to minimize the intra-cluster variance and therefore the cluster separability. This method produces, in general, very good solutions although it tends to create clusters of smaller size.

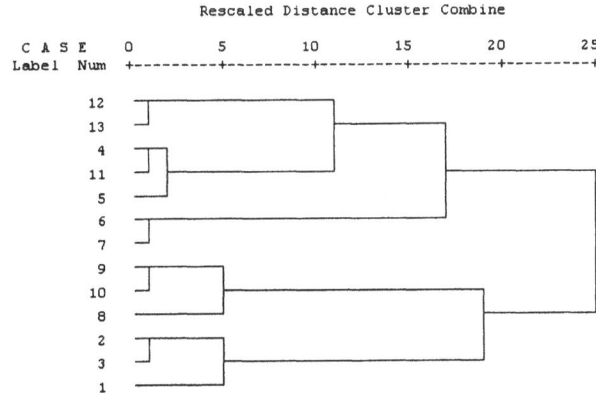

Figure 3.9. Dendrogram of the +*Cross* data clustering using the *UWGMA* rule.

3.3.2 Tree Clustering Experiments

As with any clustering method, when performing tree-clustering experiments it is important to choose appropriate metrics and linkage rules guided by the inspection of the scatter diagram of the data. Let us consider, as an illustration, the crimes data, which is shown in the scatter diagram of Figure 3.6a. Euclidian or squared

Euclidian metrics seem appropriate, given the somewhat globular aspect of the data. Using the *Ward*'s method with the Euclidian metric the solution shown in Figure 3.10 is obtained, which clearly identifies two clusters that are easy to interpret: high and low crime rates against property. The city-block metric could also be used with similar results. A single linkage rule, on the contrary, would produce drastically different solutions, as it would tend to leave aside singleton clusters ({Coimbra} and {Aveiro}), rendering the interpretation more problematic.

Clustering can also be used to assess the "data-support" of a supervised classification. As a matter of fact, if a supervised classification uses distance measures in a "natural" way we would expect that a data-driven approach would also tend to reproduce the same classification as the supervised one. Let us refer to the cork stoppers data of Figure 3.1. In order to perform clustering it is advisable for the features to have similar value ranges and thereby contribute equally to the distance measures. We can achieve this by using the new feature PRT10 = PRT/10 (see also the beginning of section 2.3). Figure 3.11a shows the scatter plot for the supervised classification.

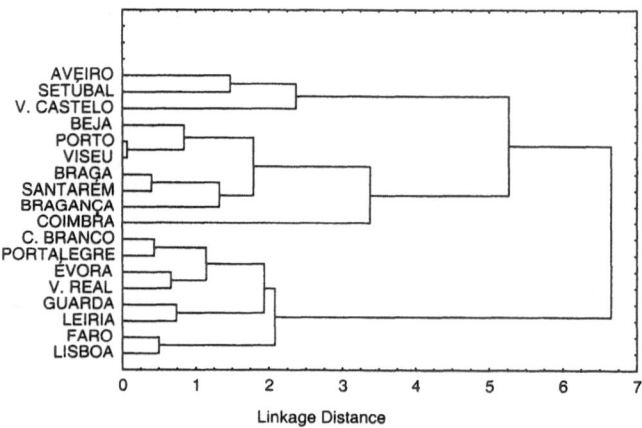

Figure 3.10. Dendrogram for the *Crimes* data using Ward's method. Two clusters are clearly identifiable.

Experimenting with the complete linkage, *UWGMA* and *Ward*'s rules we obtain the best results with *Ward*'s rule and squared Euclidian distance metrics. The respective scatter plot is shown in Figure 3.11b. The resemblance to the supervised classification is quite good (only 19 differences in 100 patterns).

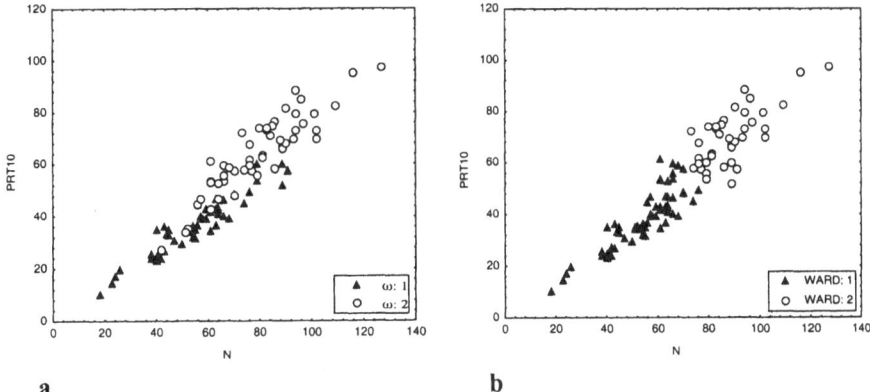

Figure 3.11. Scatter plots for the first two classes of cork stoppers. (a) Supervised classification; (b) Clusters with Ward's method.

3.4 Dimensional Reduction

In the previous sections several examples of data clustering using two features were presented. Utility and interpretation considerations could then be easily aided through visual inspection of the scatter plots of the features. The situation is not so easy when more than two features have to be considered. Visual inspection is straightforward in two-dimensional plots (scatter plots). 3-D plots are more difficult to interpret, therefore they are much less popular. Higher dimensional spaces cannot be visually inspected. In the present section we will approach the topic of obtaining data representations with a smaller number of dimensions than the original one, still retaining comparable inter-distance properties.

A popular method of obtaining two or three-dimensional representations of the data is based on the principal component analysis presented in section 2.4. Let us consider again the eigenvectors of the cork stoppers data ($c=2$) mentioned in section 2.4 and let us retain the first two principal components or *factors*[1]. The coefficients needed for the transformation in a two-dimensional space with new features (factors) *Factor1* and *Factor2*, as a linear combination of the original features are shown in Figure 3.12a. The representation of the patterns in this new space is shown in Figure 3.12b.

The relation between the factors and the original features can be appreciated through the respective correlation values, also called *factor loadings*, shown in Figure 3.13a. Significant values appear in black. A plot of the factor loadings is

---

[1] Principal components analysis is also sometimes called *factor analysis*, although in a strict sense factor analysis takes into account variance contributions shared by the features. In practice the difference is usually minimal.

shown in Figure 3.13b. It is clearly visible that *Factor1* is highly correlated with all features except N and the opposite happens with *Factor2*. These observations suggest, therefore, that the cork stoppers classification can be achieved either with these two factors or with feature N and one of the other features.

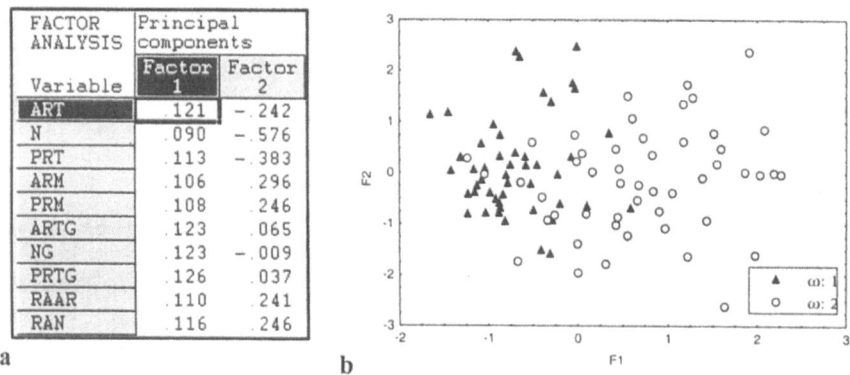

a   b

Figure 3.12. Dimensionality reduction of the first two classes of cork stoppers using two eigenvectors. (a) Eigenvector coefficients; (b) Eigenvector scatter plot.

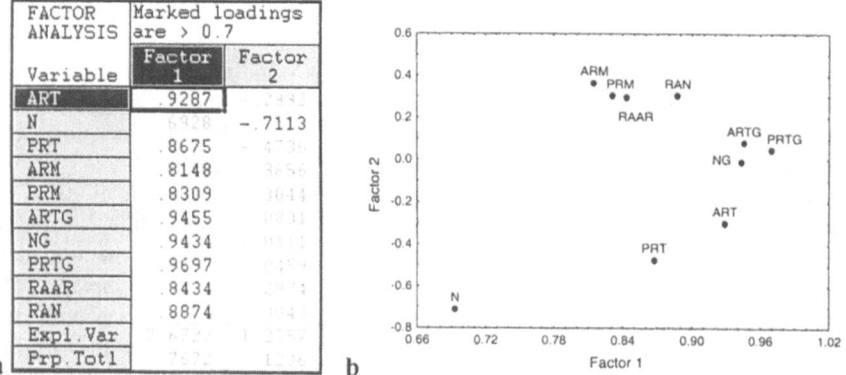

a   b

Figure 3.13. Factor loadings table (a) and graph (b) for the first two classes of cork stoppers.

Notice that the scatter plot of Figure 3.12b is in fact similar to the one that would be obtained if the data of Figure 3.11a were referred to the orthogonal system of the factors.

Multidimensional scaling is another method of representing data in a smaller number of dimensions preserving as much as possible the similarity structure of the data. Unlike factor analysis it is an iterative method. It has a broader application than the principal components analysis that we have just described, since it makes no assumptions as to the metric used for assessing similarity. It can even be used with similarity measures that do not satisfy all properties listed in (2-8).

The basic idea is to try, in an iterative way, to position the feature vectors in the reduced dimension space so that the distance or dissimilarity values among them are preserved as much as possible. For this purpose, the following quadratic error measure known as *stress*, is iteratively minimized:

$$p = \sum_{i,j} [\; d^{*}(\mathbf{x}_i, \mathbf{x}_j) - f(d(\mathbf{x}_i, \mathbf{x}_j))\;]^2 \;,$$ (3-4)

where:

- $\mathbf{x}_i$, $\mathbf{x}_j$ are any arbitrary pair of distinct patterns ($i \neq j$);
- $d(\mathbf{x}_i, \mathbf{x}_j)$ is the original dissimilarity between $\mathbf{x}_i$ and $\mathbf{x}_j$;
- $d^{*}(\mathbf{x}_i, \mathbf{x}_j)$ is the transformed dissimilarity in the lower dimensional space;
- f is a monotonic transformation function.

The details of this iterative process are beyond the scope of this book. The interested reader can refer, for instance, to (Sammon, 1969) and (Leeuw and Heisen, 1982).

NUMERIC VALUES		1 A	2 B	3 C	4 D	5 E	6 F	7 G	8 H
	A	.0	33.8	10.3	12.3	98.1	25.3	8.6	25.
	B	33.8	.0	36.4	31.7	76.7	35.4	34.7	50.
	C	10.3	36.4	.0	15.5	95.9	27.6	11.6	24.
	D	12.3	31.7	15.5	.0	96.2	20.9	9.6	21.
	E	98.1	76.7	95.9	96.2	.0	101.4	101.4	115.
	F	25.3	35.4	27.6	20.9	101.4	.0	20.9	26.
	G	8.6	34.7	11.6	9.6	101.4	20.9	.0	18.
	H	25.0	50.3	24.7	21.8	115.6	26.6	18.2	.
	I	86.8	79.6	78.2	84.4	77.1	85.8	85.2	90.
	J	23.5	49.8	17.3	27.6	109.8	33.8	20.1	20.
	K	79.1	75.7	70.1	76.7	80.2	78.5	77.6	82.
	L	25.1	32.3	22.5	29.0	90.9	36.3	25.1	38.

Figure 3.14. Dissimilarity matrix for the Food dataset. Dissimilarity values correspond to Euclidian distances.

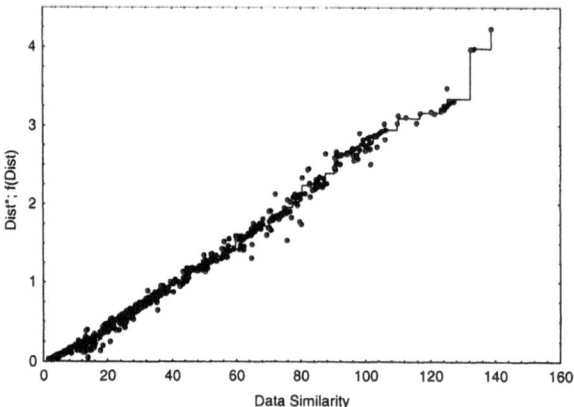

Figure 3.15. Shepard diagram for the *Food* dataset, showing the target distance d^* (dots) and the transformed distance $f(d)$ (step function) against the original data similarity.

We illustrate the application of this technique using the *Food* dataset. In order to have comparable features in terms of their contribution to the dissimilarity measure, the following standardized features were computed: Cal10 = Cal/10; P10 = P/10; Ca10 = Ca/10; B10 = B1B2x10.

When using *Statistica* for multidimensional scaling, the first step is the creation of a dissimilarity matrix for all patterns, which can be done during the cluster analysis process. The elements of the dissimilarity matrix are the distances $d(\mathbf{x}_i, \mathbf{x}_j)$. Figure 3.14 shows this matrix using Euclidian distances. For notation simplicity, food cases have been named from A to Z and then from AA to AJ.

Next, the iterative multidimensional scaling is performed on this matrix, after setting the desired number of dimensions ($d=2$ for this example). After convergence of the iterative process the user has the option to evaluate the goodness of fit of the solution by looking at the *Shepard diagram* shown in Figure 3.15. This diagram shows the target distances $d^*(\mathbf{x}_i, \mathbf{x}_j)$ and the transformed distances $f(d(\mathbf{x}_i, \mathbf{x}_j))$ against the original ones. The transformed distances are represented by a step-line. As Figure 3.15 shows the target distances are very close to the step-function, indicating a good fit to the monotone transformation.

Figure 3.16 shows the *Food* data represented in the two derived dimensions with a four cluster solution. When tree clustering is performed with the Ward method and a Euclidian metric, the solution shown by the vertical icicle of Figure 3.17 is obtained, which shows a good agreement with the scatter plot in the reduced two-dimensional space.

The interpretation of the clusters can be a problem when using multidimensional scaling alone. With principal components analysis we can derive two factors distinguishing the following sets of features: {Cal10}, {Ca10}, {Fe, B10}, {Prot, P10}. The previous four cluster solution can also be interpreted in terms of these sets. For instance the {AA, AD, AE}={butter, fat, oil} cluster is the high calory food cluster.

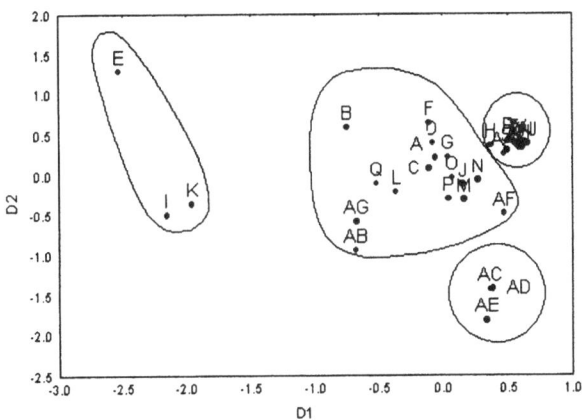

Figure 3.16. Scatter plot of the food data in a two-dimensional space obtained by multidimensional scaling.

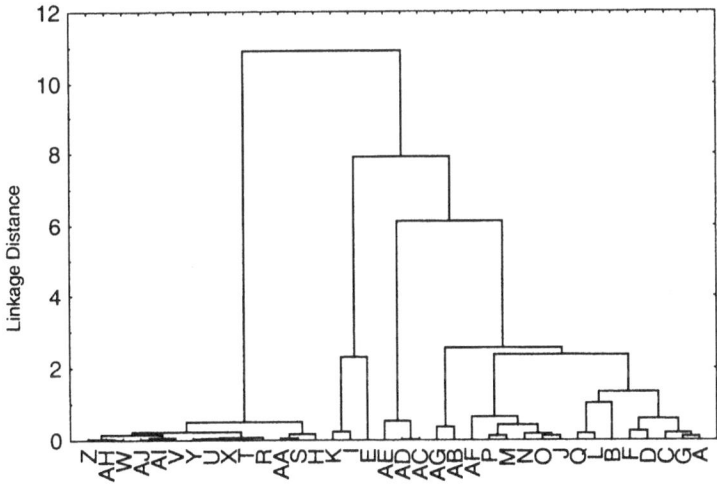

Figure 3.17. Icicle plot for the *Food* data using the reduced two-dimensional space. Four clusters can be easily identified at a linkage distance of 4.

3.5 K-Means Clustering

The *k-Means* or *ISODATA* clustering algorithm is the most popular example of an algorithm that performs iterative adjustment of c (k in the original algorithm version) cluster centroids. It has a distinct application from the tree clustering methods since it is intended to yield a clustering solution for an arbitrarily large number of patterns and for a previously defined number of clusters. The choice of the number of clusters can be made by performing tree clustering either in a smaller set of data or in a reduced dimension space obtained for instance by multidimensional scaling.

The central idea of the algorithm is to minimize an overall within-cluster distance from the patterns to the centroids. Usually, except in the case of a quite small number of patterns, an exhaustive search in all partitions of n patterns in c clusters is prohibitive. Instead, a local minimum of the overall within-cluster distance is searched by iteratively adjusting c cluster centroids, $\mathbf{m}_j$, and by assigning each pattern to the closest centroid:

$$E = \sum_{j=1}^{c} \sum_{x_i \in \omega_j} \left\| \mathbf{x}_i - \mathbf{m}_j \right\|^2 . \tag{3-5}$$

Notice that E can also be viewed as the error (sum of squared deviations) of the cluster partition.

The algorithm, in a simple formulation, is as follows:

1. Denote: c, the number of clusters; *maxiter*, the maximum number of iterations allowed; Δ, a minimum threshold for the allowed error deviation in consecutive iterations. Assume c initial centroids $\mathbf{m}_j^{(k)}$ for the iteration $k=1$.
2. Assign each $\mathbf{x}_i$ in the dataset to the cluster represented by the nearest $\mathbf{m}_j^{(k)}$.
3. Compute for the previous partition the new centroids $\mathbf{m}_j^{(k+1)}$ and the error $E^{(k+1)}$.
4. Repeat steps 2 and 3 until $k=maxiter$ or $\left| E^{(k+1)} - E^{(k)} \right| < \Delta$.

There are several variants of this algorithm depending on the choice of the initial cluster centroids, the pattern assignment rule, the centroid computation (often computed as the cluster mean) and the stop criteria. Usually the algorithm stops after a small number of iterations (<10). As for the initial choice of centroids, which may have a strong influence on the final solution, it can be done in several ways. *Statistica* and *SPSS* provide the following alternatives:

1. Specify which patterns are used as initial centroids. Tree clustering in a reduced number of patterns may be performed for this purpose.
2. Choose the first c patterns as initial centroids.

3. Sort the distances between all patterns and choose patterns at constant intervals of these distances as initial centroids.
4. Choose patterns that maximize between-cluster distance, as follows: start by selecting the first c patterns as centroids; a subsequent pattern replaces the closest centroid if its distance from the centroid is greater than the distance between the two closest centroids or the smallest distance between that centroid and any of the others.

Clustering solutions are usually evaluated using the overall within-cluster distance of formula (3-5) as well as using the within-cluster distance for each feature j:

$$E_j = \sum_{i=1}^{n} \sum_{x \in \omega_i} \left\| x_j - m_{ij} \right\|^2 . \qquad (3\text{-}6)$$

Let $E_j^{(c)}$ and $E^{(c)}$ denote the errors for c clusters for feature j and for all features, respectively. If the pattern features follow a normal distribution, it can be shown that:

$$R_j^{(c+1)} = \left(\frac{E_j^{(c)}}{E_j^{(c+1)}} - 1 \right)(n-c-1) \approx F_{1,n-c-1} ; \qquad (3\text{-}7a)$$

$$R^{(c+1)} = \left(\frac{E^{(c)}}{E^{(c+1)}} - 1 \right)(n-c-1) \approx F_{d,(n-c-1)d} . \qquad (3\text{-}7b)$$

where $F_{a,b}$ is the distribution F (Fisher) with (a,b) degrees of freedom.

When the normality assumption is not satisfied, the *cluster merit indexes R and R_j* are still useful since they measure the decrease in overall within-cluster distance when passing from a solution with c clusters to one with $c+1$ clusters. A high value of the merit indexes indicates a substantial decrease in overall within-cluster distance.

Let us consider the *Rocks* dataset with 134 cases, characterized by physical and chemical features. Performing a factor analysis produces the factor loadings graph shown in Figure 3.18. Factor 1 is highly correlated with chemical features such as the CaO and SiO_2 contents, which determine important categorizations of the rocks (e.g. silicate vs. non-silicate rocks). Factor 2 is highly correlated with physical features such as PAOA (apparent porosity), AAPN (water absorption) and MVAP (volumetric weight).

We now perform several experiments of k-means clustering using the factors as features, for c between 2 and 8. Using 10 iterations and rule 4 for the initial choice of centroids, we compute for each solution the cluster merit indexes. Using *Statistica*, one can use for this purpose the computed values of the within sum of squared deviations, per variable. Notice that $E_j^{(1)}$ is just the variance of feature j multiplied by $(n-1)$.

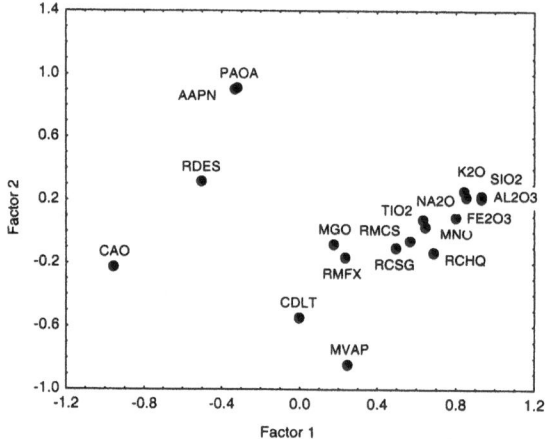

Figure 3.18. Factor loadings graph for the *Rocks* dataset. Factor 1 is highly correlated with chemical features and Factor 2 with physical features.

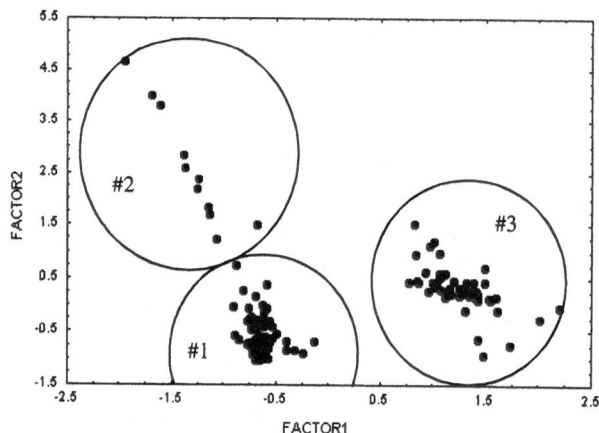

Figure 3.19. Scatter plot of the *Rocks* data in the factor space with three identified clusters.

Figure 3.20 shows the cluster merit indexes for the several values of c, computed with formula (3-7a). Factor 1 has the most important contribution in terms of the decrease of the within-cluster error. Inspection of Figure 3.20 suggests that the values c = 3, 5, 8 are sensible choices for the number of clusters. In particular, the solution with 3 clusters looks quite attractive since it corresponds to high values of the merit indexes. This solution is shown in Figure 3.19. Cluster #1 has 74 cases corresponding to calcium carbonate rocks, such as limestones and marbles. Cluster #2 has 11 cases that correspond to the same type of rocks but with higher porosity. Finally, cluster #3 has 49 cases, which correspond to silicate stones such as granites and diorites.

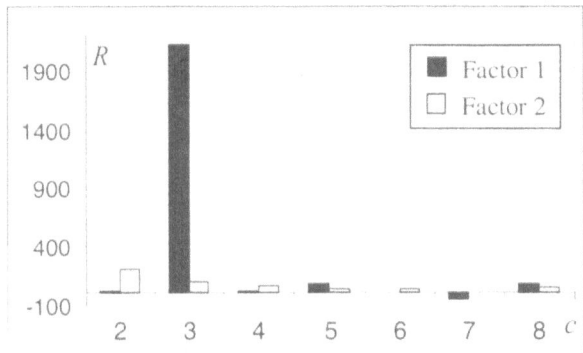

Figure 3.20. Variation of the cluster index R for the two features Factor 1 and Factor 2, with the number of clusters c (*Rocks* dataset).

The solution with 5 clusters is also an interesting solution. It divides the calcium carbonate rocks into three clusters corresponding to "high", "medium" and "low" porosity. The silicate rocks are divided into two clusters, also according to the porosity. The solution with 8 clusters is not interesting, since it contains a singleton cluster.

Notice that in all these experiments we are using a Euclidian distance, therefore imposing a circular shape onto the cluster boundaries. Another metric for measuring distances, such as the Mahalanobis metric, could be more appropriate in some cases.

3.6 Cluster Validation

Clustering results assessment is usually performed by some kind of measure of within-cluster dissimilarity. In the previous section we used cluster merit indexes that reflect such dissimilarity. Other statistical indexes have been proposed (see e.g. Milligan, 1996). As a simple validation test, one could also apply the Kruskal-Wallis test to the cluster solution and consider it acceptable if the corresponding test probability is below a certain confidence level.

A different approach to cluster validation is to perform a *replication analysis*, developed by McIntyre and Blashfield (1980). This is essentially a cross-validation process, where the results on a subset of the data are cross-validated with the results obtained on another subset. In the following we describe the main steps of the replication analysis, illustrating it with the application to the k-means cluster solution of the *Rocks* dataset derived in the previous section.

1. Divide the original dataset into two datasets.

The original dataset is randomly split into two sets. Statistical software such as *SPSS* or *Statistica* make this possible by using filter variables filled in with zeros and ones. With the *Rocks* dataset, two samples $S1$ and $S2$ with 66 and 68 cases respectively, were obtained in this way.

2. Cluster the first dataset and determine the centroids.

Performing the k-means clustering on $S1$ the centroids shown in Table 3.1 were found.

Table 3.1. Centroids of the first *Rocks* dataset, $S1$.

	Cluster #1	Cluster #2	Cluster #3
Factor 1	-0.64	-1.51	1.24
Factor 2	-0.53	3.37	0.31

3. Assign the data of the second dataset to the nearest centroids.

The distances between the patterns of the second dataset, $S2$, and the centroids previously determined on $S1$ are computed. Each $S2$ pattern is assigned to the nearest centroid. *SPSS* makes it possible to save the previously determined centroids, making them available for "classification" (assignment) alone in this step.

Table 3.2. Centroids of the second *Rocks* dataset, $S2$.

	Cluster #1	Cluster #2	Cluster #3
Factor 1	-0.64	-1.24	1.27
Factor 2	-0.65	2.29	0.29

4. Cluster the second dataset.

The second dataset is clustered using the k-means algorithm in the same conditions as in step 2. The centroids derived in this step for the *Rocks* dataset *S2* are shown in Table 3.2. Notice the proximity to the centroids of Table 3.1.

5. Compute a measure of agreement between the clustering of *S2* based on the nearest centroid of *S1* and the direct clustering of *S2*.

For the *Rocks* dataset *S2* only two patterns changed their assignments: from cluster #1 according to the centroids of *S1*, to the neighbour cluster #2 (see Figure 3.19).

Table 3.3. Agreement table for the two clustering methods of the *Rocks* dataset.

Cluster #1	Cluster #2	Cluster #3	Nr of occurrences
2	0	0	33
1	1	0	1
1	1	0	1
0	2	0	6
0	0	2	27

The agreement between the two clustering methods (using the centroids of *S1* or via directly clustering *S2*) is shown in Table 3.3. The entries in this table under a cluster column are the number of times a pattern was assigned to that cluster. The "Nr of occurrences" column indicates how many times this event occurred. For instance, both methods unanimously assigned a pattern to cluster #1 thirty-three times.

A measure of agreement can be computed using Cohen's κ statistic. As this method is of interest in a broad class of pattern recognition situations, namely for comparing classifiers, we will describe here the major aspects of this statistical method whose details can be found in e.g. Siegel and Castellan (1988).

Consider an "agreement table" such as Table 3.3 with n objects assigned by k judges (classifiers, methods) to one of c categories (clusters, classes). In the *Rocks* example we have $n=68$, $k=2$ and $c=3$. Instead of filling in a table with 68 rows we condensed it by adding the extra "Nr of occurrences" column. Let us denote n_{ij} the number of times an object i is assigned to category j.

The κ statistic is given by the formula:

$$\kappa = \frac{P(A) - P(E)}{1 - P(E)} , \tag{3-8}$$

where $P(A)$ is the proportion of times the k judges agree and $P(E)$ is the proportion of times that we would expect the k judges to agree by chance. If there is complete agreement among the judges, then $\kappa=1$ ($P(A)=1$, $P(E)=0$). If there is no agreement among the judges other than what would be expected by chance, then $\kappa=0$ ($P(A)=P(E)$). The values of $P(A)$ and $P(E)$ are computed as follows:

$$P(A) = \frac{1}{nk(k-1)} \sum_{i=1}^{n} \sum_{j=1}^{c} n_{ij}^2 - \frac{1}{k-1} ; \qquad (3\text{-}8a)$$

$$P(E) = \sum_{j=1}^{c} \left(\sum_{i=1}^{n} n_{ij} / nk \right)^2 . \qquad (3\text{-}8b)$$

For the *Rocks* example these quantities are computed as $P(A)=0.971$ and $P(E)=0.418$, resulting in a high value of κ, $\kappa=0.95$. In order to test the significance of κ, the following statistic, approximately normally distributed for large n with zero mean and unit standard deviation, is used:

$$z = \frac{\kappa}{\sqrt{\operatorname{var}(\kappa)}} , \text{ with}$$

$$\operatorname{var}(\kappa) \approx \frac{2}{n\kappa(\kappa-1)} \frac{P(E) - (2\kappa-3)[P(E)]^2 + 2(\kappa-2)\sum p_j^3}{[1-P(E)]^2} . \qquad (3\text{-}8c)$$

The value of $z = 9.5$ is obtained for the present example, allowing us to conclude significantly high agreement at a $\alpha = 0.01$ significance level ($z_{\alpha=0.01} = 2.32$).

Bibliography

Andrews HC (1972) Introduction to Mathematical Techniques in Pattern Recognition. John Wiley & Sons, Inc.

Barnett S (1979) Matrix Methods for Engineers and Scientists. McGraw Hill Book Co.

Borg I, Groenen P (1997) Modern Multidimensional Scaling. Springer-Verlag.

Chambers JM, Kleiner B (1982) Graphical Techniques for Multivariate Data and for Clustering. In: Krishnaiah PR, Kanal LN (eds), Handbook of Statistics vol.2, North Holland Pub. Co., 209-244.

Chien, Yi Tzuu (1978) Interactive Pattern Recognition. Marcel Dekker Inc.

De Leeuw J, Heiser W (1982) Theory of Multidimensional Scaling. In: Krishnaiah PR, Kanal LN (eds), Handbook of Statistics vol.2, North Holland Pub. Co., 285-316.

Duda R, Hart P (1973) Pattern Classification and Scene Analysis. Wiley, New York.

Gordon A (1996) Hierarchical Classification. In: Arabie P, Hubert LJ, De Soete G (eds) Clustering and Classification. World Scientific Pub. Co., Singapore.

Hartigan JA (1975) Clustering Algorithms. John Wiley & Sons, New York.

Kaufman L, Rousseeuw PJ (1990) Finding Groups in Data. An Introduction to Cluster Analysis. John Wiley & Sons, Inc.

Mc Intyre RM, Blashfield RK (1980) A Nearest-Centroid Technique for Evaluating the Minimum-Variance Clustering Procedure. Multivar. Behavioral Research, 15:225-238.

Milligan GW (1996) Clustering Validation: Results and Implications for Applied Analyses. In: Arabie P, Hubert LJ, De Soete G (eds) Clustering and Classification. World Scientific Pub. Co., Singapore.

Pipes A, Hovanessian SA (1977) Matrix-Computer Methods in Engineering. Robert E. Krieger Pub. Co., Malabar, Florida.

Rohlf FJ (1982) Single-Link Clustering Algorithms. In: Krishnaiah PR, Kanal LN (eds), Handbook of Statistics vol.2, North Holland Pub. Co., 267-284.

Sammon Jr JW (1969) A Nonlinear Mapping for Data Structure Analysis. IEEE Tr Comp, 18: 401-409.

Siegel S, Castellan Jr NJ (1988) Nonparametric Statistics for the Behavioural Sciences. Mc Graw Hill Book Co.

Späth H (1980) Cluster Analysis Algorithms. Ellis Horwood, Ltd., England.

Exercises

3.1 Determine the tree clustering solutions of the *+Cross* data (*Cluster.xls*), using the UWGMA linkage rule with the city-block and Chebychev norms. Explain the results.

3.2 Determine the tree clustering solutions of the *xCross* data (*Cluster.xls*), using the UWGMA linkage rule with the city-block and Chebychev norms. Explain the results, comparing them with those obtained in the previous exercise.

3.3 Determine the tree clustering solutions of the *Globular* data (*Cluster.xls*), using the UPGMA and UWGMA linkage rules with the Euclidian norm. Compare the results with those obtained using complete linkage in section 3.3.

3.4 Determine the tree clustering solutions of the *Filamentary* data (*Cluster.xls*), using the Ward method with the city-block norm. Compare the results with those obtained using single linkage in section 3.3.1.

3.5 Perform a factor analysis of the *Food* data and determine the K-means cluster solutions for $c=3$, 4 and 5 in a two-dimensional space. Compare the results with those obtained by multidimensional scaling (section 3.4).

3.6 Repeat the experiments on the *Food* data described in section 3.4 using a city-block norm. Compare the results with those obtained using Ward method.

3.7 Perform a factor analysis of the *Cork Stoppers* data and determine the k-means cluster solution for $c=3$ in a two-dimensional space. Compare the cluster results with the supervised classification. Which class is in least agreement with the cluster solution and why?

3.8 Perform a factor analysis of the *CTG* data. Determine which k-means clustering solutions most resemble the supervised classification in three classes, *N*, *S* and *P*.

3.9 Repeat the experiment of the previous exercise for the other values of c between 2 and 5. Compute the cluster merit factors and determine the most adequate cluster solutions.

3.10 Perform a replication analysis for the clustering solution of the *Cork Stoppers* data with $c=3$.

3.11 Apply multidimensional scaling to the *Rocks* dataset and compare with the results obtained using factor analysis (section 3.5). Perform k-means clustering and assess with cluster merit factors what are the most adequate solutions.

3.12 Determine the tree clustering solutions of the Rocks data in a two-dimensional factor space, using single and complete linkage with the Euclidian norm. Compare the results with those obtained in section 3.5.

4 Statistical Classification

4.1 Linear Discriminants

In previous chapters, several distance metrics were presented and used to assess pattern similarity relative to a prototype. In the present chapter, we further explore this way of thought, taking into account the specificity of the pattern distributions.

4.1.1 Minimum Distance Classifier

Let us consider the cork stoppers classification problem (see the *Cork Stoppers.xls* dataset description in Appendix A). Assume that the main goal was to design a classifier for classes 1 (ω_1) and 2 (ω_2), having only feature N (number of defects) available (see A.3). Therefore, a feature vector with only one element represents each pattern: $\mathbf{x} = [N]$.

Let us first inspect the pattern distributions in the feature space ($d=1$) represented by the histograms of Figure 4.1. The distributions have a similar shape with some amount of overlap. The sample means are $m_1=55.28$ for ω_1 and $m_2=79.74$ for ω_2.

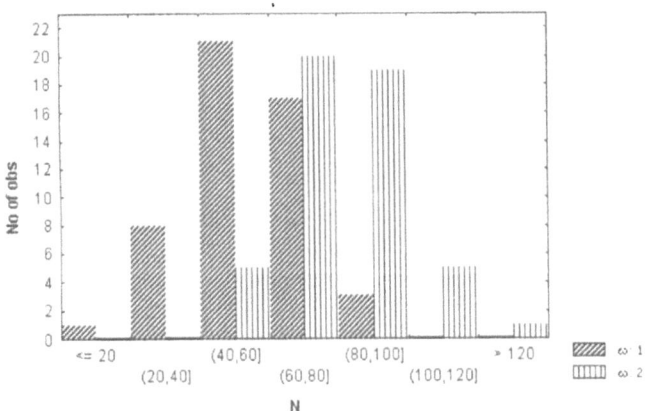

Figure 4.1. Feature N histograms for the first two classes of the cork stoppers data.

As seen in previous chapters, it seems reasonable to take those sample means as class prototypes and assign each cork stopper to its nearest prototype. This is the essence of what is called the *minimum distance* or *template matching classification*. The classification rule is then:

$$\text{If} \quad \left\| \mathbf{x} - [55.28] \right\| < \left\| \mathbf{x} - [79.74] \right\| \quad \text{then} \quad \mathbf{x} \in \omega_1 \quad \text{else} \quad \mathbf{x} \in \omega_2{}^{'}. \tag{4-1}$$

We assume, for the moment, that a Euclidian metric is used. Using the value at half distance from the means, we can rewrite (4-1) as:

$$\text{If} \quad \mathbf{x} < 67.51 \quad \text{then} \quad \mathbf{x} \in \omega_1 \quad \text{else} \quad \mathbf{x} \in \omega_2. \tag{4-1a}$$

The separating "hyperplane" is simply the point 67.51. Note that in the equality case ($\mathbf{x}$=67.51) the class assignment is arbitrary (ω_2 is a possibility, as in 4-1a).

Let us now evaluate the performance of this simple classifier by computing the error rate in the training set of n=50 cases per class. Figure 4.2 shows the classification matrix (obtained with *Statistica*) with the predicted classifications along the columns and the true (observed) classifications along the rows.

DISCRIM. ANALYSIS	Rows: Observed classifications Columns: Predicted classifications		
Group	Percent Correct	G_1:1 p=.50000	G_2:2 p=.50000
G_1:1	82.00000	41	9
G_2:2	72.00000	14	36
Total	77.00000	55	45

Figure 4.2. Classification matrix of two classes of cork stoppers using only one feature, N. Both classes have equal probability of occurrence ("p=.5" in the listed classification matrix).

We see that for this simple classifier the overall percentage of correct classification in the training set is 77%, or equivalently, the overall training set error is 23% (18% for ω_1 and 28% for ω_2). For the moment we will not assess how the classifier performs with independent patterns, i.e., we will not assess its test set error.

Let us now use one more feature: PRT10 = PRT/10. The feature vector is:

' We assume an underlying real domain for the ordinal feature N. Conversion to an ordinal will be performed when needed. For instance, the practical threshold of the classifier in (4-1a) would be 68.

$$x = \begin{bmatrix} N \\ PRT10 \end{bmatrix} \quad \text{or} \quad x = \begin{bmatrix} N & PRT10 \end{bmatrix}'. \tag{4-2}$$

We use PRT10 instead of PRT for the scaling reason already explained at the beginning of section 2.3. There is also another reason: although statistical classification is in principle independent of the feature measurement scales, as we will have to compute later the inverse of a covariance matrix, numerical considerations recommend that, for this calculation to be performed in the best conditions, the value ranges should not be too different. The scatter diagram of the feature vectors is shown in Figure 4.3.

In this two-dimensional feature space, the minimum distance classifier using Euclidian metrics is implemented as follows:

1. Draw the straight line (decision surface) equidistant from the sample means (see Figure 4.3), i.e., perpendicular to the segment linking the means and passing at half distance.
2. Any pattern above the straight line is assigned to ω_2. Any sample below is assigned to ω_1. The assignment is arbitrary if the pattern falls on the straight line boundary.

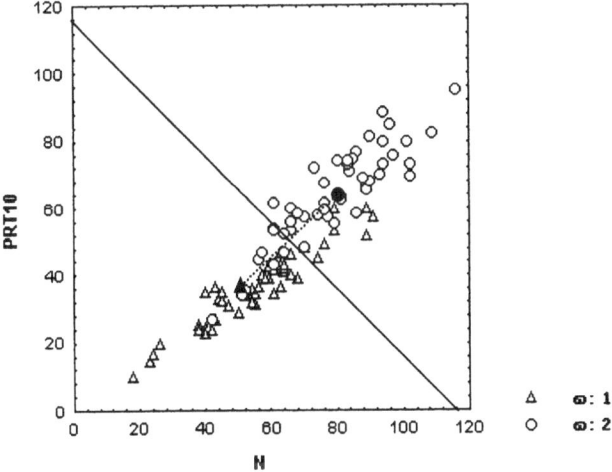

Figure 4.3. Scatter diagram for two classes of cork stoppers (features N, PRT10) with the linear discriminant at half distance from the means (solid line).

Counting the number of training set cases wrongly classified, it is observed that the overall error falls to 18%. The addition of PRT10 seems beneficial.

In general, the minimum distance classifier (using any distance metric) has the structure represented in Figure 4.4, where **x** is the input feature vector to be assigned to one of c classes ω_k ($k=1, ..., c$) represented by the respective prototypes $\mathbf{m}_k$.

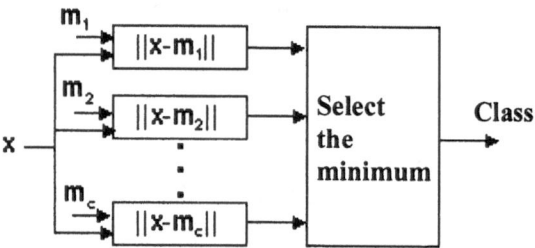

Figure 4.4. Minimum distance classifier system for a feature vector **x** as input.

4.1.2 Euclidian Linear Discriminants

The previous minimum distance classifier for two classes and a two-dimensional feature vector, using a Euclidian metric, has a straightforward generalization (Figure 4.4) for any d-dimensional feature vector **x** and any number of classes, ω_k ($k=1, ..., c$), represented by their prototypes $\mathbf{m}_k$. The square of the Euclidian distance between a feature vector **x** and a prototype $\mathbf{m}_k$ is expressed as follows:

$$d_k^2(\mathbf{x}) = \left\| \mathbf{x} - \mathbf{m}_k \right\|^2 = (\mathbf{x} - \mathbf{m}_k)'(\mathbf{x} - \mathbf{m}_k) = \mathbf{x}'\mathbf{x} - \mathbf{m}_k'\mathbf{x} - \mathbf{x}'\mathbf{m}_k + \mathbf{m}_k'\mathbf{m}_k . \quad (4\text{-}3)$$

We choose class ω_k, therefore the $\mathbf{m}_k$, which minimizes $d_k^2(\mathbf{x})$. Grouping together the terms dependent on $\mathbf{m}_k$, we obtain:

$$d_k^2(\mathbf{x}) = -2(\mathbf{m}_k'\mathbf{x} - 0.5\mathbf{m}_k'\mathbf{m}_k) + \mathbf{x}'\mathbf{x} . \quad (4\text{-}3a)$$

Let us assume $c=2$. The decision boundary between the classes corresponds to:

$$d_1^2(\mathbf{x}) = d_2^2(\mathbf{x}) . \quad (4\text{-}3b)$$

Thus, using (4-3a):

$$\mathbf{m}_1'\mathbf{x} - 0.5 \left\| \mathbf{m}_1 \right\|^2 = \mathbf{m}_2'\mathbf{x} - 0.5 \left\| \mathbf{m}_2 \right\|^2$$
$$\Rightarrow (\mathbf{m}_1 - \mathbf{m}_2)'[\mathbf{x} - 0.5(\mathbf{m}_1 + \mathbf{m}_2)] = 0 . \quad (4\text{-}3c)$$

This last equation, which is linear in $\mathbf{x}$, represents a hyperplane perpendicular to $(\mathbf{m}_1 - \mathbf{m}_2)'$ and passes through the point $0.5(\mathbf{m}_1 + \mathbf{m}_2)$ halfway between the means. It is a *linear discriminant* separating ω_1 from ω_2.

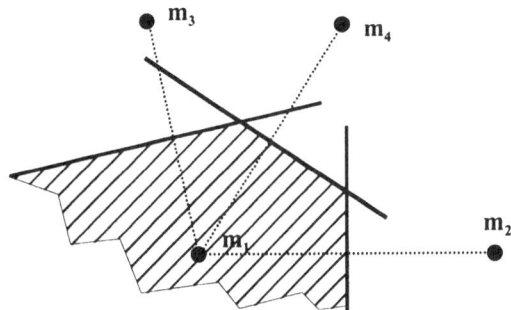

Figure 4.5. Decision region for ω_1 (hatched area) showing linear discriminants relative to three other classes.

For c classes the minimum distance discriminant is piecewise linear, composed of segments of hyperplanes with pairwise separation as discussed in 2.1.2, and illustrated in Figure 4.5 with an example of a decision region for class ω_1 in a situation of $c=4$.

Minimizing the distance $d_k^2(\mathbf{x})$, as in (4-3a), is equivalent to maximizing the following decision function:

$$g_k(\mathbf{x}) = \mathbf{m}_k'\mathbf{x} - 0.5\|\mathbf{m}_k\|^2 = \mathbf{w}_k'\mathbf{x} + \mathbf{w}_{k,0} \quad , \tag{4-3d}$$

with $\mathbf{w}_k = \mathbf{m}_k;$ $\mathbf{w}_{k,0} = -0.5\|\mathbf{m}_k\|^2.$

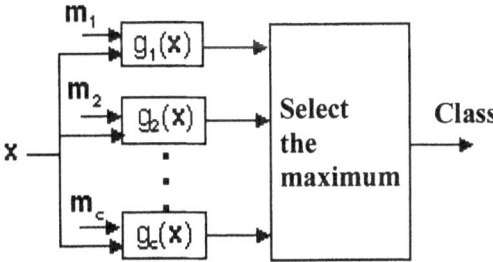

Figure 4.6. Maximum decision function classifier for an input feature vector $\mathbf{x}$.

Figure 4.6 shows the general structure of a maximum decision function classifier.

Notice that the $g_k(\mathbf{x})$ are linear decision functions (compare with 2-2) with the weight vector equal to the mean vector, and the bias term, $w_{k,0}$, dependent on the mean vector length.

We can get further insight into this linear discriminant system by referring to the previous $c=2$ situation. Consider that the coordinate axes underwent a translation so that we are now dealing with the new feature vectors $\mathbf{y} = \mathbf{x} - 0.5(\mathbf{m}_1 + \mathbf{m}_2)$. The linear discriminant functions are now expressed as:

$$h_i(\mathbf{y}) = \mathbf{m}_i'\mathbf{y} - 0.5\|\mathbf{m}_i\|^2, \quad i = 1, 2 \; ; \tag{4-4a}$$

with $\mathbf{m}_1$ and $\mathbf{m}_2$ evaluated in the new system of coordinates, we obviously have $\|\mathbf{m}_1\| = \|\mathbf{m}_2\|$, therefore the discriminant functions can be expressed simply as:

$$h_i(\mathbf{y}) = \mathbf{m}_i'\mathbf{y} . \tag{4-4b}$$

Since $\mathbf{m}_i'\mathbf{y}$ is simply the vector correlation (also known as dot product) between $\mathbf{m}_i'$ and $\mathbf{y}$, the Euclidian linear discriminant is also known as *maximum correlation classifier*. Notice that the vector correlation yields a value dependent on the angle between the vectors. It increases with decreasing angle, reaching a maximum at a zero angle. This allows an alternative interpretation (vectorial projection) of the similarity measure. The technique we have just described for assessing class membership of an unknown pattern $\mathbf{x}$ is one of the earliest known in pattern recognition, called *template matching*. Each new pattern was matched against a stored template (prototype), using a correlation measure.

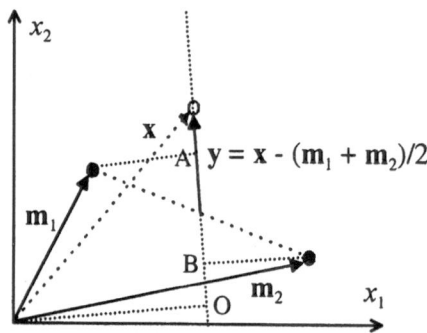

Figure 4.7. Classification of a feature vector $\mathbf{x}$ by the maximum correlation approach: $\overline{OA} > \overline{OB} \Rightarrow \mathbf{x} \in \omega_1$.

4.1.3 Mahalanobis Linear Discriminants

We know already from chapter 2 that the Mahalanobis metric is a generalization of the Euclidian metric suitable for dealing with unequal variances and correlated features. Let us assume that all classes have an identical covariance matrix $\mathbf{C}$, reflecting a similar hyperellipsoidal shape of the corresponding feature vector distributions. The generalization of (4-3) is then written as:

$$d_k^2(\mathbf{x}) = (\mathbf{x} - \mathbf{m}_k)'\mathbf{C}^{-1}(\mathbf{x} - \mathbf{m}_k),\qquad (4\text{-}5)$$

or, $d_k^2(\mathbf{x}) = \mathbf{x}'\mathbf{C}^{-1}\mathbf{x} - \mathbf{m}_k'\mathbf{C}^{-1}\mathbf{x} - \mathbf{x}'\mathbf{C}^{-1}\mathbf{m}_k + \mathbf{m}_k'\mathbf{C}^{-1}\mathbf{m}_k$.

Grouping, as we have done before, the terms dependent on $\mathbf{m}_k$, we obtain:

$$d_k^2(\mathbf{x}) = -2\left((\mathbf{C}^{-1}\mathbf{m}_k)'\mathbf{x} - 0.5\mathbf{m}_k'\mathbf{C}^{-1}\mathbf{m}_k\right) + \mathbf{x}'\mathbf{C}^{-1}\mathbf{x}.\qquad (4\text{-}5\text{a})$$

The decision functions are:

$$g_k(\mathbf{x}) = \mathbf{w}_k'\mathbf{x} + w_{k,0},\qquad (4\text{-}5\text{b})$$

with $\mathbf{w}_k = \mathbf{C}^{-1}\mathbf{m}_k$; $w_{k,0} = -0.5\mathbf{m}_k'\mathbf{C}^{-1}\mathbf{m}_k$. $(4\text{-}5\text{c})$

We again obtain linear discriminant functions in the form of hyperplanes passing through the middle point of the line segment linking the means. The only difference from the results of the previous section is that the hyperplanes separating class ω_i from class ω_j are now orthogonal to the vector $\mathbf{C}^{-1}(\mathbf{m}_i\text{-}\mathbf{m}_j)$.

In the particular case of $\mathbf{C} = s^2\mathbf{I}$ (uncorrelated features with the same variance for all classes), the Mahalanobis classifier is identical to the Euclidian classifier (as it should be).

In practice, it is impossible to guarantee that all class covariance matrices are equal. Fortunately, the decision surfaces are usually not very sensitive to mild deviations from this condition; therefore, in normal practice, one uses a pooled covariance matrix computed as an average of the individual covariance matrices. This is also done in all statistical software applications. We now exemplify the previous results for the cork stoppers problem with two classes.

One feature, N

Given the similarity of both distributions, already pointed out in 4.1.1, the Mahalanobis classifier produces the same classification results as the Euclidian classifier.

The decision function coefficients, as computed by *Statistica*, are shown in Figure 4.8.

DISCRIM. ANALYSIS	G_1:1 p=.50000	G_2:2 p=.50000
N	.19219	.2772
Constant	−6.00532	−11.7464

Figure 4.8. Decision functions coefficients for two classes of cork stoppers and one feature, N.

Let us check these results. The class means are $\mathbf{m}_1$=[55.28] and $\mathbf{m}_2$=[79.74]. The average variance is s^2=287.6296. Applying formula (4-5c) we obtain:

$$\mathbf{w}_1 = \mathbf{m}_1 / s^2 = [0.19219] \quad ; \quad w_{1,0} = -0.5\|\mathbf{m}_1\|^2 / s^2 = -6.00532. \tag{4-6a}$$

$$\mathbf{w}_2 = \mathbf{m}_2 / s^2 = [0.27723] \quad ; \quad w_{2,0} = -0.5\|\mathbf{m}_2\|^2 / s^2 = -11.7464. \tag{4-6b}$$

These results confirm the ones shown in Figure 4.8. Let us assume that a new cork stopper has arrived and we measure 65 defects. To which class is it assigned? As $g_1([65])$=6.49 is greater than $g_2([65])$=6.27 it is assigned to class ω_1.

Two features, N and PRT10

The training set classification matrix is shown in Figure 4.9. A significant improvement was obtained in comparison with the Euclidian classifier results mentioned in section 4.1.1 (namely an overall training set error of 10% instead of 18%). The Mahalanobis metric, taking into account the shape of the pattern clusters, not surprisingly, performed better. The decision function coefficients are shown in Figure 4.10. Using these coefficients we write the decision functions as:

$$g_1(\mathbf{x}) = \mathbf{w}_1'\mathbf{x} + w_{1,0} = [0.2616 \quad -0.09783]\mathbf{x} - 6.1382. \tag{4-7a}$$

$$g_2(\mathbf{x}) = \mathbf{w}_2'\mathbf{x} + w_{2,0} = [0.0803 \quad 0.27760]\mathbf{x} - 12.8166. \tag{4-7b}$$

DISCRIM. ANALYSIS	Rows: Observed classifications Columns: Predicted classifications		
Group	Percent Correct	G_1:1 p=.50000	G_2:2 p=.50000
G_1:1	98.00000	49	1
G_2:2	82.00000	9	41
Total	90.00000	58	42

Figure 4.9. Classification matrix for two classes of cork stoppers with two features, N and PRT10.

DISCRIM. ANALYSIS	G_1:1 p=.50000	G_2:2 p=.50000
N	.26160	.0803
PRT10	−.09783	.2776
Constant	−6.13820	−12.8166

Figure 4.10. Decision function coefficients for the two classes of cork stoppers with features N and PRT10.

The pooled covariance matrix of the data is:

$$C = \begin{bmatrix} 287.6296 & 204.0698 \\ 204.0698 & 172.5529 \end{bmatrix} \quad \Rightarrow \quad C^{-1} = \begin{bmatrix} 0.0216 & -0.0255 \\ -0.0255 & 0.036 \end{bmatrix}. \quad (4\text{-}8)$$

Substituting C^{-1} in formula (4-5c), the reader can verify the results shown in Figure 4.10.

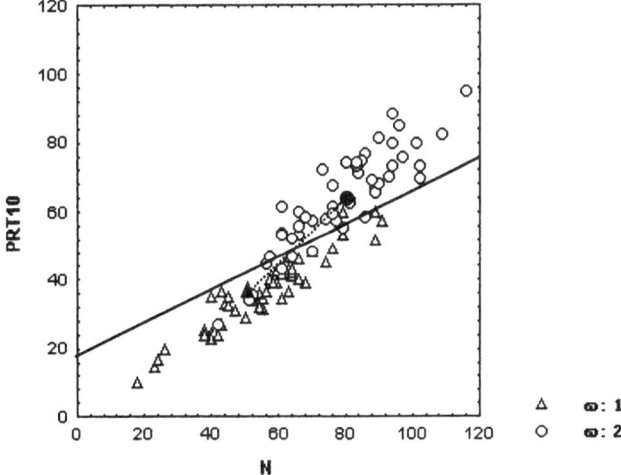

Figure 4.11. Mahalanobis linear discriminant (solid line) for the two classes of cork stoppers.

It is also straightforward to compute $C^{-1}(m_1\text{-}m_2) = [0.18 \quad -0.376]'$. The orthogonal line to this vector with slope 0.4787 and passing through the middle point between the means is shown with a solid line in Figure 4.11. As expected, the "hyperplane" leans along the regression direction of the features (see Figure 4.3 for comparison).

Let us suppose that the previously mentioned cork stopper with 65 defects, and assigned to class ω_1 based on this feature only, had a total perimeter of the defects of 520 pixels. To which class will it be assigned now? As $g_1([65\ 52]')=5.78$ is smaller than $g_2([60\ 48]')=6.84$, it is assigned to class ω_2. This cork stopper has a total perimeter of the defects that is too big to be assigned to class ω_1.

Notice that if the distributions of the feature vectors in the classes correspond to different hyperellipsoidal shapes, they will be characterized by unequal covariance matrices. The distance formula (4-5) will then be influenced by these different shapes in such a way that we will obtain quadratic decision boundaries as shown in Figure 2.12b. Table 4.1 summarizes the different types of minimum distance classifiers, depending on the covariance matrix.

Table 4.1. Summary of minimum distance classifier types.

Covariance	Classifier	Equiprobability surfaces	Discriminants
$C_i=s^2I$	Linear, Euclidian	Hyperspheres	Hyperplanes orthogonal to the segment linking the means
$C_i=C$	Linear, Mahalanobis	Hyperellipsoids	Hyperplanes leaning along the regression
C_i	Quadratic, Mahalanobis	Hyperellipsoids	Quadratic surfaces

4.1.4 Fisher's Linear Discriminant

In the previous chapter the problem of dimensionality reduction was addressed in an unsupervised context. In a supervised context, we are able to use the classification information of the training set in order to produce an optimised mapping into a lower dimensional space, easing the classification task and obtaining further insight into the class separability. The *Fisher linear discriminant* provides the necessary tool for this mapping.

Consider two classes with sample means $\mathbf{m}_1$ and $\mathbf{m}_2$ and an overall sample mean $\mathbf{m}$. We can measure the class separability in a way similar to the well-known Anova statistical test by evaluating the volume of the pooled covariance matrix of the classes relative to the separation of their means. To get a more concrete idea of this, let us consider:

$$S_w = \sum_{k=1}^{2} \sum_{x \in c_k} (\mathbf{x} - \mathbf{m}_k)(\mathbf{x} - \mathbf{m}_k)', \text{ the within-class scatter matrix, and} \qquad (4\text{-}9a)$$

$S_B = (\mathbf{m}_1 - \mathbf{m}_2)(\mathbf{m}_1 - \mathbf{m}_2)'$, the between-class scatter matrix. (4-9b)

Notice that S_w is directly related, indeed proportional, to the pooled covariance matrix. Both S_w and S_B are symmetric positive semidefinite matrices.

The goal is to choose a direction in the feature space along which the distance of the means relative to the within-class variance reaches a maximum, thereby maximizing the class separability. This corresponds to maximizing the following criterion function:

$$J(\mathbf{x}) = \frac{\mathbf{x}' S_b \mathbf{x}}{\mathbf{x}' S_w \mathbf{x}}.$$ (4-10)

The direction $\mathbf{x}$ that maximizes $J(\mathbf{x})$ can be shown to be:

$$\mathbf{x} = S_w^{-1}(\mathbf{m}_1 - \mathbf{m}_2).$$ (4-10a)

The reader may find the demonstration of this important result in Duda and Hart (1973), where the generalization for c classes, yielding $c-1$ independent directions, is also explained.

For the two class case, an important result of this many-to-one mapping is that it yields the same direction as the linear discriminant for equal covariances with Mahalanobis metric, expressed by formulas (4-5b) and (4-5c)! This discriminant is proved to be optimal, in a specific sense, for symmetric distributions of the feature vectors (e.g. normal distributions), as will be explained in the next section.

Let us compute the Fisher discriminant for the two classes of the cork stoppers data. Using $\mathbf{C}^{-1}$ as given in (4-8) and the difference of the means [-24.46 -27.78]', the Fisher discriminant is the vector computed in the previous section, x=[0.18 –0.376]', corresponding to the solid line of Figure 4.11. Projecting the points along this direction we create a new feature, FISHER = 0.18xN-0.376xPRT10. Using the Mahalanobis threshold for this new feature, the same classification results as in Figure 4.9 are obtained (see Exercise 4.6).

The Fisher linear discriminant can also be obtained through the minimization of the following mean squared error:

$$E = \frac{1}{n} \sum_{i=1}^{n} (\mathbf{w}' \mathbf{x}_i + w_0 - t_i)^2,$$ (4-11)

where t_i are the target classification values. This is equivalent to finding the linear regression surface for the dataset. As a matter of fact, it is possible to estimate posterior probabilities of feature vector assignment to a class and determine decision functions using regression techniques (see e.g. Cherkassky and Mulier, 1998). Classification and regression tasks are, therefore, intimately related to each other. In the following chapter on neural networks we will have the opportunity to use the error measure (4-11) again.

4.2 Bayesian Classification

In the previous section we presented linear classifiers based solely on the notion of similarity, which was evaluated as a distance to class prototypes, usually the class means. We did not assume anything specific regarding the pattern distributions, mentioning only the fact that the distance metrics used should reflect the shape of the pattern clusters around the means. As we saw, the Mahalanobis metric takes care of this aspect through the use of the covariance matrix.

In the present section we will take into account the specific probability distributions of the patterns in each class. Doing so, we will be able to address two important issues:

− Is our classifier optimal in any sense?
− How can we adjust our classifier to the specific risks of a classification?

4.2.1 Bayes Rule for Minimum Risk

Let us consider again the cork stoppers problem and imagine that factory production was restricted to the two classes we have been considering, denoted as: ω_1=Super and ω_2=Average. Let us assume further that the factory had a record of production stocks for a reasonably long period of time, summarized as:

Number of produced cork stoppers of class ω_1: $n_1 =$ 901 420
Number of produced cork stoppers of class ω_2: $n_2 =$ 1 352 130
Total number of produced cork stoppers: $n\ =$ 2 253 550

With this information we can readily obtain good estimates[2] of the probabilities of producing a cork stopper from either of the two classes, the so-called *prior probabilities* or *prevalences*:

$$P(\omega_1) = n_1 / n = 0.4 ; \qquad P(\omega_2) = n_2 / n = 0.6 . \tag{4-12}$$

Note that the prevalences are not entirely controlled by the factory, they depend mainly on the quality of the raw material. In the same way, a cardiologist does not control how prevalent myocardial infarction is in a given population. Prevalences can, therefore, be regarded as "states of nature".

Suppose we are asked to make a blind decision as to which class a cork stopper belongs to without looking at it. If the only available information is the prevalences, the sensible choice is class ω_2. This way, we expect to be wrong only 40% of the times.

---

[2] Deviation from the true probability values is less than 0.0006 with 95% confidence level.

Assume now that we were allowed to measure the feature vector $\mathbf{x}$ of the presented cork stopper. Let $P(\omega_i \mid \mathbf{x})$ be the conditional probability of the cork stopper represented by $\mathbf{x}$ belonging to class ω_i. If we are able to determine the probabilities $P(\omega_1 \mid \mathbf{x})$ and $P(\omega_2 \mid \mathbf{x})$, the sensible decision is now:

If $P(\omega_1 \mid \mathbf{x}) > P(\omega_2 \mid \mathbf{x})$ we decide $\mathbf{x} \in \omega_1$;

If $P(\omega_1 \mid \mathbf{x}) < P(\omega_2 \mid \mathbf{x})$ we decide $\mathbf{x} \in \omega_2$;   (4-13)

If $P(\omega_1 \mid \mathbf{x}) = P(\omega_2 \mid \mathbf{x})$ the decision is arbitrary.

We can condense (4-13) as:

If $P(\omega_1 \mid \mathbf{x}) > P(\omega_2 \mid \mathbf{x})$ then $\mathbf{x} \in \omega_1$ else $\mathbf{x} \in \omega_2$.   (4-13a)

The *posterior probabilities* $P(\omega_i \mid \mathbf{x})$ can be computed if we know the *pdf*s of the distributions of the feature vectors in both classes. We then calculate the respective $p(\mathbf{x} \mid \omega_i)$, the so-called *likelihood* of $\mathbf{x}$. As a matter of fact, the well-known Bayes law states that:

$$P(\omega_i \mid \mathbf{x}) = \frac{p(\mathbf{x} \mid \omega_i) P(\omega_i)}{p(\mathbf{x})} ,$$ (4-14)

with $p(\mathbf{x}) = \sum_{i=1}^{c} p(\mathbf{x} \mid \omega_i) P(\omega_i)$, the *total probability* of $\mathbf{x}$.

Note that $P(\omega_i)$ and $P(\omega_i \mid \mathbf{x})$ are discrete probabilities (symbolized by capital letter), whereas $p(\mathbf{x} \mid \omega_i)$ and $p(\mathbf{x})$ are values of *pdf* functions. Note also that the term $p(\mathbf{x})$ is a common term in the comparison expressed by (4-13a), therefore we may rewrite for two classes:

If $p(\mathbf{x} \mid \omega_1) P(\omega_1) > p(\mathbf{x} \mid \omega_2) P(\omega_2)$ then $\mathbf{x} \in \omega_1$ else $\mathbf{x} \in \omega_2$,   (4-15)

or,

if $v(\mathbf{x}) = \dfrac{p(\mathbf{x} \mid \omega_1)}{p(\mathbf{x} \mid \omega_2)} > \dfrac{P(\omega_2)}{P(\omega_1)}$ then $\mathbf{x} \in \omega_1$ else $\mathbf{x} \in \omega_2$.   (4-15a)

In the formula (4-15a), $v(\mathbf{x})$ is the so-called *likelihood ratio*. The decision depends on how this ratio compares with the inverse prevalence ratio or *prevalence threshold*, $P(\omega_2)/P(\omega_1)$.

Let us assume for the cork stoppers problem that we only used feature N, $\mathbf{x}=[N]$, and that a cork was presented with $\mathbf{x}=[65]$.

Figure 4.12 shows the histograms of both classes with superimposed normal curve.

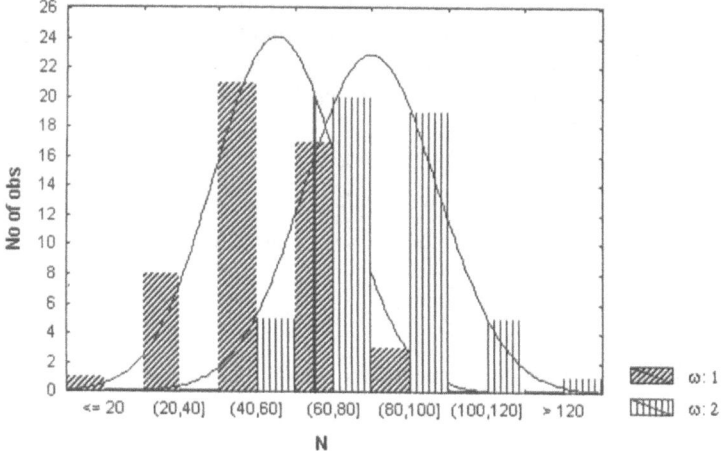

Figure 4.12. Histograms of feature N for two classes of cork stoppers. The threshold value N=65 is marked with a vertical line.

From this graphic display we can estimate the likelihoods[3]:

$$p(\mathbf{x}\,|\,\omega_1) = 20\,/\,24 = 0.833 \qquad \Rightarrow \qquad P(\omega_1)p(\mathbf{x}\,|\,\omega_1) = 0.333\;; \qquad (4\text{-}16a)$$

$$p(\mathbf{x}\,|\,\omega_2) = 16\,/\,23 = 0.696 \qquad \Rightarrow \qquad P(\omega_2)p(\mathbf{x}\,|\,\omega_2) = 0.418\;. \qquad (4\text{-}16b)$$

We then decide class ω_2, although the likelihood of ω_1 is bigger than that of ω_2. Notice how the statistical model changed the conclusions derived by the minimum distance classification (see 4.1.3).

Figure 4.13 illustrates the effect of adjusting the prevalence threshold assuming equal and normal *pdf*s:

- Equal prevalences. With equal *pdf*s, the decision threshold is at half distance from the means. The number of cases incorrectly classified, proportional to the shaded areas, is equal for both classes. This situation is identical to the minimum distance classifier.
- Prevalence of ω_1 bigger than that of ω_2. The decision threshold is displaced towards the class with smaller prevalence, therefore decreasing the number of cases of the class with higher prevalence that are wrongly classified, as it seems convenient.

---

[3] The normal curve fitted by *Statistica* is multiplied by the factor (number of cases)x(histogram interval width), which is 100 in the present case. This constant factor is of no importance and is neglected in the computations (4-16).

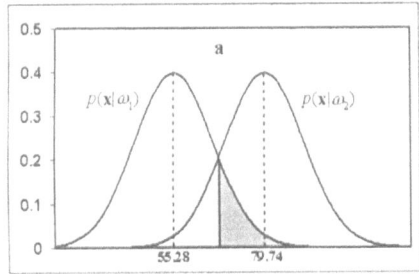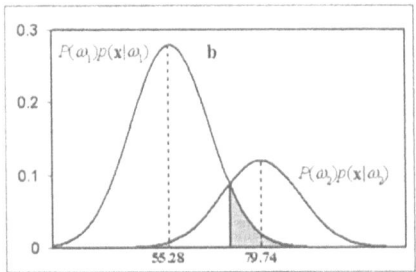

Figure 4.13. Influence of the prevalence threshold on the classification errors, represented by the shaded areas (dark grey represents the errors for class ω_1). (a) Equal prevalences; (b) Unequal prevalences.

Figure 4.14 shows the classification matrix obtained with the prevalences computed in (4-12), which are indicated in the *Group* row.

We see that indeed the decision threshold deviation led to a better performance for class ω_2 than for class ω_1. This seems reasonable since class ω_2 now occurs more often. Since the overall error has increased, one may wonder if this influence of the prevalences was beneficial after all. The answer to this question is related to the topic of *classification risks*, which we will present now.

Let us assume that the cost of a ω_1 ("super") cork stopper is 0.025 € and the cost of a ω_2 ("average") cork stopper is 0.015 €. Suppose that the ω_1 cork stoppers are to be used in special bottles whereas the ω_2 cork stoppers are used in normal bottles.

A wrong classification of a super quality cork stopper will amount to a loss of 0.025-0.015=0.01 € (see Figure 4.15). A wrong classification of an average cork stopper leads to its rejection with a loss of 0.015 €.

Denote:

SB – Action of using a cork stopper in *special bottles*.
NB - Action of using a cork stopper in *normal bottles*.
$\omega_1=S$ (class super); $\omega_2=A$ (class average)

DISCRIM. ANALYSIS	Rows: Observed classifications Columns: Predicted classifications		
Group	Percent Correct	G_1:1 p=.40000	G_2:2 p=.60000
G_1:1	64.00000	32	18
G_2:2	82.00000	9	41
Total	73.00000	41	59

Figure 4.14. Classification results of the cork stoppers with unequal prevalences: 0.4 for class ω_1 and 0.6 for class ω_2.

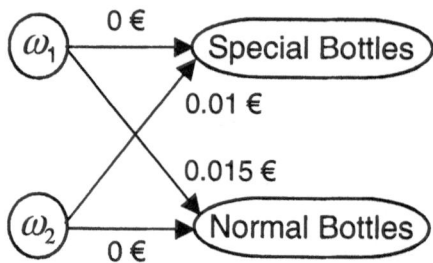

Figure 4.15. Loss diagram for two classes of cork stoppers. Correct decisions have zero loss.

Define:

$\lambda_{ij} = \lambda(\alpha_i \mid \omega_j)$ as the loss associated with an action α_i when the correct class is ω_j. In the present case, $\alpha_i \in \{SB, NB\}$.

We can arrange the λ_{ij} in a loss matrix Λ, which in the present case is:

$$\Lambda = \begin{bmatrix} 0 & 0.015 \\ 0.01 & 0 \end{bmatrix}. \tag{4-17}$$

Therefore, the risk (loss) associated with the action of using a cork, characterized by the feature vector $\mathbf{x}$, in special bottles, can be expressed as:

$$R(\alpha_1 \mid \mathbf{x}) = R(SB \mid \mathbf{x}) = \lambda(SB \mid S)P(S \mid \mathbf{x}) + \lambda(NB \mid M)P(A \mid \mathbf{x}); \tag{4-17a}$$
$$R(\alpha_1 \mid \mathbf{x}) = 0.015 P(A \mid \mathbf{x}).$$

And likewise for normal bottles:

$$R(\alpha_2 \mid \mathbf{x}) = R(NB \mid \mathbf{x}) = \lambda(NB \mid S)P(S \mid \mathbf{x}) + \lambda(NB \mid A)P(A \mid \mathbf{x}); \tag{4-17b}$$
$$R(\alpha_2 \mid \mathbf{x}) = 0.01 P(S \mid \mathbf{x}).$$

We assume that in the risk evaluation the only influence is from wrong decisions. Therefore, correct decisions have zero loss, $\lambda_{ii}=0$, as in (4-17). If instead of two classes we have c classes, the risk associated with a certain action α_i is expressed as follows[4]:

$$R(\alpha_i \mid \mathbf{x}) = \sum_{j=1}^{c} \lambda(\alpha_i \mid \omega_j)P(\omega_j \mid \mathbf{x}). \tag{4-17c}$$

---

[4] It is assumed without loss of generality that only one action corresponds to each class.

We are obviously interested in minimizing an average risk computed for an arbitrarily large number of cork stoppers. The *Bayes rule for minimum risk* achieves this through the minimization of the individual conditional risks $R(\alpha_i \mid \mathbf{x})$.

Let us assume first that wrong decisions imply the same loss, which can be scaled to a unitary loss:

$$\lambda_{ij} = \lambda(\alpha_i \mid \omega_j) = \begin{cases} 0 & \text{if} \quad i = j \\ 1 & \text{if} \quad i \neq j \end{cases}. \tag{4-18a}$$

In this situation, since all posterior probabilities add up to one, we have to minimize:

$$R(\alpha_i \mid \mathbf{x}) = \sum_{j \neq i} P(\omega_j \mid \mathbf{x}) = 1 - P(\omega_i \mid \mathbf{x}). \tag{4-18b}$$

This corresponds to maximizing $P(\omega_i \mid \mathbf{x})$, i.e., the Bayes decision rule for minimum risk corresponds to the generalized version of (4-13a):

$$\text{Decide} \quad \omega_i \quad \text{if} \quad P(\omega_i \mid \mathbf{x}) > P(\omega_j \mid \mathbf{x}), \quad \forall j \neq i. \tag{4-18c}$$

In short:

> *The Bayes decision rule for minimum risk, when correct decisions have zero loss and wrong decisions have equal losses, corresponds to selecting the class with maximum posterior probability.*

The decision function for class ω_i is therefore:

$$g_i(\mathbf{x}) = P(\omega_i \mid \mathbf{x}). \tag{4-18d}$$

Let us now consider the situation of different losses for wrong decisions, assuming first, for the sake of simplicity, that $c=2$. Taking into account expressions (4-17a) and (4-17b), it is readily concluded that we will decide ω_1 if:

$$\lambda_{21} P(\omega_1 \mid \mathbf{x}) > \lambda_{12} P(\omega_2 \mid \mathbf{x}) \quad \Rightarrow \quad \frac{p(\mathbf{x} \mid \omega_1)}{p(\mathbf{x} \mid \omega_2)} > \frac{\lambda_{12} P(\omega_2)}{\lambda_{21} P(\omega_1)}. \tag{4-19}$$

Therefore, the decision threshold with which the likelihood ratio is compared is inversely weighted by the losses (compare with 4-15a). This decision rule can be implemented as shown in Figure 4.16 (see also Figure 4.6).

Equivalently, we can use the following *adjusted prevalences*:

$$P^*(\omega_1) = \frac{\lambda_{21} P(\omega_1)}{\lambda_{21} P(\omega_1) + \lambda_{12} P(\omega_2)} \; ; \quad P^*(\omega_2) = \frac{\lambda_{12} P(\omega_2)}{\lambda_{21} P(\omega_1) + \lambda_{12} P(\omega_2)}. \tag{4-19a}$$

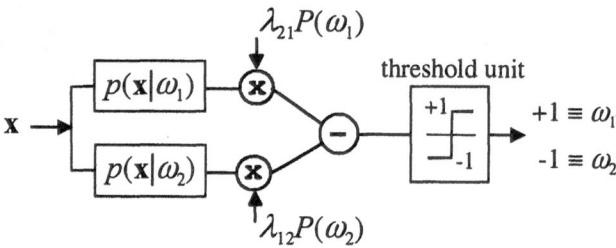

Figure 4.16. Implementation of the Bayesian decision rule for two classes with different loss factors for wrong decisions.

For the cork stopper losses $\lambda_{12}=0.015$ and $\lambda_{21}=0.01$, using the previous prevalences, one obtains $P^*(\omega_1)=0.308$ and $P^*(\omega_2)=0.692$. The higher loss associated with a wrong classification of a ω_2 cork stopper leads to an increase of $P^*(\omega_2)$ compared with $P^*(\omega_1)$. The consequence of this adjustment is the decrease of the number of ω_2 cork stoppers wrongly classified as ω_1. This is shown in the classification matrix of Figure 4.17.

DISCRIM. ANALYSIS	Rows: Observed classifications Columns: Predicted classifications		
Group	Percent Correct	G_1:1 p=.30800	G_2:2 p=.69200
G 1:1	54.00000	27	23
G_2:2	90.00000	5	45
Total	72.00000	32	68

Figure 4.17. Classification matrix of two classes of cork stoppers with adjusted prevalences.

We can now compute the average risk for the 2-class situation, as follows:

$$R = \int_{R_1} \lambda_{12} P(\omega_2 \mid \mathbf{x}) p(\mathbf{x}) d\mathbf{x} + \int_{R_2} \lambda_{21} P(\omega_1 \mid \mathbf{x}) p(\mathbf{x}) d\mathbf{x} = \lambda_{12} Pe_{12} + \lambda_{21} Pe_{21}, \quad (4\text{-}20)$$

where R_1 and R_2 are the decision regions for ω_1 and ω_2 respectively, and Pe_{ij} is the error probability of deciding class ω_i when the true class is ω_j.

Let us use the training set estimates of these errors, $Pe_{12}=0.1$ and $Pe_{21}=0.46$ (see Figure 4.17). The average risk per cork stopper is now computed as $R = 0.015Pe_{12} + 0.01Pe_{21} = 0.0061$ €. If we had not used the adjusted prevalences we would have obtained the higher risk of 0.0063 €.

For a set of classes, Ω, formula (4-20) generalizes to:

$$R = \sum_{\omega_i \in \Omega} \int_X \lambda(\alpha(\mathbf{x})| \omega_i) P(\omega_i, \mathbf{x}) d\mathbf{x} = \sum_{\omega_i \in \Omega} \int_X \lambda(\alpha(\mathbf{x})| \omega_i) P(\omega_i | \mathbf{x}) p(\mathbf{x}) d\mathbf{x} . \quad (4\text{-}20a)$$

The Bayes decision rule is not the only alternative in statistical classification. It is, however, by far the most popular rule. The interested reader can find alternative methods to the Bayes rule for accounting for action losses in Fukunaga (1990).

Note also that, in practice, one tries to minimize the average risk by using estimates of *pdf*s computed from a training set, as we have done above for the cork stoppers. If we have grounds to believe that the *pdf*s satisfy a certain parametric model, we can instead compute the appropriate parameters from the training set, as discussed next. In either case, we are using an *empirical risk minimization* (ERM) principle: minimization of an empirical risk instead of a true risk.

4.2.2 Normal Bayesian Classification

Until now we have assumed no particular distribution model for the likelihoods. Frequently, however, the normal model is a reasonable assumption. The wide spread applicability of the normal model has a justification related to the well-known Central Limit Theorem, according to which the sum of independent and identically distributed random variables has (under very general conditions) a distribution converging to the normal law with an increasing number of variables. In practice, one frequently obtains good approximations to the normal law, even for a relatively small number of added random variables (say, above 5). For features that can be considered the result of the addition of independent variables, the normal assumption is often an acceptable one.

A normal likelihood for class ω_i is expressed by the following *pdf*:

$$p(\mathbf{x}|\omega_i) = \frac{1}{(2\pi)^{d/2}|\Sigma_i|^{1/2}} \exp\left(-\frac{1}{2}(\mathbf{x}-\mu_i)'\Sigma_i^{-1}(\mathbf{x}-\mu_i) \right), \qquad (4\text{-}21)$$

with:

$\mu_i = E_i[\mathbf{x}];$ mean vector for class ω_i (4-21a)

$\Sigma_i = E_i[(\mathbf{x}-\mu_i)(\mathbf{x}-\mu_i)']$ covariance for class ω_i .   (4-21b)

Note that μ_i and Σ_i, the *distribution parameters*, are the theoretical or true mean and covariance, whereas until now we have used the sample estimates $\mathbf{m}_i$ and $\mathbf{C}_i$, respectively. Figure 4.18 illustrates the normal distribution for the two-dimensional situation.

Given a training set with n patterns $T=\{\mathbf{x}_1, \mathbf{x}_2, .., \mathbf{x}_n\}$ characterized by a distribution with $pdf\, p(T|\theta)$, where θ is a parameter vector of the distribution (e.g. the mean vector of a normal distribution), an interesting way of obtaining sample estimates of the parameter vector θ is to maximize $p(T|\theta)$, which viewed as a function of θ is called the *likelihood of θ for the given training set*. Assuming that each pattern is drawn independently from a potentially infinite population, we can express this likelihood as:

$$p(T|\theta) = \prod_{i=1}^{n} p(\mathbf{x}_i | \theta). \tag{4-22}$$

When using the *maximum likelihood estimation* of distribution parameters it is often easier to compute the maximum of $\ln[p(T|\theta)]$, which is equivalent (the logarithm is a monotonic increasing function). For Gaussian distributions, the sample estimates given by formulas (4-21a) and (4-21b) are maximum likelihood estimates and will converge to the true values with an increasing number of cases. The reader can find a detailed explanation of the parameter estimation issue in Duda and Hart (1973).

As can be seen from (4-21), the surfaces of equal probability density for normal likelihood satisfy the Mahalanobis metric already discussed in sections 2.2, 2.3 and 4.1.3.

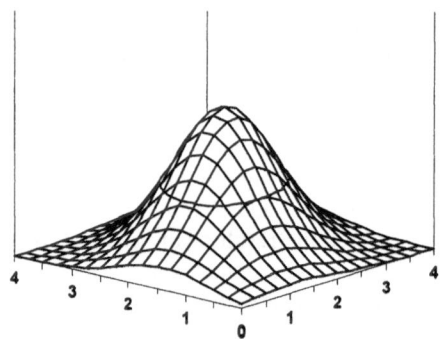

Figure 4.18. The bell-shaped surface of a two-dimensional normal distribution. An ellipsis with equal probability density points is also shown.

Let us now proceed to compute the decision function (4-18d) for normally distributed features:

$$g_i(\mathbf{x}) = P(\omega_i | \mathbf{x}) = P(\omega_i) p(\mathbf{x}|\omega_i). \tag{4-23}$$

We may apply a monotonic logarithmic transformation (see 2.1.1), obtaining:

$$h_i(\mathbf{x}) = \ln(g_i(\mathbf{x})) = \ln(P(\omega_i)p(\mathbf{x}\,|\,\omega_i))\,;\qquad\qquad (4\text{-}23a)$$

$$h_i(\mathbf{x}) = -\frac{1}{2}(\mathbf{x}-\boldsymbol{\mu}_i)'\,\boldsymbol{\Sigma}_i^{-1}(\mathbf{x}-\boldsymbol{\mu}_i)-\frac{d}{2}\ln 2\pi -\frac{1}{2}\log|\boldsymbol{\Sigma}_i|+\ln P(\omega_i)\,.\qquad (4\text{-}23b)$$

Using these decision functions, clearly dependent on the Mahalanobis metric, one can design a minimum risk Bayes classifier, usually called an *optimum classifier*. In general, one obtains quadratic discriminants.

Notice that formula (4-23b) uses the true value of the Mahalanobis distance, whereas before we have used estimates of this distance.

For the situation of equal covariance for all classes ($\Sigma_i=\Sigma$), neglecting constant terms, one obtains:

$$h_i(\mathbf{x}) = -\frac{1}{2}(\mathbf{x}-\boldsymbol{\mu}_i)'\,\boldsymbol{\Sigma}^{-1}(\mathbf{x}-\boldsymbol{\mu}_i)+\ln P(\omega_i)\,.\qquad\qquad (4\text{-}23c)$$

For a two-class problem, the discriminant $d(\mathbf{x})=h_1(\mathbf{x})-h_2(\mathbf{x})$ is easily computed as:

$$d(\mathbf{x}) = \mathbf{w}'\mathbf{x}+w_0\,,\qquad\qquad (4\text{-}24)$$

where,

$$\mathbf{w} = \boldsymbol{\Sigma}^{-1}(\boldsymbol{\mu}_1-\boldsymbol{\mu}_2);\quad w_0 = -\frac{1}{2}\left(\boldsymbol{\mu}_1'\boldsymbol{\Sigma}^{-1}\boldsymbol{\mu}_1-\boldsymbol{\mu}_2'\boldsymbol{\Sigma}^{-1}\boldsymbol{\mu}_2\right)+\ln\frac{P(\omega_1)}{P(\omega_2)}\,.\qquad (4\text{-}24a)$$

Therefore, one obtains linear decision functions (notice the similarity to formulas (4-5b) and (4-5c)).

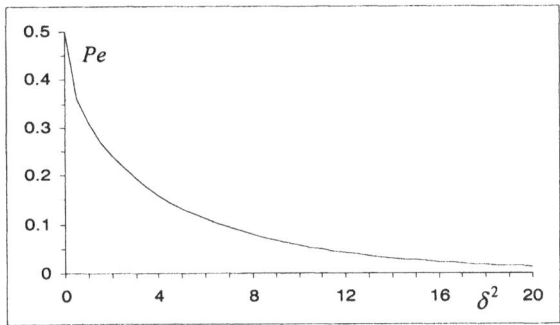

Figure 4.19. Error probability of a Bayesian two-class discrimination with normal distributions and equal prevalences and covariance.

For a two-class discrimination with normal distributions and equal prevalences and covariance, there is also a simple formula for the probability of error of the classifier (see e.g. Fukunaga, 1990) :

$$Pe = 1 - erf(\delta / 2),\qquad\qquad (4\text{-}25)$$

with:

$$erf(x) = \frac{1}{\sqrt{2\pi}} \int_{-\infty}^{x} e^{-t^2/2} dt ,\qquad (4\text{-}25a)$$

known as error function[5], and

$$\delta^2 = (\mu_1 - \mu_2)' \Sigma^{-1} (\mu_1 - \mu_2),\qquad\qquad (4\text{-}25b)$$

the square of the so-called *Bhattacharyya distance*, a Mahalanobis distance of the difference of the means, reflecting the class separability.

Figure 4.19 shows the behaviour of *Pe* with increasing squared Bhattacharyya distance. After an initial quick, exponential-like decay, *Pe* converges asymptotically to zero. It is, therefore, increasingly difficult to lower a classifier error when it is already small.

Note that even when the pattern distributions are not normal, as long as they are symmetric and obey the Mahalanobis metric, we will obtain the same decision surfaces as for a normal optimum classifier, although with different error rates and posterior probabilities. As an illustration of this topic, let us consider two classes with equal prevalences and one-dimensional feature vectors following three different types of symmetric distributions, with the same unitary standard deviation and means 0 and 2.3, as shown in Figure 4.20:

Normal distribution: $\quad p(x \mid \omega_i) = \dfrac{1}{\sqrt{2\pi}\, s} e^{-\frac{(x-m_i)^2}{2s^2}} .\qquad (4\text{-}26a)$

Cauchy distribution: $\quad p(x \mid \omega_i) = 1/\pi s \left\{ 1 + \left(\dfrac{x - m_i}{s} \right)^2 \right\} .\qquad (4\text{-}26b)$

Logistic distribution: $\quad p(x \mid \omega_i) = \dfrac{1}{s} \dfrac{e^{-\frac{(x-m_i)}{s}}}{\left(1 + e^{-\frac{(x-m_i)}{s}} \right)^2} .\qquad (4\text{-}26c)$

---

[5] The error function is the cumulative probability distribution function of $N(0,1)$.

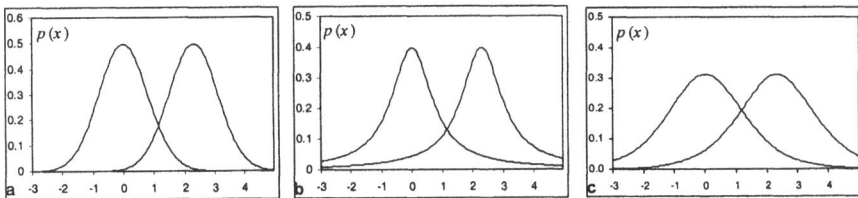

Figure 4.20. Two classes with symmetric distributions and the same standard deviation. (a) Normal; (b) Cauchy; (c) Logistic.

The optimum classifier for the three cases uses the same decision threshold value: 1.15. However, the classification errors are different:

Normal: $Pe = 1 - erf(2.3/2) = 12.5\%$
Cauchy: $Pe = 22.7\%$
Logistic: $Pe = 24.0\%$

As previously mentioned, statistical software products use a pooled covariance matrix when performing discriminant analysis. The influence of this practice on the obtained error, compared with the theoretical optimal Bayesian error, is discussed in detail in Fukunaga (1990). Experimental results show that when the covariance matrices exhibit limited deviations from the pooled covariance matrix, then the designed classifier has a performance similar to the optimal performance with equal covariances. This is reasonable, since for covariance matrices that are not very distinct, the difference between the optimum quadratic solution and the sub-optimum linear solution should only be noticeable for the patterns that are far away from the prototypes, as shown in Figure 4.21.

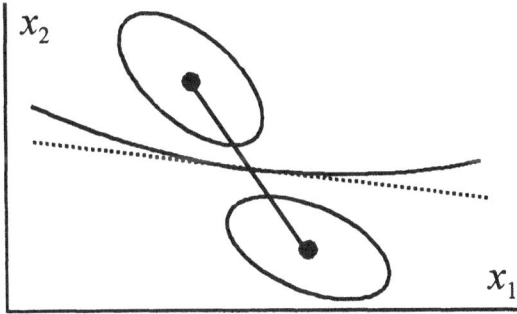

Figure 4.21. Discrimination of two classes with optimum quadratic classifier (solid line) and sub-optimum linear classifier (dotted line).

Let us illustrate this issue using the *Norm2c2d* dataset (see Appendix A). The theoretical error for this two-class, two-dimensional, dataset is:

$$\delta^2 = \begin{bmatrix} 2 & 3 \end{bmatrix} \begin{bmatrix} 0.8 & -0.8 \\ -0.8 & 1.6 \end{bmatrix} \begin{bmatrix} 2 \\ 3 \end{bmatrix} = 8 \quad \Rightarrow \quad Pe = 1 - erf(\sqrt{2}) = 7.9\%$$

The training set error estimate for this dataset is 5%. By introducing deviations of ±0.1 into the values of the transforming matrix **A** of this dataset, with corresponding deviations between 15% and 42% of the covariance values, training set errors of 6% were obtained, a mild deviation from the previous 5% error rate for the equal covariance situation (see Exercise 4.9).

DISCRIM. ANALYSIS	Incorrect classifications are marked with *		
Case	Observed Classif.	G_1:1 p=.50000	G_2:2 p=.50000
50	G_1:1	.964	.036
51	G_2:2	.128	.872
52	G_2:2	.272	.728
53	G_2:2	.113	.887
54	G_2:2	.157	.843
* 55	G_2:2	.782	.218
56	G_2:2	.095	.905
57	G_2:2	.065	.935

Figure 4.22. Partial listing of the posterior probabilities for two classes of cork stoppers.

Let us go back to the cork stoppers classification problem using two features, N and PRT, with equal prevalences. The classification matrix is shown in Figure 4.8. Note that statistical classifiers are, apart from numerical considerations, invariant to scaling operations, therefore the same results are obtained using either PRT or PRT10.

A partial listing of the posterior probabilities, useful for spotting classification errors, is shown in Figure 4.22.

The covariance matrices are shown in Table 4.2. The deviations of the covariance matrices elements compared with the central values of the pooled matrix are between 5 and 30%. The cluster shapes are also similar. Therefore, there are good reasons to believe that the designed classifier is near the optimum one.

Table 4.2. Covariances per class and pooled covariance for the cork stoppers (two classes).

C_1		C_2		Pooled C	
272.859	1729.17	302.400	2352.22	287.630	2040.70
1729.17	12167.8	2352.22	22343.0	2040.70	17255.3

As already mentioned in section 2.2, using decision functions based on the individual covariance matrices, instead of a pooled covariance matrix, will produce quadratic decision boundaries. However, a quadratic classifier is less robust (more sensitive to parameter deviations) than a linear one, especially in high dimensional spaces, and needs a much larger training set for adequate design (see e.g. Fukunaga and Hayes, 1989).

4.2.3 Reject Region

In practical applications of pattern recognition, it often happens that simply using a decision rule such as (4-13a) or (4-18c) will produce many borderline decisions, very sensitive to noise present in the data and to the numerical accuracy of the classifiers. For instance, for the cork stoppers data with the decision border depicted in Figure 4.11, many patterns lying near the border can change the assigned class by only a slight adjustment. This means that, in fact, such patterns largely share the characteristics of both classes. For such patterns, it is often more advisable to place them in a special class for further inspection. This is certainly a must in some applications, e.g., in the medical field, where borderline cases between normal and abnormal states deserve further analysis. One way to do this is to attach qualifications to the computed posterior probabilities $P(\omega_i|\mathbf{x})$ for the decided class ω_i. We could, for instance, attach the qualitative "definite" if the probability is bigger than 0.9, "probable" if it is between 0.9 and 0.8 and "possible" if it is below 0.8. In this way, the cork stopper case 55 (Figure 4.22) would be classified as a "possible" cork of class "super", and case 54 as a "probable" cork of class "average".

Instead of attaching qualitative descriptions to the obtained classifications, a method used in certain circumstances is to stipulate the existence of a special class, the *reject class* or *region*.

Let us denote:

ω^*:   the decided class;

ω_i :   the class with maximum posterior probability, i.e., $P(\omega_i|\mathbf{x}) = \max P(\omega_j|\mathbf{x})$ for all classes $\omega_j \neq \omega_i$.

The Bayes rule can then be written simply $\omega^*=\omega_i$.

Let us now stipulate that the posterior probabilities of a cork stopper must be higher than a certain *reject threshold* λ_r, otherwise it is classified in a special reject class ω_r. The Bayes rule is now reformulated as:

$$\omega^* = \begin{cases} \omega_i & \text{if} & P(\omega_i \mid \mathbf{x}) \geq \lambda_r \\ \omega_r & \text{if} & P(\omega_i \mid \mathbf{x}) < \lambda_r \end{cases} . \tag{4-27}$$

When comparing the likelihood ratio with the prevalence ratio, one now has to multiply this ratio by $(1 - \lambda_r)/\lambda_r$. Notice that for a c class problem there is never a rejection if $\lambda_r < (c-1)/c$, therefore $\lambda_r \in [(c-1)/c, 1]$.

Let us illustrate the concept of a reject class using the cork stoppers data. Suppose that a reject threshold of $\lambda_r = 0.7$ is stipulated. In order to compute decision borders for the reject class, it is enough to determine the discriminant function for the new prevalences $P(\omega_1) = (1 - \lambda_r) = 0.3$, $P(\omega_2) = \lambda_r = 0.7$ and vice-versa. The decision lines have the same slope, and intersect the vertical axis at PRT10=15.5 and PRT10=20.1, respectively. Notice that these lines are therefore symmetrically disposed around the decision line determined in section 4.1.3. (crossing at 17.8). Figure 4.23 shows the scatter plot with the new decision lines. The area between the solid lines is the reject region.

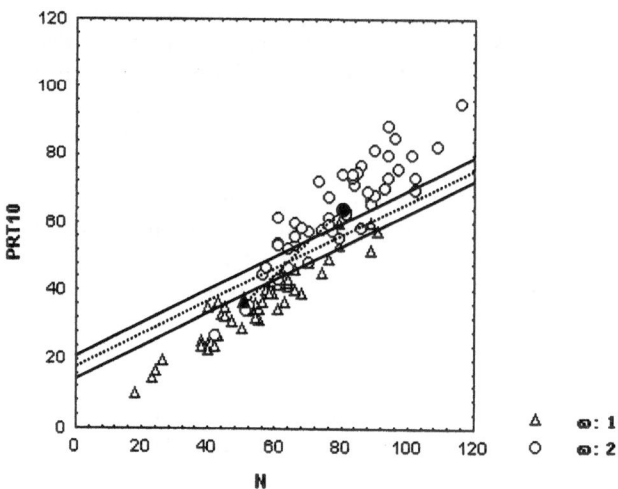

Figure 4.23. Discriminant analysis for two classes of cork stoppers with reject region between the solid lines corresponding to reject threshold $\lambda_r = 0.7$.

Let us look now to the classification matrices shown in Figure 4.24. A bit of thought will reveal that 4 patterns of class 1, and 5 patterns of class 2 fall into the reject region, i.e., 9% of the patterns. The misclassifications are now 1 pattern for class 1 (2%) and 5 patterns for class 2 (10%), therefore an overall error of 6%.

a	Rows: Observ. classif. Cols: Pred. classif.		
Group	% Correct	G_1:1 p=.70	G_2:2 p=.30
G_1:1	98.0	49	1
G_2:2	80.0	10	40
Total	89.0	59	41

b	Rows: Observ. classif. Cols: Pred. classif.		
Group	% Correct	G_1:1 p=.30	G_2:2 p=.70
G_1:1	90.0	45	5
G_2:2	90.0	5	45
Total	90.0	50	50

Figure 4.24. Classification matrices of two classes of cork stoppers with prevalences adjusted for the reject region boundaries.

4.2.4 Dimensionality Ratio and Error Estimation

As already pointed out in section 2.7 the dimensionality ratio issue is an essential one when designing a classifier. An adequately high dimensionality ratio will guarantee that the designed classifier has reproducible results, i.e., it performs equally well when presented with new patterns. Looking at the Mahalanobis and the Bhattacharyya distance formulas, it is clear that they can only increase when adding more and more features. This would certainly be the case if we had the true values of the means and the covariances available, which, in practical applications, we do not.

When using a large number of features, as already pointed out in sections 2.3 and 2.7, we will have numeric troubles in obtaining a good estimate of C^{-1}, given the finiteness of the training set. Surprising results can then be expected; for instance, the performance of the classifier can degrade when more features are added, instead of improving.

a	Rows: Observ. classif. Cols: Pred. classif.		
Group	% Correct	G_1:1 p=.50	G_2:2 p=.50
G_1:1	98.0	49	1
G_2:2	86.0	7	43
Total	92.0	56	44

b	Rows: Observ. classif. Cols: Pred. classif.		
Group	% Correct	G_1:1 p=.50	G_2:2 p=.50
G_1:1	98.0	49	1
G_2:2	88.0	6	44
Total	93.0	55	45

Figure 4.25. Classification results of two classes of cork stoppers using: (a) Ten features; (b) Four features.

Figure 4.25a shows the classification matrix for the two-class cork stoppers problem using the whole ten-feature set and equal prevalences. The performance did not increase significantly compared with the two-feature solution presented previously, and is worse than the solution using the four-feature vector [ART PRM NG RAAR]', as shown in Figure 4.25b.

There are, however, further compelling reasons for not using a large number of features. As a matter of fact, when using estimates of means and covariance derived from a training set, we are designing a biased classifier, fitted to the training set (review section 2.6 again). Therefore, we should expect that our training set error estimates are, on average, optimistic. On the other hand, error estimates obtained in independent test sets are expected to be, on average, pessimistic.

The bibliography at the end of the present chapter includes references explaining the mathematical details of this issue. We present here some important results as an aid for the designer to choose sensible values for the dimensionality ratio, n/d. Later, when we discuss the topic of classifier evaluation, we will come back to this issue from another perspective.

Let us denote:

Pe –   Probability of error of an optimum Bayesian classifier.
$Pe_d(n)$ –   Training (design) set estimate of Pe for n patterns.
$Pe_t(n)$ –   Test set estimate of Pe for n patterns.

Thus, the quantity $Pe_d(n)$ represents an estimate of Pe influenced only by the finite size of the design set, i.e., the classifier error is measured exactly and its deviation from Pe is due solely to the finiteness of the design set; the quantity $Pe_t(n)$ represents an estimate of Pe influenced only by the finite size of the test set, i.e., the error of the Bayesian classifier is estimated by counting how many of n patterns are misclassified. These quantities verify that $Pe_d(\infty)=Pe$ and $Pe_t(\infty)=Pe$, i.e., they converge to the theoretical value Pe with increasing values of n.

In normal practice, these error probabilities are not known exactly. Instead, we compute estimates of these probabilities, $\widehat{Pe}_d$ and $\widehat{Pe}_t$, as percentages of misclassified patterns, in exactly the same way as we have done in the classification matrices presented so far. The probability of obtaining k misclassified patterns out of n for a classifier with a theoretical error Pe, is given by the binomial law:

$$P(k) = C(n,k)Pe^k (1-Pe)^{n-k} .$$

$$(4-28)$$

The maximum likelihood estimation of Pe under this binomial law is precisely:

$$\widehat{Pe} = \frac{k}{n}.$$

$$(4-29)$$

The standard deviation of this estimate is simply:

$$s = \sqrt{\frac{Pe(1-Pe)}{n}} \ .$$

(4-30)

Formula (4-30) allows the computation of confidence interval estimates for $\hat{Pe}$, by substituting $\hat{Pe}$ in place of Pe and using the normal distribution approximation for sufficiently large n (say, $n \geq 25$). Notice that they are zero for the extreme cases of $Pe=0$ or $Pe=1$. Furthermore, as this formula is independent of the classifier model, its value is to be considered a worst-case value, yielding in many circumstances unrealistically large intervals.

In normal practice we compute $\hat{Pe}_d$ by designing and evaluating the classifier in the same set with n patterns, $\hat{Pe}_d(n)$. This error estimate is related to an empirical risk, mentioned already in section 4.2.1. As for $\hat{Pe}_t$, we may compute it using an independent set of n patterns, $\hat{Pe}_t(n)$. In order to have some guidance on how to choose an appropriate dimensionality ratio, we would like to know the deviation of the expected values of these estimates from the Bayes error, where the expectation is computed on a population of classifiers of the same type and trained in the same conditions. Formulas for these expectations, $E[\hat{Pe}_d(n)]$ and $E[\hat{Pe}_t(n)]$, are quite intricate and can only be computed numerically. Like formula (4-25), they depend on the Bhattacharyya distance. The bibliography section includes references where these formulas for two classes with normal distributions can be found, namely Foley (1972) and Raudys and Pikelis (1980). A software tool, *PR Size*, computing these formulas for the linear discriminant case is included in the CD distributed with the book. *PR Size* also allows the computation of confidence intervals of these estimates, using (4-30).

Figure 4.26 is obtained with *PRSize* and illustrates how the expected values of the error estimates evolve with n patterns (assumed here to be the number of patterns in each class), in the situation of equal covariance. Both curves have an asymptotic behaviour with $n \to \infty$[6], with the average design set error estimate converging to the Bayes error (related to the optimal risk) from below and the average test set error estimate converging from above.

Both standard deviations, which can be inspected in text boxes for a selected value of n/d, are initially high for low values of n and converge slowly to zero with $n \to \infty$. For the situation shown in Figure 4.26, the standard deviation of $\hat{Pe}_d(n)$ changes from 0.089 for $n=d$ (14 patterns, 7 per class) to 0.033 for $n=10d$ (140 patterns, 70 per class).

Based on the behaviour of the $E[\hat{Pe}_d(n)]$ and $E[\hat{Pe}_t(n)]$ curves some criteria can be established for the dimensionality ratio. As a general rule of thumb, using dimensionality ratios above 3 is recommended.

---

[6] Numerical approximations in the computation of the average test set error may result in a deviation from this asymptotic behaviour, for sufficiently large n.

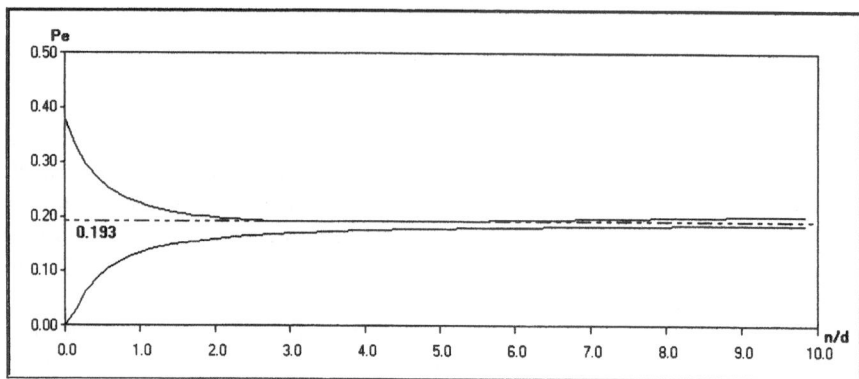

Figure 4.26. Two-class linear discriminant $E[\hat{Pe}_d(n)]$ and $E[\hat{Pe}_t(n)]$ curves, for $d=7$ and $\delta^2=3$, below and above the dotted line, respectively. The dotted line represents the Bayes error (0.193).

For precise criteria concerning the deviation of the expected values of $\hat{Pe}_d(n)$ and $\hat{Pe}_t(n)$ from Pe, the magnitude of the standard deviations, and therefore the 95% confidence interval of the estimates, it is advisable to use the *PRSize* program. If the patterns are not equally distributed by the classes it is advisable to use the smaller number of patterns per class as value of n. Notice also that a multi-class problem with absolute separation of the classes can be seen as a generalization of a two-class problem (see section 2.1.2). Therefore, the total number of needed training samples, for a given deviation of the expected error estimates from the Bayes error can be estimated as cn^*, where n^* is the particular value of n that achieves such a deviation in the most unfavourable two-class dichotomy of the multi-class problem. If a hierarchical approach is followed, one can use the estimate $(c-1)n^*$ instead.

4.3 Model-Free Techniques

The classifiers presented in the previous sections assumed particular shapes of the pattern clusters and sometimes also particular distributions of the feature vectors. Briefly, a certain model of the distribution of the feature vectors in the feature space was assumed. In the present section we will present three important model-free techniques to design classifiers. These methods do not make any assumptions about the underlying pattern distributions. They are often called *non-parametric* methods, however, at least some of them could be better called semi-parametric. Although all of these methods are model-free, their tuning to the particular distributions of the feature vectors is still based on statistical considerations.

The Parzen window and k-nearest neighbour methods, to be explained in the following sections, are both based on the idea of estimating the *pdf* of the pattern distributions. The ROC curve method is a completely model-free method for two-class situations, which simply addresses the problem of choosing the best discriminating thresholds as a compromise in conflicting cost requirements.

The methods incorporating *pdf* estimation assume well-behaved, smooth distributions, such that the probability density $p(\mathbf{x})$ at point $\mathbf{x}$ can be estimated by considering a sufficiently small region R with volume V, centred at $\mathbf{x}$, as follows:

$$p(\mathbf{x})V \approx \int_R p(\mathbf{u})\,d\mathbf{u} \ . \tag{4-31}$$

Imagine that one has a training set of n patterns and that k of these patterns fall in the region R. The second hand integral of (4-31) then represents the number of patterns falling inside R, therefore we obtain the estimate:

$$\hat{p}(\mathbf{x}) \approx \frac{k\,/\,n}{V} \ . \tag{4-32}$$

If the volume is too small compared to the number of samples, we will obtain quite erratic estimates with a high variance. If it is too big so that it encloses a large number of samples, we will obtain a smoothing effect since our point estimate will depend on distant samples. These conflicting requirements can be addressed in two ways:

1. Fix the volume so that it is inversely dependent on the number of available points, i.e., the more points there are, the smaller is the volume. Compute k from the data. This leads to the so-called *kernel-based approaches* such as the *Parzen window* method.
2. Fix k depending on the number of points and compute V from the data. This leads to the *k-nearest neighbour* method.

Usually the model-free techniques are only used in low dimensional situations. Estimation of a *pdf* is a rather difficult issue in high-dimensional spaces, and ROC analysis in this situation also requires burdensome computations for a large number of combinations of thresholds.

It is worth noting that *pdf* estimation in high dimensional spaces suffers from the *curse of dimensionality* already discussed in section 2.6. Going back to the argument presented in that section, concerning the partitioning of the feature space into m^d hypercubes, it is understandable that in order to obtain a reliable *pdf* estimate we need to select a sufficiently high number m of intervals along each dimension, and have at least one point in each hypercube. Hence, the training set size required for accurate *pdf* estimation will grow exponentially with d.

Model-free techniques come at a cost. First of all, no design formulas are available; therefore, a trial and error strategy often has to be employed in order to obtain a "best" solution. Second, dimensionality ratio, performance and reproducibility are less accessible to formal analysis, and in practice they have to be assessed in a purely experimental way.

4.3.1 The Parzen Window Method

As explained previously, in order to estimate $p(\mathbf{x})$ we will choose a sufficiently small region R centred at $\mathbf{x}$. Let us select R as a d-dimensional hypercube whose edge $h(n)$ varies with n. By varying $h(n)$ we are able to select an appropriate hypercube size depending on how many training patterns we have available. The volume of R is:

$$V(n) = h^d(n).$$

(4-33)

Let us define the following counting function:

$$\varphi(\mathbf{x}) = \begin{cases} 1 & \text{if} \quad |x_k| \le 1/2, \quad k = 1, \ldots, d\,; \\ 0 & \text{otherwise.} \end{cases}$$

(4-34)

Therefore, if a point falls inside the unit hypercube centred at the origin, it is counted; otherwise, it is not counted. Using this function we can express compactly the number $k(n)$ of points $\mathbf{x}_i$ falling inside any hypercube centred at $\mathbf{x}$, as:

$$k(n) = \sum_{i=1}^{n} \varphi\left(\frac{\mathbf{x} - \mathbf{x}_i}{h(n)}\right).$$

(4-35)

In this formula function φ is scaled by the hypercube edge length $h(n)$, and the counting criterion depends on the difference vector $\mathbf{x} - \mathbf{x}_i$, between a feature vector $\mathbf{x}$ and a training set feature vector $\mathbf{x}_i$.

With this $k(n)$ we can now express equation (4-32) as:

$$\hat{p}(\mathbf{x}, n) = \frac{1}{nV(n)} \sum_{i=1}^{n} \varphi\left(\frac{\mathbf{x} - \mathbf{x}_i}{h(n)}\right).$$

(4-36)

From formula (4-36) we see that if there is a large agglomeration of points in the immediate neighbourhood of $\mathbf{x}$ one obtains a high value of $\hat{p}(\mathbf{x}, n)$. If the number of such points is small, the value of $\hat{p}(\mathbf{x}, n)$ is also small.

Figure 4.27 illustrates the Parzen window method applied to a one-dimensional distribution and using a rectangular window. The *pdf* estimates at the regularly spaced marks are given by the height of the solid bars, proportional to the number of points (circles) that fall inside the window associated with a specific position.

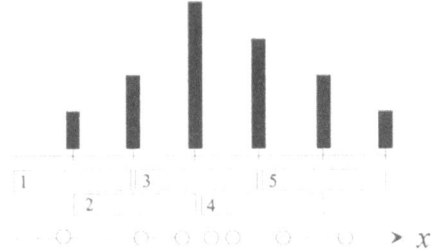

Figure 4.27. Parzen window estimation of a one-dimensional distribution, using a rectangular window.

The Parzen window method is a generalization of this formula, such that, instead of a hard-limiting hypercube window φ, we use any smooth window satisfying simple conditions of positiveness and unitary volume. The multivariate normal function is a frequently used window function. The role of this smoothing window, known as *interpolating kernel*, is to weight the contribution of each training set vector $\mathbf{x}_i$ to the *pdf* estimate at $\mathbf{x}$, in accordance with its deviation from $\mathbf{x}$. As for the smoothing parameter $h(n)$, which must vary inversely with n, Duda and Hart (1973) suggest $1/\sqrt{n}$. This can be taken as a first guess to be adjusted experimentally. Concerning the choice of kernel function φ, the normal function with estimated covariance is in fact the optimal choice for a large family of symmetric distributions that include the normal *pdf* itself (see Fukunaga, 1990).

Let us consider the *LogNorm* dataset in the *Parzen.xls* file (see Appendix A), which has a lognormal distribution characterized by a left asymmetry. Figure 4.28 illustrates the influence of the number of points and the smoothing factor $h(n)$ on the density estimate. Notice also the difficulty in obtaining a good adjustment of the peaked part of the distribution, requiring a high number of training samples. Even for smoother distributions, such as the normal one, we may need a large training set size (see Duda and Hart, 1973) in order to obtain an estimate that follows the true distribution closely. The problem is even worse when there is more than one dimension, due to the curse of dimensionality already referred to previously. The large datasets necessary for accurate *pdf* estimation may be a difficulty in the application of the method.

Let us now see how the Parzen window method can be applied to real data. For this purpose let us use the cork stoppers data (two classes) and feature ARM. This feature has an unknown asymmetrical distribution with a clear deviation from the normal distribution. The Parzen window method seems, therefore, a sensible alternative to the Bayesian approach. Figure 4.29 shows the Parzen window estimates of the distributions, also included in the *Parzen.xls* file. From these distributions it is possible to select a threshold for class discrimination. Choosing the threshold corresponding to the distribution intersection point, and assuming equal prevalences, the overall training set error is 24%. This is in fact a very reasonable error rate compared to the 23% obtained in 4.1.1 for the much more discriminating feature N.

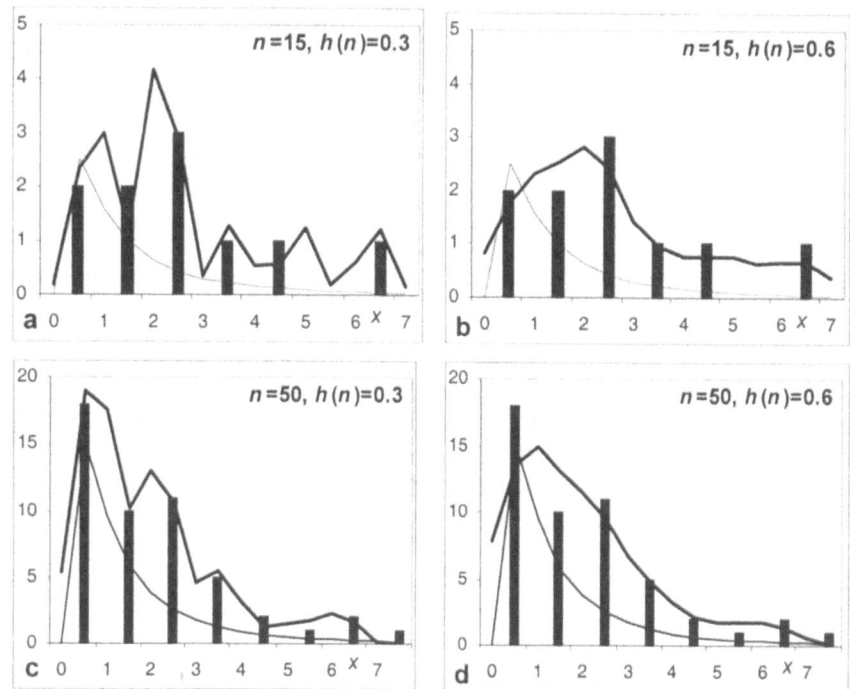

Figure 4.28. Parzen window *pdf* estimates (thick black line) of the lognormal distribution for *n*=15 and *n*=50 training set points, with the histograms represented by the black bars. The true distribution is the superimposed hairline curve (multiplied by a scale factor).

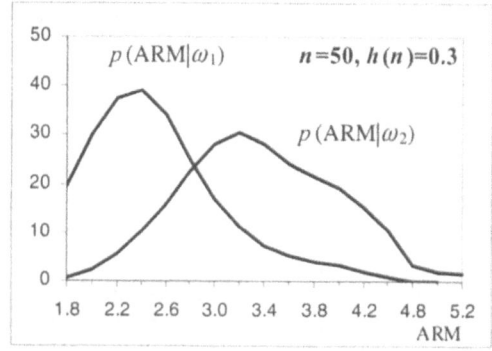

Figure 4.29. Parzen window estimate of feature ARM *pdf* (multiplied by 50) for two classes of cork stoppers.

An implementation of the Parzen window method developed by Specht (1990) is worth mentioning, since it constitutes an efficient way of obtaining estimates of the conditional probabilities of feature vector distributions and, therefore, lets us proceed to their classification, once we have a representative training set available. Assuming a Gaussian kernel function let us rewite equation(4-36) as:

$$p(\mathbf{x}, n) = \frac{1}{nV(n)} \sum_{i=1}^{n} \exp\left(\frac{(\mathbf{x} - \mathbf{x}_i)'(\mathbf{x} - \mathbf{x}_i)}{2\sigma^2} \right). \tag{4-37}$$

The summation terms can be computed, except for a scaling factor, in the following way:

1. Normalize $\mathbf{x}$ and $\mathbf{x}_i$ to unit length: $\mathbf{x}/\|\mathbf{x}\|$, $\mathbf{x}_i/\|\mathbf{x}_i\|$;
2. Compute the normalized dot products $\mathbf{z}_i = \mathbf{x}' \mathbf{x}_i / (\|\mathbf{x}\|.\| \mathbf{x}_i \|)$;
3. Apply the kernel function $\exp((\mathbf{z}_i - 1)/\sigma^2)$.

Summing all the exponential terms results in conditional probabilities estimates to which we can then apply the decision device illustrated in Figure 4.16.

The computational flow-diagram of this method resembles the connectionist structure of a neural network, hence the name of *probabilistic neural network* given to this method. However, it lacks any non-trivial learning capability, which, as we will see later, is a key aspect of neural nets. *Statistica* makes this method available in its Neural Networks tool. For the two-class cork stoppers data with features N and PRT10, a training set error of 5% is achieved with this method, which is very good compared to the previous result. Notice, however, that this is a training set estimate, which is usually optimistic. For a more accurate error estimate, the classifier would have to be evaluated using one of the methods that will be described in section 4.5.

It is also worth mentioning that Statistical Learning Theory teaches us that *pdf* estimation is a more difficult type of problem than pattern classification. Therefore, when using the Parzen window method for pattern classification, we are violating a commonsense principle: do not attempt to solve a specified problem by indirectly solving a harder problem as an intermediate step (see e.g. Cherkassky and Mulier, 1998).

4.3.2 The K-Nearest Neighbours Method

This method of *pdf* estimation is based on fixing the number of points $k(n)$ that exist in a certain region centred on a feature vector $\mathbf{x}$. This is done by growing a region around $\mathbf{x}$, with a suitable metric, until k points are captured. These are the $k(n)$ nearest neighbours of $\mathbf{x}$. The region then has a volume $V(n)$ and the *pdf* estimate is given by:

$$\hat{p}(\mathbf{x}, n) = \frac{k(n)/n}{V(n)} .$$

(4-38)

If there are few points around $\mathbf{x}$, the region grows large and the volume $V(n)$ will also be large, therefore yielding a low density value. If there are many points around $\mathbf{x}$, in which case $\mathbf{x}$ is a high density point, the volume $V(n)$ will be small.

The smoothing parameter in this case is $k(n)$ which must grow with n. Fukunaga and Hostetler (1973) derived an expression for $k(n)$, which for normal distributions is $k_0 n^{4/(d+4)}$. The constant k_0, initially 1.0 for $d=1$, decreases with d, to 0.75 for $d=4$ and to 0.42 for $d=32$. For instance, the two-class cork stoppers classification with 100 patterns would need about 7 neighbours when using 4 features. As we have done with the $h(n)$ factor in Parzen window estimation, the $k(n)$ factor also has to be adjusted experimentally.

When used as a *pdf* estimator the k-nearest neighbours method, or k-NN method for short, has the folowing shortcomings: the divergence to infinite of the integral of the density estimate and the computational burden of the method. Rather than using this method for *pdf* estimation, we will use it simply as a classification method, according to the following nearest neighbour rule: consider the $k(n)$ points that are nearest neighbours of $\mathbf{x}$, using a certain distance metric; the classification of $\mathbf{x}$ is then the class label that is found in majority among the $k(n)$ neighbours. The distance metric used results in different decision boundaries.

When applying the k-NN method, we are interested in knowing its attainable performance in terms of its error rate $Pe(k)$ for an arbitrarily large population, i.e., for $n \to \infty$, compared with the optimal Bayes error Pe. Bounds on $Pe(k)$ are studied and presented in Duda and Hart (1973) and can be expressed, for two classes and odd $k(n)$, as:

$$Pe \le Pe(k) \le \sum_{i=0}^{(k-1)/2} C(k,i) \left[Pe^{i+1} (1-Pe)^{k-i} + Pe^{k-i} (1-Pe)^{i+1} \right] .$$

(4-39)

In this formula Pe is the Bayes error. In particular, for the 1-NN case, the error has the following upper bound:

$$Pe(k) \le 2Pe(1-Pe).$$

(4-40)

These bounds are shown in Figure 4.30. As can be seen, $Pe(k)$ approaches Pe for increasing values of k, also demanding large numbers of points, and is never worse than $2Pe$. Even in the case of $k=1$, the *nearest neighbour rule*, the performance of the technique is quite remarkable. Bear in mind, however, that $Pe(k)$ is the asymptotic value of the overall error rate when the number of available points grows towards infinity. A training set estimate of $Pe(k)$ can have a significant bias relative to this asymptotic value. This issue is discussed in detail in Fukunaga and Hummels (1987) where the effects of dimensionality and metric are presented. An important conclusion of this study is that the bias tends to decay rather slowly with n, approximately as a/n^2, particularly for high dimensions. Therefore, the number of patterns required to lower the bias significantly may be quite prohibitive, especially for high dimensions.

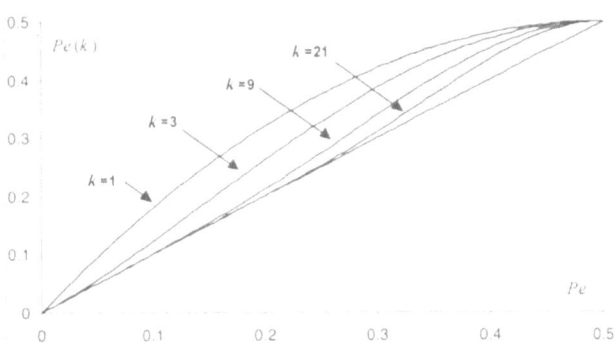

Figure 4.30. Bounds on the asymptotic k-NN error rate, $Pe(k)$, as a function of the Bayes error Pe.

Another difficulty with the k-NN method is which patterns to keep in the training set as "prototypes" for assessing the neighbourhoods. The *edition method* has the goal of reducing the number of training set patterns, therefore the number of distances to be computed, and at the same time improving the discrimination, by discarding unreliable patterns from the training set. The method consists of the following steps:

1. First, each pattern in the training set is classified using k neighbours from the other training set patterns.
2. If the obtained classification is different from the original one, the pattern is discarded from the training set. In this way a new, smaller training set, is obtained.
3. The test patterns are classified using the 1-NN rule and the new training set derived in step 2.

With the edition method, the patterns that are near the boundaries and have unreliable assignments based on the k-NN rule are eliminated. The error probability of this method was shown, by Devijver and Kittler (1980), to decrease asymptotically after each successive edition in a suite of editions.

The *KNN* program allows one to perform k-NN experiments for two-class situations. It was used to perform 50 runs of k-NN classification for the cork stoppers data, with features N and PRT10, using the leave-one-out method (see section 4.5). An average error rate of 9% was obtained, near the value reported previously for the normal classifier and with a similar 95% confidence interval.

Performing edition in half of the samples, the best result was obtained for k=1, with 18% overall error rate. The edition process kept 22 out of 25 patterns from the first class and 23 out of 25 from the second class, in the training set. Using the edition method many important borderline patterns were discarded, which contributed to a degradation of the performance.

In spite of the difficulties posed by the k-NN method it can still be an interesting model-free technique for application in some situations. We will see in chapter five how some ideas of this method are incorporated in certain neural network approaches.

4.3.3 The ROC Curve

The concept of a *Receiver Operating Characteristic* curve, popularly named ROC curve, appeared in the fifties as a means of selecting the best voltage threshold discriminating pure noise from signal plus noise, in signal detection applications such as radar. Since the seventies, the concept has been used in the areas of medicine and psychology, namely for diagnostic test assessment purposes.

The ROC curve is an interesting analysis tool in two-class problems, especially in situations where one wants to detect rarely occurring events such as a signal, a disease, etc. Let us call the absence of the event the *normal* situation (N) and the occurrence of the rare event the *abnormal* situation (A). Figure 4.31 shows the classification matrix for this situation, with true classes along the rows and decided (predicted) classifications along the columns.

Figure 4.31. The canonical classification matrix for two-class discrimination of an abnormal event (A) from the normal event (N).

From the classification matrix of Figure 4.31, the following parameters are defined:

- True Positive Ratio $\equiv$ TPR = $a/(a+b)$. Also known as *sensitivity*, this parameter tells us how sensitive our decision method is in the detection of the abnormal event. A classification method with high sensitivity will rarely miss the abnormal event when it occurs.

- True Negative Ratio $\equiv$ TNR $= d/(c+d)$. Also known as *specificity*, this parameter tells us how specific our decision method is in the detection of the abnormal event. A classification method with a high specificity will have a very low rate of false alarms, caused by classifying a normal event as abnormal.
- False Positive Ratio $\equiv$ FPR $= c/(c+d) = 1$ - specificity.
- False Negative Ratio $\equiv$ FNR $= b/(a+b) = 1$ - sensitivity.

Both the sensitivity and specificity are usually given in percentages. A decision method is considered good if it simultaneously has a high sensitivity (rarely misses the abnormal event when it occurs) and a high specificity (has a low false alarm rate).

The ROC curve depicts the sensitivity versus the FPR (complement of the specificity). Let us illustrate the application of the ROC curve using the *Signal Noise* dataset (see Appendix A). This set presents 100 signal+noise samples $s(n)$ consisting of random noise plus signal impulses with random amplitude, occurring at random times according to the Poisson law. The signal+noise is shown in Figure 4.32.

The signal+noise amplitude is often greater than the average noise amplitude, therefore revealing the presence of the signal impulses (e.g. at time instants 53 and 85). Imagine that we decide to discriminate between signal and noise simply by using an amplitude threshold, Δ, such that we decide "impulse" (our abnormal event) if $s(n) > \Delta$, and "noise" (the normal event) otherwise. For a given threshold value one can establish the signal vs. noise classification matrix and compute the sensitivity and specificity values. By varying the threshold (easily done in the *Signal Noise.xls* file), the corresponding sensitivity and specificity values can then be obtained, as shown Table 4.3.

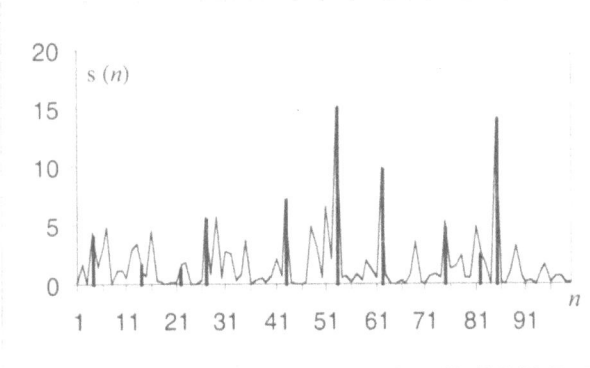

Figure 4.32. One hundred samples of a signal consisting of noise plus signal impulses (bold lines) occurring at random times.

Table 4.3. Sensitivity and specificity in impulse detection (100 signal values).

Threshold	Sensitivity	Specificity
1	0.90	0.66
2	0.80	0.80
3	0.70	0.87
4	0.70	0.93

As shown in Table 4.3, there is a compromise to be made between sensitivity and specificity. This compromise is made more patent in the ROC curve, which was obtained with the *SPSS*, and corresponds to eight different threshold values, as shown in Figure 4.33a. Notice that given the limited number of values the ROC curve has a stepwise aspect, with different values of the FPR corresponding to the same sensitivity, as also appearing in Table 4.3 for the specificity value of 0.7. With a large number of signal samples and threshold values one would obtain a smooth ROC curve, as represented in Figure 4.33b.

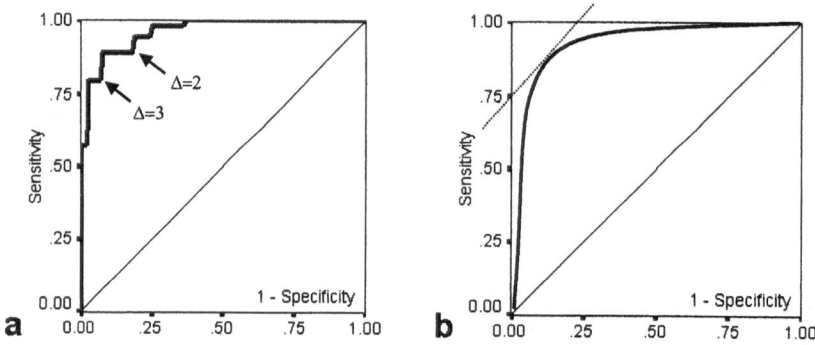

Figure 4.33. ROC curve (bold line) for the *Signal Noise* data: (a) Eight threshold values (the values for Δ=2 and Δ=3 are indicated); b) A large number of threshold values (expected curve) with the 45° slope point.

The following characteristic aspects of the ROC curve are clearly visible:

– The ROC curve graphically depicts the compromise between sensitivity and specificity. If the sensitivity increases, the specificity decreases, and vice-versa.
– All ROC curves start at (0,0) and end at (1,1) (see Exercise 4.16).
– A perfectly discriminating method corresponds to the point (0,1). The ROC curve is then a horizontal line at a sensitivity =1.

A non-informative ROC curve corresponds to the diagonal line of Figure 4.33, with sensitivity = 1 - specificity. In this case, the true detection rate of the abnormal situation is the same as the false detection rate. The best compromise decision of sensitivity=specificity=0.5 is then as good as flipping a coin.

One of the uses of the ROC curve is related to the issue of choosing the best decision threshold that discriminates both situations, in the case of the example, the presence of the impulses from the presence of the noise alone. Let us address this discriminating issue as a cost decision issue as we have done in section 4.2.1. Representing the sensitivity and specificity of the method for a threshold Δ by $s(\Delta)$ and $f(\Delta)$ respectively, and using the same notation as in (4-17), we can write the total risk as:

$$R = \lambda_{aa}P(A)s(\Delta) + \lambda_{an}P(A)(1 - s(\Delta))$$
$$+ \lambda_{na}P(N)f(\Delta) + \lambda_{nn}P(N)(1 - f(\Delta)),$$
(4-41)

or,

$$R = s(\Delta)\left(\lambda_{aa}P(A) - \lambda_{an}P(A)\right) + f(\Delta)\left(\lambda_{na}P(N) - \lambda_{nn}P(N)\right) + \text{constant}.$$
(4-41a)

In order to obtain the best threshold we minimize the risk R by differentiating and equalling to zero, obtaining then:

$$\frac{ds(\Delta)}{df(\Delta)} = \frac{(\lambda_{nn} - \lambda_{na})P(N)}{(\lambda_{aa} - \lambda_{an})P(A)}.$$
(4-42)

The point of the ROC curve where the slope has the value given by formula (4-42) represents the optimum operating point or, in other words, corresponds to the best threshold for the two-class problem. Notice that this is a model-free technique of choosing a feature threshold for discriminating two classes, with no assumptions concerning the specific distributions of the patterns.

Let us now assume that, in a given situation, we assign zero cost to correct decisions, and a cost that is inversely proportional to the prevalences to a wrong decision. Then the slope of the optimum operating point is at 45°, as shown in Figure 4.33b. For the impulse detection example the best threshold would be somewhere between 2 and 3.

Another application of the ROC curve is in the comparison of classification methods. Let us consider the *FHR Apgar* dataset, containing several parameters computed from foetal heart rate (FHR) tracings obtained previous to birth, as well as the so-called Apgar index. This is a ranking index, measured on a one-to-ten scale, and evaluated by obstetricians taking into account several clinical observations of a newborn baby. Imagine that two FHR parameters are measured, ABLTV and ABSTV (percentage of abnormal long term and short term variability, respectively), and one wants to elucidate which of these parameters is better in clinical practice for discriminating an Apgar > 6 (normal situation) from an Apgar ≤ 6 (abnormal or suspect situation).

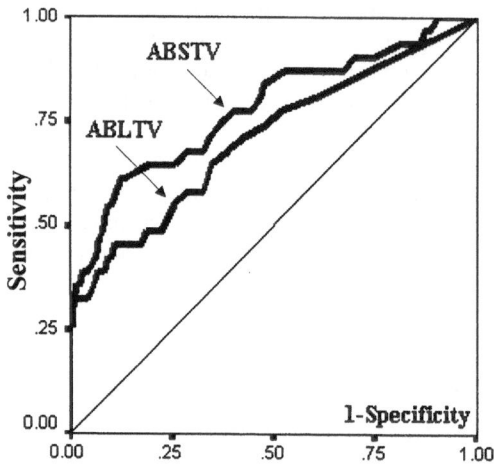

Figure 4.34. ROC curves for the *FHR Apgar* dataset, corresponding to features ABLTV and ABSTV.

We have already seen in 4.2.1 how prevalences influence classification decisions. As illustrated in Figure 4.13, for a two-class situation, the decision threshold is displaced towards the class with the smaller prevalence. Consider that the test with any of the FHR parameters is applied to a population where the prevalence of the abnormal situation is low. Then, for the mentioned reason, the decision maker should operate in the lower left part of the ROC curve in order to keep FPR as small as possible, otherwise, given the high prevalence of the normal situation, a high rate of false alarms would be obtained. Conversely, if the test is applied to a population with a high prevalence of the abnormal situation, the decision maker should adjust the decision threshold to operate on the FPR high part of the curve.

Briefly, in order for our classification method to perform optimally for a large range of prevalence situations, we would like to have an ROC curve very near the perfect test curve, i.e., with an underlying area of 1. It seems, therefore, reasonable to select from among the candidate classification methods the one that has an ROC curve with the highest underlying area, which, for the FHR-Apgar example, would amount to selecting the ABSTV parameter as the best diagnostic method.

The area under the ROC curve represents the probability of correctly answering the two-alternative-forced-choice problem, where an observer, when confronted with two objects, one randomly chosen from the normal class and the other randomly chosen from the abnormal class, must decide which one belongs to the abnormal class. For a perfect classification method, this area is one (the observer always gives the correct answer). For a non-informative classification method, the area is 0.5. The higher the area, the better the method is.

The area under the ROC curve is computed by the *SPSS* with a 95% confidence interval. For the FHR-Apgar data these areas are 0.709 ± 0.11 and 0.781± 0.10 for ABLTV and ABSTV, respectively.

Despite some shortcomings, the ROC curve area method is a popular method of assessing classifier performance. This and an alternative method based on information theory are described in Metz *et al.* (1973).

4.4 Feature Selection

As already seen in sections 2.7 and 4.2.3, great care must be exercised in reducing the number of features used by a classifier, in order to maintain a high dimensionality ratio and therefore reproducible performance, with error estimates sufficiently near the theoretical value. For this purpose, several feature assessment techniques were already explained in chapter 2 with the aim of discarding features that are clearly non-useful at an initial stage of the PR project.

The feature assessment task, while assuring that an information-carrying feature set is indeed used in a PR project, does not guarantee that a given classifier needs the whole set. Consider, for instance, that we are presented with a set of two-dimensional patterns described by feature vectors consisting of 4 features, x_1, x_2, x_3 and x_4, with x_3 and x_4 being the eigenvectors of the covariance matrix of x_1 and x_2. Assuming that the true dimension of the patterns is not known, statistical tests find that all features contribute to pattern discrimination. However, this discrimination could be performed equally well using the alternative sets $\{x_1, x_2\}$ or $\{x_3, x_4\}$. Briefly, discarding features with no aptitude for pattern discrimination is no guarantee against redundant features, and it is, therefore, good practice to attempt some sort of feature selection.

There is abundant literature on the topic of feature selection. Important references are included in the bibliography. The most popular methods of feature selection use a search procedure of a feature subset obeying a stipulated merit criterion. Let F_t be the original set of t features and F be any subset whose cardinality $|F|$ is the desired dimensionality d, $|F| = d$. Furthermore, let $J(F)$ represent the merit criterion used in the selection. The problem of feature selection is to find a subset F^* such that:

$$J(F^*) = \max_{F \subseteq F_t, |F|=d} J(F) .$$

(4-43)

A possible choice for $J(F)$ is 1-Pe, with the disadvantage that the feature selection process depends on the chosen type of classifier. More often, a class separability criterion such as the Bhattacharyya distance or the Anova F statistic is used.

As for the search method, there is a broad scope of possibilities. In the following we mention several relevant methods, many of which can be found in available software products.

Optimal methods

1. Exhaustive search
The exhaustive search of all subsets F of F_t will certainly yield an optimum subset. This is rarely done, however, given the computational burden usually implied by such a search.

2. Branch and bound search
The branch and bound algorithm is a well-known method of finding optimal solutions in combinatorial problems with a monotonic criterion. In the present case, it will guarantee the optimal solution if the used criterion $J(F)$ is monotonic (e.g. the Bhattacharyya distance). We will now explain the most important aspects of this powerful search method, whose implementation details can be found in Narendra and Fukunaga (1977).

Let D be a set of discarded features, which at the end of the search will have $m=t-d$ discarded features. We will arbitrarily enumerate these features from 1 to m and represent the search process depending on $J(D)$ as a tree. Figure 4.35 represents this tree for $t=5$ and $d=2$, with values of $J(D)$ for some nodes. Each path in the tree represents a sequence of discarded features. Notice that for building the tree, we only have to enumerate features with higher indices at each node, since the order of the discarded features is of no importance. Furthermore, given the monotonicity of the class separability criterion, it can only decrease when going downwards in the tree (increasing the number of discarded features).

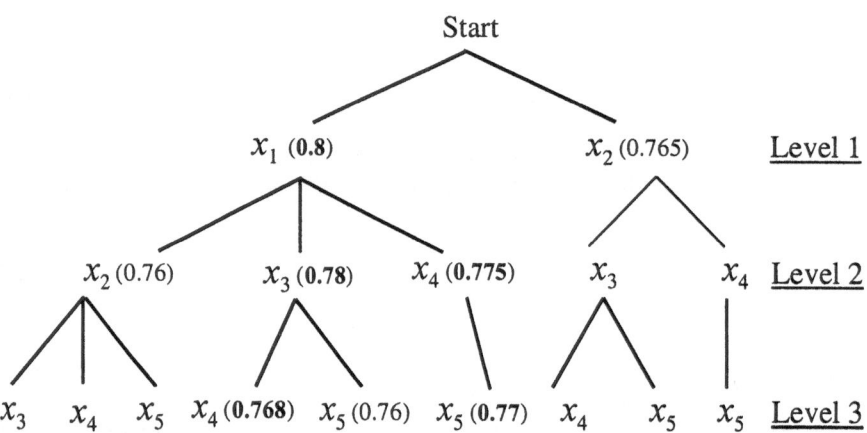

Figure 4.35. Branch-and-bound tree for $t=5$ and $d=2$. Followed optimal paths have the criterion values in bold.

Imagine that at the start of the search process (level 1 of the tree) we measure $J(x_1)$ and $J(x_2)$, corresponding to discarding features x_1 and x_2, respectively, and obtain the values shown in Figure 4.35. We then proceed on the path below x_1 (larger J), and continue in the same way until level 3, resulting in the solution of discarding $D=\{x_1, x_3, x_4\}$, with $J(D)=0.768$. At this time we have a lower bound for our search process, $B=0.768$, therefore we can immediately eliminate the sub-trees starting at $\{x_2\}$ and at $\{x_1, x_2\}$, from our search process, since $J(\{x_2\})<B$ and $J(\{x_1, x_2\})<B$. We still have to consider the sub-tree starting at $\{x_1, x_4\}$. We therefore *backtrack* to this node and find a better solution, where $D=\{x_1, x_4, x_5\}$ is discarded, and we end up with $F=\{x_2, x_3\}$.

The process described here for $t=5$ and $d=2$ has an obvious generalization for any value of t and d. As can be appreciated, this search algorithm avoids the computational burden of the exhaustive search by neglecting sub-trees that are not of interest, those that do not satisfy a bound criterion.

Sub-optimal methods

1. Genetic algorithm search
This is a stochastic search in the feature space guided by the idea of inheriting, at each search step, good properties of parent subsets found in previous steps. This search method can be combined with the probabilistic neural networks described in section 4.3.1. We will describe this search method in section 5.8.

2. Sequential search (direct)
The direct sequential search corresponds to following just one path of the complete search tree.
    In a *backward search* the process starts with the whole feature set and, at each step, the feature that contributes the least to class discrimination is removed. The process goes on until the merit criterion for any candidate feature is above a specified threshold. Backward search is therefore similar to following just one path of the branch-and-bound tree (ending up with solution $\{x_2, x_5\}$ in Figure 4.35).
    In a *forward search* one starts with the feature of most merit and, at each step, all the features not yet included in the subset are revised; the one that contributes the most to class discrimination is evaluated through the merit criterion. This feature is then included in the subset and the procedure advances to the next search step. The process goes on until the merit criterion for any candidate feature is below a specified threshold.
    Direct sequential search is therefore faster than the branch-and-bound algorithm, but can miss "nested" feature subsets (like $\{x_4, x_5\}$ in Figure 4.35).

3. Sequential search (dynamic)
The problem of "nested" feature subsets is tackled in a dynamic search by performing a combination of forward and backward searches at each level. Also known as "plus *l*-take away *r*" selection, it represents a compromise in terms of computational effort between the branch and bound method and the direct sequential search. A version of the "plus *l*-take away *r*" selection known as

sequential forward floating search uses *l* and *r* determined automatically and updated dynamically. It was found to perform almost as well as the branch and bound method with much less computational effort (see Jain and Zongker, 1997).

```
Stepwise Analysis - Step 0

Number of variables in the model: 0
Wilks' Lambda: 1.000000

Stepwise Analysis - Step 1

Number of variables in the model: 1
Last variable entered:     ART   F (  1,   99) = 136.5565   p < .0000
Wilks' Lambda: .4178098   approx. F (  1,   98) = 136.5565   p < .0000

Stepwise Analysis - Step 2

Number of variables in the model: 2
Last variable entered:     PRM   F (  1,   98) = 3.880044   p < .0517
Wilks' Lambda: .4017400   approx. F (  2,   97) = 72.22485   p < .0000

Stepwise Analysis - Step 3

Number of variables in the model: 3
Last variable entered:     NG    F (  1,   97) = 2.561449   p < .1128
Wilks' Lambda: .3912994   approx. F (  3,   96) = 49.77880   p < .0000

Stepwise Analysis - Step 4

Number of variables in the model: 4
Last variable entered:     RAAR  F (  1,   96) = 1.619636   p < .2062
Wilks' Lambda: .3847401   approx. F (  4,   95) = 37.97999   p < .0000

Stepwise Analysis - Step 4 (Final Step)

Number of variables in the model: 4
Last variable entered:     RAAR  F (  1,   95) = .3201987   p < .5728
```

Figure 4.36. Feature selection using a forward search for two classes of the cork stoppers data.

Direct sequential search methods can be applied using *Statistica* and *SPSS*, the latter affording a dynamic search procedure that is in fact a "plus 1-take away 1" selection. As merit criterion, *Statistica* uses the Anova F (for all selected features at a given step) with default value of one. *SPSS* allows the use of other merit criteria such as the squared Bhattacharyya distance.

It is also common to set a lower limit to the so-called *tolerance level*, $T = 1 - R^2$, which must be satisfied by all features, where R is the multiple correlation factor of one candidate feature with all the others. Highly correlated features, which could raise problems in the computation of the inverse covariance matrix, are therefore removed. One must be quite conservative, however, in the specification of the tolerance. A value at least as low as 1% is standard practice.

Figure 4.36 shows the summary of a forward search for the first two classes of the cork stoppers data obtained with *Statistica*, using default values for the tolerance (0.01) and F (1.0). The *Wilks' lambda* indicated in Figure 4.36 is equal to the determinant of the pooled covariance divided by the determinant of the total covariance. Physically, it can be interpreted as the ratio between the average class volume and the total volume of the cluster constituted by all the patterns. Therefore, it reflects the class separability. The F statistic is computed from the Wilks' lambda.

The four-feature solution shown in Figure 4.36 corresponds to the classification matrix shown before in Figure 4.24b.

Using a backward search, the solution presented previously with only two features (N and PRT) was obtained (see Figure 4.8). Notice that the backward search usually needs to start with a very low tolerance value (in the present case T=0.002 is sufficient).

It was already shown that this classifier solution uses a pooled covariance not too far from the individual covariance matrices. Also, the dimensionality ratio is comfortably high: $n/d=25$. One can therefore be confident that this classifier performs in a nearly optimal way.

	Entered	Removed	Min. D Squared		Exact F			
			Statistic	Between Groups	Statistic	df1	df2	Sig.
Step								
1	PRT		2.401	1.00and 2.00	60.015	1	147.000	1.176E-12
2	PRM		3.083	1.00and 2.00	38.279	2	146.000	4.330E-14
3	N		4.944	1.00and 2.00	40.638	3	145.000	.000
4	ARTG		5.267	1.00and 2.00	32.248	4	144.000	7.438E-15
5		PRT	5.098	1.00and 2.00	41.903	3	145.000	.000
6	RAAR		6.473	1.00and 2.00	39.629	4	144.000	2.316E-22

Figure 4.37. Feature selection using a dynamic search on the cork stoppers data (three classes).

Figure 4.37 shows the listing produced by *SPSS* in a dynamic search performed on the cork stoppers data (three classes), using the squared Bhattacharyya distance of the two closest classes as a merit criterion. Furthermore, features were only entered or removed from the selected set if they contributed significantly to the Anova F. The solution corresponding to Figure 4.37 used a 5% level for the statistical significance of a candidate feature to enter the selected set and 10% to remove it. Notice that PRT, which had entered at step 1, was later removed, at step 5. The nested solution {PRM, N, ARTG, RAAR} would not have been found by a direct forward search.

4.5 Classifier Evaluation

The determination of reliable estimates of a classifier error rate is obviously an essential task in order to assess its usefulness and to compare it with alternative solutions.

As explained in section 4.2.3 design set estimates are on average optimistic and the same can be said about using an error formula such as (4-25), when true means and covariance are replaced by their sample estimates. It is, therefore, mandatory that the classifier be empirically tested, using a test set of independent cases. As mentioned already in section 4.2.3, these test set estimates are on average pessimistic.

We describe in the following the influence of the finite sample sizes of the design and test sets on the classifier performance. For this purpose, we consider a two-class classifier with Bayes error:

$$Pe = P_1 Pe_1 - P_2 Pe_2 . \tag{4-44}$$

The influence of the finite sample sizes can be summarized as follows (for details, consult Fukunaga, 1990).

Influence of finite test set

Let $Pe_t(n)$ be the test set estimate, influenced only by the finiteness of the test set, and consider the ensemble average of all such estimates, $E[Pe_t(n)]$, of a given classifier with Bayes error Pe. The expectation $E[Pe_t(n)]$ can be computed with arbitrarily large accuracy for a growing number of these estimates, with independent sets of size n. The following results for the expectation and variance are verified:

$$E[Pe_t(n)] = Pe \; ; \tag{4-45a}$$

$$v[Pe_t(n)] = P_1^2 \frac{Pe_1(1 - Pe_1)}{n_1} + P_2^2 \frac{Pe_2(1 - Pe_2)}{n_2} . \tag{4-45b}$$

Therefore, test set estimates are unbiased, but have a variance inversely proportional to the number of test samples (n_1 for ω_1 and n_2 for ω_2).

Influence of finite design set

The estimate of the design set error will depend on the particular sample distributions in both classes. For normal distributions, the design set error is influenced by the deviation of the sample means and covariances, computed with n design samples, from the true values, resulting in:

$$E[Pe_d(n)] \cong Pe + \frac{\upsilon}{n} \; ; \tag{4-46a}$$

$$v[Pe_d(n)] \cong 0 \; . \tag{4-46b}$$

Therefore, the variance is zero, but there is a bias υ/n, where υ is constant for the same classifier and n is the number of design samples used. For the linear normal classifier the bias is approximately proportional to d/n. For the quadratic normal classifier the bias is approximately proportional to d^2/n, therefore it grows quite fast with d. This makes the quadratic classifier more sensitive to parameter estimation errors than the linear one.

When influences from both the finite design set and the finite test set are taken into account, it is verified that the bias is only influenced by the design set as stated in (4-46a), and the variance is given by:

$$v[Pe(n)] = P_1^2 \frac{Pe_1(n)(1 - Pe_1(n))}{n_1} + P_2^2 \frac{Pe_2(n)(1 - Pe_2(n))}{n_2} + v[Pe_d(n)]. \tag{4-47}$$

The last term on the right hand side is nearly zero for the linear classifier. The variance is thus dominated by the first two terms. These are influenced by the bias of the design set. However, this influence is minimal and can be neglected. Briefly:

- The bias is predominantly influenced by the finiteness of the design set;
- The variance is predominantly influenced by the finiteness of the test set.

In normal practice we only have a pattern set X with n samples available. The problem arises of how to divide the available patterns into design set and test set. The following alternatives are possible:

Resubstitution method

The whole set X is used for design, and also for testing the classifier. As a consequence of the non-independence of design and test sets, the method yields, on average, an optimistic estimate of the error, corresponding to the estimate $E[\hat{Pe}_d(n)]$ mentioned in section 4.2.4. For the two-class linear discriminant with normal distributions, an example of such an estimate for various values of n is plotted in Figure 4.26 (lower curve).

Holdout method

The available n samples of X are randomly divided into two disjointed sets (traditionally with 50% of the samples each), X_d and X_t used for design and test, respectively. The error estimate is obtained from the test set, and therefore suffers from the bias and variance effects previously described. By taking the average over many partitions of the same size, a reliable estimate of the design set error with the bias of (4-46a) can be obtained, which is an upper bound of the Bayes error and corresponds to the estimate $E[\hat{Pe}_t(n)]$, mentioned to in section 4.2.4. For the two-class linear discriminant with normal distributions, an example of such an estimate for various values of n is plotted in Figure 4.26 (upper curve).

Partition methods

Partition methods divide the available set X into a certain number of subsets, which rotate in their use of design and test, as follows:

1. Divide X into $k>1$ subsets of randomly chosen patterns, with each subset having n/k patterns.
2. Design the classifier using the patterns of $k-1$ subsets and test it on the remaining one. A test set estimate Pe_{ti} is thereby obtained.
3. Repeat the previous step rotating the position of the test set, obtaining thereby k estimates Pe_{ti}.
4. Compute the average test set estimate $Pe_t = \sum_{i=1}^{k} Pe_{ti} / k$ and the variance of the Pe_{ti}.

For $k=2$, the method is similar to the traditional holdout method. For $k=n$, the method is called the *leave-one-out method*, with the classifier designed with $n-1$ samples and tested on the one remaining sample. Since only one sample is being used for testing, the variance of the error estimate is large. However, the samples are being used independently for design in the best possible way, therefore the average test set error estimate will be a good estimate of the classifier error for sufficiently high n, since the bias contributed by the finiteness of the design set will be low. For other values of k there is a compromise between the high bias-low variance of the holdout method, and the low bias-high variance of the leave-one-out method, with less computational effort.

Bootstrap method

Bootstrap methods are based on the generation of artificial samples (bootstrap samples) by randomly drawing the existing samples with uniform distribution within each class. The error estimate is computed in the original set with the classifier designed using large sets of the bootstrap samples. It can be shown that the expected value of this error estimate is similar to the one obtained with the leave-one-out method, with a variance similar to the one obtained with the resubstitution method. The bootstrap method combines, therefore, the best qualities of both methods.

Statistical software products such as *SPSS* and *Statistica* allow the selection of the cases used for training and for testing linear discriminant classifiers. With *SPSS* it is possible to use a selection variable, easing the task of specifying randomly selected samples. With *Statistica*, one can initially select the cases used for training (*Select* option in the toolbar *Options* menu), and once the classifier is designed, specify test cases (*Select Cases* button in the results form).

For the two-class cork stoppers classifier, with two features, presented in section 4.1.3 (classification matrix shown in Figure 4.9), using a partition method with $k=3$, a test set estimate of $Pe_t= 9.9$ % was obtained, which is near the training set error estimate of 10%. The leave-one-out method also produces $Pe_t = 10$ %. The closeness of these figures is an indication of reliable error estimation.

It is also possible to assess whether there is a significant difference between test set and design set estimates of the class errors by using a standard statistical test based on 2x2 contingency tables.

For this purpose let us denote:

n_d: number of design patterns;
n_t: number of test patterns;
k_d: number of wrongly classified patterns in the design set;
k_t: number of wrongly classified patterns in the test set.

Let us now compute the following quantity:

$$a = \frac{\left| (n_t + n_d)(n_t k_d - n_d k_t) \right|}{n_t n_d (k_d + k_t)(n_t + n_d - k_d - k_t)} . \tag{4-48}$$

Then, provided that n_d, n_t, $n_d - k_d$, $n_t - k_t$ are all greater than 5, the quantity a has a chi-square distribution with one degree of freedom. The test must be applied to the classes individually, unless the same number of patterns and error rates occur. Let us see how this works for the cork stoppers classification with errors estimated by the previous partition method, with n_d=67 patterns for design and n_t=33 patterns for testing. For class ω_2, in one run of the partition method k_d=6 patterns of the design set were misclassified and, k_t=3 patterns of the test set were misclassified. The value of a=0.00017 is therefore obtained, which, looking at the chi-square tables, indicates a non-significant difference at a 95% confidence level.

When presenting error estimates, it is convenient to also present the respective confidence intervals. For the two-class cork stoppers classifier, a 95 % confidence interval of [4%, 16%] is obtained using formula (4-30). As already discussed in section 4.2.4, this formula usually yields intervals that are too large. More realistic intervals can be obtained using the variance of the Pe_{ti} computed by a partition method for a reasonable number of partitions (say, above 5).

4.6 Tree Classifiers

4.6.1 Decision Trees and Tables

In multi-class classification tasks one is often confronted with the problem that reasonable performances can only be achieved through the use of a large number of features. This requires a very large design set for proper training, probably much larger than what we have available. Also, the feature subset that is the most discriminating set for some classes can perform rather poorly for other classes. As an attempt to overcome these difficulties, a "divide and conquer" principle through the use of multistage classification has been proposed, the so-called *decision tree* classifiers, also known as *hierarchical classifiers*, where an unknown pattern is classified into a class using decision functions in successive stages.

At each stage of the tree classifier a simpler problem with a smaller number of features is solved. This has an additional benefit: in practical multi-class problems it is rather difficult to guarantee normal or even symmetric distributions with similar covariance matrices for all the classes, but it may be possible that by using a multistage approach these conditions are approximately met, affording optimal classifiers at each stage.

Figure 4.38 shows an example of a simple decision tree with two levels of classification, l_1 and l_2. At the first level, l_1, a set of four classes $\Omega=\{\omega_1, \omega_2, \omega_3, \omega_4\}$ is available for classification. However, instead of allowing the assignment of pattern $\mathbf{x}$ to any of the four classes, we limit the assignment to a dichotomic partition of Ω, denoted as $\Omega(l_1)=\{\omega_3, \Omega(l_2)\}$. At level l_2, the classifier then has to decide which class of $\Omega(l_2)$ the unknown pattern $\mathbf{x}$ belongs to, with $\Omega(l_2)=\{\omega_1, \omega_2, \omega_4\}$.

Let us study the tree classification performance following the work of Kulkarni (1978), assuming for simplicity that the features used along a path of the tree, in order to reach a certain node, have independent distributions. The *pdf* relative to a class ω_k can then be expressed as:

$$p(\mathbf{x} \mid \omega_k) = \prod_{j=1}^{l} p(\mathbf{x}_j \mid \omega_k), \qquad (4\text{-}49)$$

where $\mathbf{x}_j$ are the subvectors corresponding to the l independent feature subsets used to classify ω_k, along a certain tree path.

Denoting the probability of a correct classification of ω_k by $Pc(\omega_k)$, with the assumption that the feature subsets used in the classification are independent, one has, in the same way:

$$P_c(\omega_k) = \prod_{l_i \in T(\omega_k)} P_c(\omega_k \mid l_i), \qquad (4\text{-}50)$$

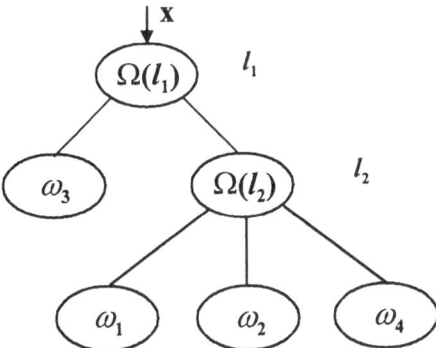

Figure 4.38. Example of a decision tree classifier for four classes and two levels of decision.

where $Pc(\omega_k \mid l_i)$ are the probabilities of a correct decision at each traversed node l_i in the path leading to ω_k, denoted $T(\omega_k)$. Averaging these $Pc(\omega_k)$ with the prevalences, one obtains the correct recognition rate of the tree:

$$P_c(T) = \sum_{k=1}^{c} P(\omega_k) \prod_{l_i \in T(\omega_k)} P_c(\omega_k \mid l_i) . \tag{4-51}$$

At the same time, the correct recognition rate at a node l_i, averaged across all the classes that can be reached from it, is written as:

$$P_c(l_i) = \frac{\sum\limits_{k \in \omega(l_i)} P(\omega_k) P_c(\omega_k \mid l_i)}{\sum\limits_{k \in \omega(l_i)} P(\omega_k)} . \tag{4-52}$$

This last formula shows that the node performance is a linear function of the class recognition rates, whereas the total performance expressed by (4-51) is a nonlinear function. Therefore, contrary to common sense, optimizing the tree performance at each level does not guarantee that the overall tree performance is also optimal. The determination of the optimal structure of the tree is an additional complication. We see, therefore, that designing an optimal tree is not an easy task, and would require, in general, a prohibitively exhaustive search in the space of all structures and feature combinations. Search techniques such as dynamic programming and branch-and-bound methods have been used for this purpose. Descriptions of these methods can be found in the bibliography.

Keeping in mind that optimizing node performance is no guarantee of optimal tree performance it must be said, that in practical applications one usually follows this "manual" method of tree design, selecting the best solutions of tree structure and node classification based on the separability properties of the features. Notice from (4-50) that in order to obtain a class classification performance that is better than the one obtained by a non-hierarchical approach, one must have very high performances at each node. For instance, if for the tree in Figure 4.38, both $Pc(\Omega(l_2)|\ l_1)$ and $Pc(\omega_2|\ l_2)$ have a value of 0.94, then $Pc(\omega_2) = 0.94^2 = 0.88$. With a larger tree if this 0.94 correct classification rate is iterated 4 times one obtains an error of 22%! The error can therefore degrade drastically along a tree path.

Let us now illustrate a practical tree classifier design using the *Breast Tissue* dataset (electric impedance measurements of freshly excized breast tissue) with 6 classes denoted *car* (carcinoma), *fad* (fibro-adenoma), *gla* (glandular), *mas* (mastopathy), *con* (connective) and *adi* (adipose). Some features of this dataset can be well modeled by a normal distribution in some classes, namely I0, AREA_DA and IPMAX. Performing a Kruskal-Wallis analysis, it is readily seen that all the features have discriminative capabilities and that it is practically impossible to discriminate between classes *gla, fad* and *mas*. The low dimensionality ratio of this dataset for the individual classes (e.g. only 14 cases for class *con*) strongly suggests a decision tree approach, with the use of merged classes and a greatly reduced number of features at each node.

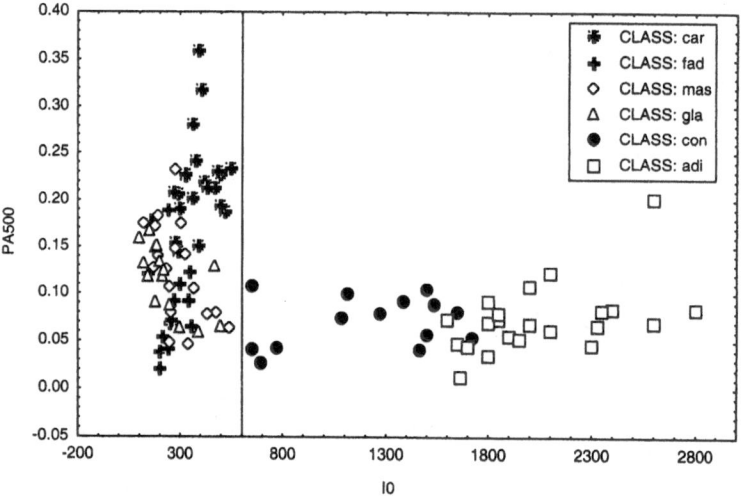

Figure 4.39. Scatter plot of six classes of breast tissue using features I0 and PA500.

As I0 and PA500 are promising features, it is worthwhile to look at the respective scatter diagram shown in Figure 4.39. Two clusters are visually identified: one corresponding to {*con, adi*}, the other to {*mas, gla, fad, car*}.

Factor analysis also reveals the existence of a factor strongly correlated with PA500, the other correlated with I0. Briefly, the data structure and the results of the feature assessment phase strongly suggest using a first stage that separates the mentioned clusters. The best results for this discrimination use I0 alone with a threshold of I0=600, achieving zero errors.

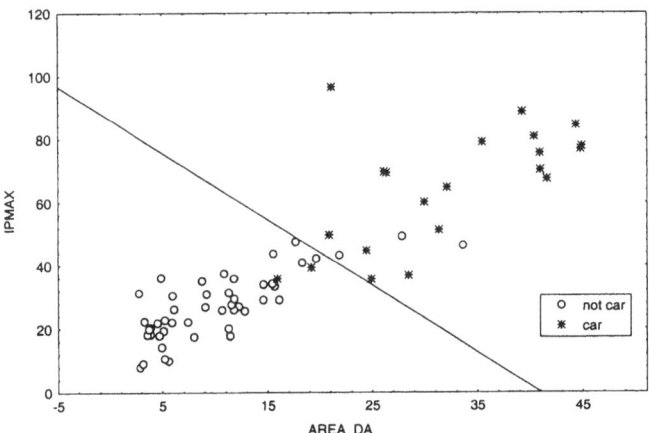

Figure 4.40. Scatter plot of breast tissue classes *car* and {*mas, gla, fad*} (denoted *not car*) using features AREA_DA and IPMAX, showing the linear discriminant separating the two classes.

At stage two we attempt the most useful discrimination from the medical point of view: class *car* (carcinoma) vs. {*fad, mas, gla*}. Using discriminant analysis this can be performed with an overall training set error of about 8%, using features AREA_DA and IPMAX.

Figure 4.40 shows the corresponding linear discriminant. Performing two randomized runs using the partition method in halves (half of the samples for design and the other half for testing), an average test set error of 8.6% was obtained, quite near the design set error. At level 2 the discrimination *con* vs. *adi* can also be performed with feature I0 (threshold I0=1550), with zero errors for *adi* and 14% errors for *con*.

With these results we can establish the decision tree shown in Figure 4.41. At each level of the decision tree a decision function is used, shown in Figure 4.41 as a *decision rule* to be satisfied. The left descendent tree branch corresponds to compliance with a rule, i.e., to a "Yes" answer; the right descendent tree branch corresponds to a "No" answer.

Since a small number of features is used at each level, one for the first level and two for the second level, respectively, we maintain a reasonably high dimensionality ratio at both levels, and therefore we obtain reliable estimates of the errors with narrow 95% confidence intervals (less than 2% for the first level and about ±3% for the *car* vs. {*fad, mas, gla*} level).

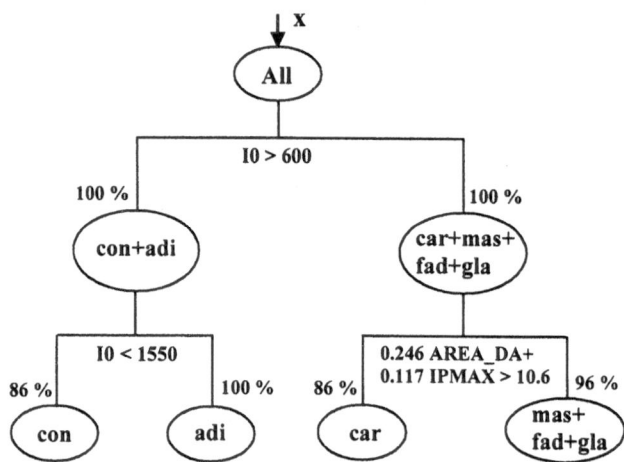

Figure 4.41. Hierarchical tree classifier for the breast tissue data with percentages of correct classifications and decision functions used at each node. Left branch = "Yes"; right branch = "No".

DISCR.	Rows: Observed classific.			
ANAL.	Columns: Predicted classific.			
Group	% Corr.	car p=.198	con p=.132	adi p=.208	fad+ p=.462
car	52.4	11	0	0	10
con	64.3	0	9	2	3
adi	95.5	0	1	21	0
fad+	98.0	1	0	0	48
Total	84.0	12	10	23	61

Figure 4.42. Classification matrix of four classes of breast tissue using three features and linear discriminants. Class *fad+* is actually the class set {*fad, mas, gla*}.

For comparison purposes the same 4 classes discrimination was carried out with only one linear classifier using the same three features I0, AREA_DA and IPMAX as in the hierarchical approach. Figure 4.42 shows the classification matrix. Given that the distributions are roughly symmetric although with some deviations in the covariance matrices, the optimal error achieved with linear discriminants should be close to what is shown in the classification matrix. The degraded performance compared with the decision tree approach is evident.

On the other hand, if our only interest is to discriminate class *car* from all other ones, a linear classifier with only one feature can achieve this discrimination with a performance of about 86% (see Exercise 4.8), a comparable result to the one previously obtained with the tree classififer.

Rules

		1	2	3	4
Conditions	I0 > 600	Y	Y	N	N
	I0 > 1550	N	Y		
	0.246AREA_DA+0.117 IPMAX > 10.6			Y	N
Actions	con	X			
	adi		X		
	car			X	
	mas+gla+fad				X

Figure 4.43. Decision table corresponding to the decision tree shown in Figure 4.41. The "Y", "N" in the rules columns correspond to the "Yes", "No" branches followed in the tree.

A formalism often used to represent decision trees is that of *decision tables*. A decision table has the layout shown in Figure 4.43 for the breast tissue hierarchical classification . The three main sectors of the table are:

– The "conditions" rows, corresponding to the decision functions or to any other type of condition (e.g. categorical conditions such as "colour = red").
– The "actions" rows, corresponding to classifications or to any other type of actions (e.g. "sound alarm" or "go to Exceptions").
– The "rules" columns, corresponding to the path followed in the decision tree.

The formalism of decision tables is especially suitable when designing a PR application that needs to incorporate previous expertise from the area where it will be applied. It provides, then, an easy formalism for the PR designer and the domain expert to interact. A good example is the design of diagnostic systems in the medical field.

Details concerning tree-table conversion, choice of rule sets and equivalence of subtables can be found in (Bell, 1978).

4.6.2 Automatic Generation of Tree Classifiers

The decision tree used for the *Breast Tissue* dataset is an example of a *binary tree*: at each node a dichotomic decision is made. Binary trees are the most popular type of trees, namely when a single feature is used at each node, resulting in linear discriminants that are parallel to the feature axes, and easily interpreted by human experts. They also allow categorical features to be easily incorporated, with node splits based on a yes/no answer to the question of whether or not a given pattern belongs to a set of categories. For instance, this type of trees is frequently used in medical applications, often built as a result of statistical studies of the influence of individual health factors in a given population.

The design of decision trees can be automated in many ways, depending on the *split criterion* used at each node, and the type of search used for best group discrimination. A split criterion has the form:

$$d(\mathbf{x}) \geq \Delta, \tag{4-53}$$

where $d(\mathbf{x})$ is a decision function of the feature vector $\mathbf{x}$ and Δ is a threshold. Usually, linear decision functions are used. In many applications, the split criteria are expressed in terms of the individual features alone (the so-called *univariate splits*).

A key concept regarding split criteria is the concept of *node impurity*. The node impurity is a function of the fraction of patterns belonging to a specific class at that node.

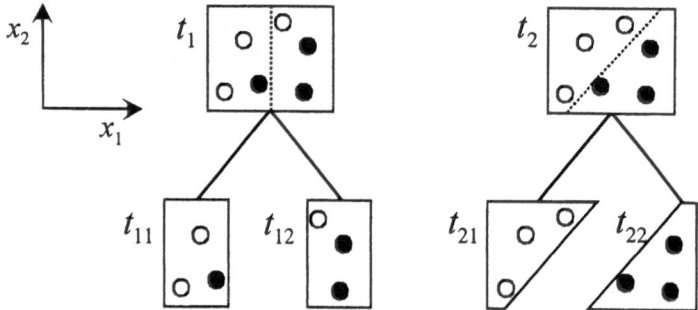

Figure 4.44. Splitting a node with maximum impurity. The left split ($x_1 \geq \Delta$) decreases the impurity, which is still non-zero; the right split ($w_1x_1 + w_2x_2 \geq \Delta$) achieves pure nodes.

Consider the two-class situation shown in Figure 4.44. Initially, we have a node with equal proportions of patterns belonging to the two classes. We say that its impurity is maximal. The right split results in nodes with zero impurity, since they contain patterns from only one of the classes. The left split, on the contrary, increases the proportion of cases from one of the classes, therefore decreasing the impurity, although some impurity is still present.

A convenient way to measure the impurity of a node t in the interval $[0, 1]$ is by using the following function:

$$i(t) = -\sum_{k=1}^{c} P(k \mid t)\log_2 P(k \mid t), \qquad (4\text{-}54)$$

where $P(k \mid t)$ is the proportion of patterns of class k at node t. This is the well-known definition of *entropy*, which measures the "disorder" of the patterns at each node. For the situation shown in Figure 4.44, we have:

$$i(t_1) = i(t_2) = -\frac{1}{2}\log_2\frac{1}{2} - \frac{1}{2}\log_2\frac{1}{2} = 1$$

$$i(t_{11}) = i(t_{12}) = -\frac{2}{3}\log_2\frac{2}{3} - \frac{1}{3}\log_2\frac{1}{3} = 0.918$$

$$i(t_{21}) = i(t_{22}) = -1\log_2 1 - 0\log_2 0 = 0$$

A popular tree-generation algorithm called *ID3* generates a binary tree using the entropy as split criterion. The algorithm starts at the root node, which corresponds to the whole training set, and progresses along the tree by searching for the feature and threshold level combination that achieve the maximum decrease of the impurity/entropy at each node. The generation of splits stops when no significant decrease of the impurity is achieved. It is common practice to use the individual feature values of the training set patterns as candidate threshold values. Often, after generating a tree in an automatic way, some sort of *tree pruning* must be performed in order to remove branches of no interest.

The method of exhaustive search for the best univariate splits is usually called the *CART* method, pioneered by Breiman, Friedman, Olshen, and Stone (see Breiman et al., 1993). Instead of the entropy measure one can use other ways to measure node impurity, for instance methods based on the ANOVA statistic.

Using the *CART* approach with the ANOVA statistic, available in *Statistica*, the following univariate splits were found for the *Breast Tissue* dataset:

– First level node: {*adi, con*} vs. others. Feature I0 was used, with the threshold I0=600.62. This split is achieved with zero misclassified cases.
– Second level, left node: *adi* vs. *con*. Feature PERIM was used, with the threshold PERIM=1563.8. This split is achieved with one misclassified case (2.8%).

- Second level, right node: *car* vs. {*mas*, *gla*, *fad*}. Feature AREA was used, with the threshold AREA=1710.5. This split is achieved with four misclassified cases (5.7%).
- Third level node: *gla* vs. {*mas*, *fad*}. Feature DA was used, with the threshold DA=36.5. This split is achieved with eight misclassified cases (17%).

Notice how the *CART* approach achieves a tree solution with similar structure to the one manually derived and shown in Figure 4.41. The classification performance is somewhat better than previously obtained. Notice the gradual increase of the errors as one progresses through the tree. Node splitting stops when no significant classification is found, in this case when reaching the {*mas*, *fad*}, as expected.

4.7 Statistical Classifiers in Data Mining

A current trend in database technology applied to large organizations (e.g. enterprises, hospitals, credit card companies), involves the concept of *data warehousing*, and sophisticated data search techniques known collectively as *data mining*. A data warehouse is a database system involving large tables whose contents are periodically updated, containing detailed history of the information, supporting advanced data description and summarizing tools as well as metadata facilities, i.e., data about the location and description of the system components (e.g. names, definitions, structures).

Data mining techniques are used to extract relevant information from data warehouses and are applied in many diverse fields, such as:

- Engineering, e.g. equipment failure prediction, web search engines.
- Economy, e.g. prediction of revenue of investment, detection of consumer profiles, assessment of loan risk.
- Biology and medicine, e.g. protein sequencing in genome mapping, assessment of pregnancy risk.

These techniques use pattern recognition approaches such as data clustering, statistical classification and neural networks, as well as artificial intelligence approaches such as knowledge representation, causality models and rule induction.

We will discuss here some issues concerning the application of statistical classifiers to data mining applications. In section 5.14 the application of neural networks is presented. Important aspects to consider in data mining applications of pattern recognition techniques are:

- The need to operate with large databases, in an on-line decision support environment, therefore imposing strict requirements regarding algorithmic performance, namely in terms of speed.

- The ill-posed nature of the data mining problems, usually with many available solutions but no clear means of judging their relative quality This is due to: the curse of dimensionality already mentioned in section 2.6, which is definitely a relevant phenomenon in many data mining applications; the incorrect inferences from correlation to causality; the difficulty in measuring the usefulness of the inferred relations.

The most important statistical classifier approach in data mining is the decision tree approach. As a matter of fact, tree classification can be achieved in a very efficient way, e.g., by using the previously described *CART* approach, and can also provide important semantic information, especially when using univariate splits. The contribution of individual features to the target classification, which is a top requirement in data mining applications, is then easily grasped.

In order to get a taste of the application of tree classification to a typical data mining problem, and to discuss some of the issues that have just been enumerated, we will consider the problem of assessing foetal heart rate (FHR) variability indexes in the diagnostic of a pathological foetal state responsible for a "flat-sinusoidal" (FS) tracing. For this purpose, we will use the *CTG* dataset with 2126 cases (see Appendix A). Four variability indexes are used (MLTV, MSTV, ALTV, ASTV), which measure the average short-term (beat to beat) and average long-term (in 1 minute sliding window) variability of the heart rate, as well as the percentage of time they are abnormal (i.e., below a certain threshold).

Using the *CART* design approach available in *Statistica*, we obtain the decision tree of Figure 4.45, which uses only two variability indexes (percentage of time the short-term and long-term variabilities are abnormal).

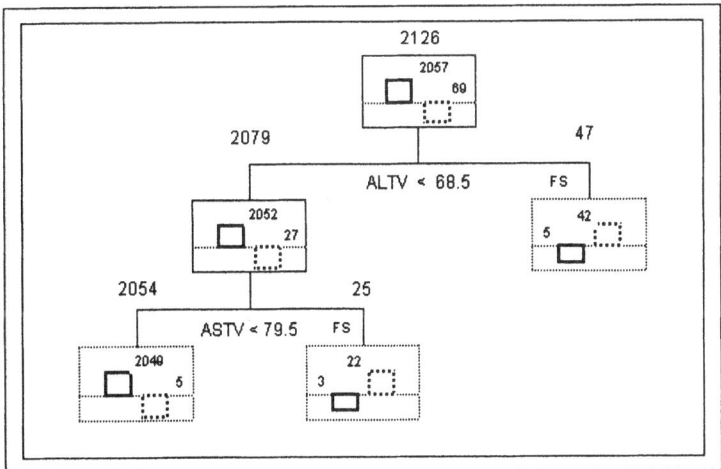

Figure 4.45. Decision tree for the flat-sinusoidal class (FS) in 2126 FHR tracings. FS cases correspond to the dotted rectangles, non-FS to the solid ones.

This decision tree provides useful insight concerning individual contributions to the target classification, especially when accompanied by an easy to read graphical display. In the present case, the clinician is able to appreciate that only two of the four variability features are required to distinguish FS from non-FS situations. Feature ALTV (abnormal long-term variability) is the one that contributes most to this distinction with a low percentage of false positives (5 in 2057). The overall classification error is achieved with remarkably high sensitivity 92.8 % (64/69) and specificity 99.6 % (2049/2057).

The decision tree design and results are obtained very quickly (*Statistica* processing time about 1 second on a 733 MHz Pentium) making this approach adequate for data mining applications.

In a more realistic data mining application in the same medical area, one would want to apply this tool for the determination of the binary tree that best discriminates the three major classes of foetal well-being, normal, suspect and pathologic, based on foetal heart rate features. Again, this can be achieved in an effective and efficient way with the *CART* approach (see Exercise 4.26).

Bibliography

Argentiero P, Chin R, Baudet P (1982) An Automated Approach to the Design of Decision Tree Classifiers. IEEE Tr Patt An Mach Intel, 4:51-57.

Batchelor BG (1974) Practical Approach to Pattern Classification. Plenum Pub. Co., New York.

Bell DA (1978) Decision Trees, Tables and Lattices. In: Batchelor BG (ed) Pattern Recognition. Ideas in Practice. Plenum Press, New York, pp. 119-141.

Breiman L, Friedman JH, Olshen RA, Stone CJ (1993) Classification and Regression Trees. Chapman & Hall / CRC.

Centor RM (1991) Signal Detectability: The Use of ROC Curves and Their Analyses. Medical Decision Making, 11:102-106.

Chang CY (1973) Dynamic Programming as Applied to Feature Subset Selection in a Pattern Recognition System. IEEE Tr Syst Man and Cybern 3:166-171.

Chen CH (1982) Application of Pattern Recognition to Seismic Wave Interpretation. In: Fu KS (ed) Applications of Pattern Recognition, CRC Press Inc., Boca Raton, pp. 107-120.

Cherkassky V, Mulier F (1998) Learning from Data. John Wiley & Sons, Inc.

Chien YT (1978) Interactive Pattern Recognition. Marcel Dekker Inc., New York.

Dattatreya GR, Sarma VV (1981) Bayesian and Decision Tree Approaches for Pattern Recognition Including Feature Measurement Costs. IEEE Tr Patt An Mach Intel 3:293-298.

Devijver PA (1982) Statistical Pattern Recognition. In: Fu KS (ed) Applications of Pattern Recognition, CRC Press Inc., Boca Raton, pp. 15-35.

Devijver PA, Kittler J (1980) On the Edited Nearest Neighbor Rule. Proc. 5th Int. Conf. on Pattern Recognition, 72-80.

Dubuisson B (1990) Diagnostic et Reconaissance des Formes. Éditions Hermes, Paris.

Duda R, Hart P (1973) Pattern classification and scene analysis. Wiley, New York.

Friedman M, Kandel A (1999) Introduction to Pattern Recognition. Imperial College Press, London.

Foley DH (1972) Considerations of sample and feature size. IEEE Tr Info Theory 18:618-626.

Fu KS (1982) Introduction. In: Fu KS (ed) Applications of Pattern Recognition. CRC Press Inc., Boca Raton, pp. 2-13.

Fu KS (1982) Application of Pattern Recognition to Remote Sensing. In: Fu KS (ed) Applications of Pattern Recognition. CRC Press Inc., Boca Raton, pp. 65-106.

Fukunaga K (1969) Calculation of Bayes' Recognition Error for Two Multivariate Gaussian Distributions. IEEE Tr Comp 18:220-229.

Fukunaga K, Hostetler LD (1973) Optimization of K-Nearest Neighbor Density Estimates, IEEE Tr Info Th 19:320-326.

Fukunaga K, Hummels DM (1987) Bias of Nearest Neighbor Error Estimates. IEEE Tr Patt An Mach Intel, 9:103-112.

Fukunaga K, Hayes RR (1989a) Effects of Sample Size in Classifier Design. IEEE Tr Patt Anal Mach Intel 11:873-885.

Fukunaga K, Hayes RR (1989b) Estimation of Classifier Performance. IEEE Tr Patt Anal Mach Intel 11:1087-1101.

Fukunaga K (1990) Introduction to Statistical Pattern Recognition. Academic Press, New York.

Holmström L, Koistinen P, Laaksonen J (1997) Neural and Statistical Classifiers – Taxonomy and Two Case Studies. IEEE Tr Neural Networks, 8:5-17.

Jain AK, Chandrasekaran B (1982) Dimensionality and Sample Size Considerations in Pattern Recognition. In: Krishnaiah PR, Kanal LN (eds) Handbook of Statistics, 2, North Holland Pub. Co., pp. 835-855.

Jain A, Zongker D (1997) Feature Selection: Evaluation, Application and Small Sample Performance. IEEE Tr Patt An Mach Intel 19:153-158.

Jain AK, Duin RPW, Mao J (2000). Statistical Pattern Recognition: A Review. IEEE Tr Patt An Mach Intel 1:4-37.

Kittler J (1978) Feature Set Search Algorithms. In (Chen CH ed): Pattern Recognition and Signal Processing, Noordhoff Pub. Co., Leyden.

Kulkarni AV (1978) On the Mean Accuracy of Hierarchical Classifiers. IEEE Tr Comp 27:771-776.

Loizou G, Maybank SJ (1987) The Nearest Neighbor and the Bayes Error Rates. IEEE Tr Patt Anal Mach Intel 9:254-262.

Lusted L (1978) General Problems in Medical Decision Making with Comments on ROC Analysis. Seminars in Nuclear Medicine, 8:299-306.

Meisel WS (1972) Computer-oriented Approaches to Pattern Recognition. Academic Press, London.

Mendel JM, Fu KS (1970) Adaptive, Learning and Pattern Recognition Systems. Academic Press, London.

Metz CE, Goodenough DJ, Rossmann K (1973) Evaluation of Receiver Operating Characteristic Curve Data in Terms of Information Theory, with Applications in Radiography. Radiology, 109:297-304.

Metz CE (1978) Basic Principles of ROC Analysis. Seminars in Nuclear Medicine, 8:283-298.

Mitchell TM (1997) Machine Learning. McGraw Hill Book Co.

Mucciardi AN, Gose EE (1971) A Comparison of Seven Techniques for Choosing Subsets of Pattern Recognition Properties. IEEE Tr Comp 20:1023-1031.

Narendra P, Fukunaga K (1977) A Branch and Bound Algorithm for Feature Subset Selection. IEEE Tr Comp 26:917-922.

Niemann H (1990) Pattern Analysis and Understanding. Springer Verlag.

Pipes LA (1977) Matrix-Computer Methods in Engineering. Krieger Pub. Co.

Raudys S, Pikelis V (1980) On dimensionality, sample size, classification error and complexity of classification algorithm in pattern recognition. IEEE Tr Patt Anal Mach Intel 2:242-252.

Schalkoff R (1992) Pattern Recognition. Wiley, New York.

Swets JA (1973) The Relative Operating Characteristic in Psychology. Science, 182:990-1000.

Shapiro SS, Wilk SS, Chen SW (1968) A comparative study of various tests for normality. J Am Stat Ass, 63:1343-1372.

Siegel S, Castellan NJ Jr (1988) Nonparametric Statistics for the Behavioral Sciences. Ms Graw Hill, New York.

Specht DF (1990) Probabilistic Neural Networks. Neural Networks, 3:109-118.

Swain PH (1977) The decision tree classifier: Design and potential. IEEE Tr Geosci Elect, 15:142-147.

Toussaint GT (1974) Bibliography on Estimation of Misclassification. IEEE Tr Info Theory, 20:472-479.

Exercises

4.1 Consider the first two classes of the *Cork Stoppers* dataset, described by features ART and PRT.

   a) Determine the Euclidian and Mahalanobis classifiers using feature ART alone, then using both ART and PRT.

   b) Compute the Bayes error using a pooled covariance estimate as the true covariance for both classes.

   c) Determine whether the Mahalanobis classifiers are expected to be near the optimal Bayesian classifier.

   d) Using *PR Size* determine the average deviation of the training set error estimate from the Bayes error, and the 95% confidence interval of the error estimate.

   e) Determine the classification of one cork stopper using the correlation approach.

4.2 Consider the first two classes of the *Cork Stoppers* dataset, described by features ART and PRT. Compute the linear discriminant corresponding to the Euclidian classifier using formula 4-3c.

4.3 Repeat the previous exercises for the three classes of the *Cork Stoppers* dataset, using features N, PRM and ARTG. Compute the pooled covariance matrix and determine the influence of small changes in its values on the classifier performance.

4.4 Consider the problem of classifying cardiotocograms (*CTG* dataset) into three classes: N (normal), S (suspect) and P (pathological).

   a) Determine which features are most discriminative and appropriate for a Mahalanobis classifier approach for this problem.

b) Design the classifier and estimate its performance using a partition method for the test set error estimation.

4.5 Repeat the previous exercise using the *Rocks* dataset and two classes: {granites} vs. {limestones, marbles}.

4.6 Apply a linear discriminant to the projections of the cork stoppers two-dimensional data (first two classes) along the Fisher direction as explained in section 4.1.4. Show that the same results, found with the linear discriminant, are obtained.

4.7 Consider the *Fruits* images dataset. Process the images in order to obtain interesting colour and shape features (a popular picture processing program, such as the *Micrografx Picture Publisher* can be used for this purpose). Design a Bayesian classifier for the 3-class fruit discrimination. Comment the results obtained.

4.8 A physician would like to have a very simple rule available for screening out the carcinoma situations from all other situations, using the same diagnostic means and measurements as in the *Breast Tissue* dataset.

a) Using the *Breast Tissue* dataset, find a linear Bayesian classifier with only one feature for the discrimination of carcinoma versus all other cases (relax the normality and equal variance requirements). Use forward and backward search and estimate the priors from the training set sizes of the classes.

b) Obtain training set and test set error estimates of this classifier and 95% confidence intervals.

c) Using the *PR Size* program, assess the deviation of the error estimate from the true Bayesian error, assuming that the normality and equal variance requirements were satisfied.

d) Suppose that the risk of missing a carcinoma is three times higher than the risk of misclassifying a non-carcinoma case. How should the classifying rule be reformulated in order to reflect these risks, and what is the performance of the new rule?

4.9 Study the influence that using a pooled covariance matrix for the *Norm2c2d* dataset has on the training set error estimate. For this purpose, perform the following computations:

a) Change the off-diagonal elements of one of the covariance matrices by a small amount (e.g. 10%).

b) Compute the training set errors using a quadratic classifier with the individual covariance matrices.

c) Compute the training set errors using a linear classifier with the pooled covariance matrix.

d) Compare the results obtained in b) and c).

4.10 Determine the reject threshold that should be used for the carcinoma classifier of Exercise 4.8, such that: a) no carcinoma is misclassified; b) only 5% of the carcinomas are misclassified. Also determine the decision rules for these situations.

4.11 Repeat exercise 4.4, considering only two classes: N and P. Determine afterwards which reject threshold best matches the S (suspect) cases.

4.12 Use the *Parzen.xls* file to repeat the experiments shown in Figure 4.28 for other types of distributions, namely the normal and the logistic distributions.

4.13 Apply the Parzen window method to the first two classes of the cork stoppers data with features N and PRT10, using the probabilistic neural network approach for pattern classification. Also use the weight values to derive the probability density estimates (limit the training set to 10 cases per class and use Microsoft Excel).

4.14 Perform a k-NN classification of the *Breast Tissue* data in order to discriminate carcinoma cases from all other cases. Use the *KNN* program in the partition and edition methods. Compare the results.

4.15 Consider the k-NN classification of the *Rocks* data, using two classes: {granites, diorites, schists} vs. {limestones, marbles, breccias}.
   a)   Give an estimate of the number of neighbours, k, that should be used.
   b)   For the previously estimated k, what is the expected deviation of the asymptotic error of the k-NN classifier from the Bayes error?
   c)   Perform the classification with the *KNN* program, using the partition and edition methods. Compare the results.

4.16 Explain why all ROC curves start at (0,0) and finish at (1,1) by analysing what kind of situations these points correspond to.

4.17 Consider the *Breast Tissue* dataset. Use the ROC curve approach to determine single features that will discriminate carcinoma cases from all other cases. Compare the alternative methods using the ROC curve areas.

4.18 Repeat the ROC curve experiments illustrated in Figure 4.34 for the *FHR Apgar* dataset, using combinations of features.

4.19 Increase the amplitude of the signal impulses by 20% in the *Signal Noise* dataset. Consider the following impulse detection rule:

An impulse is detected at time n when $s(n)$ is bigger than $\alpha \sum_{i=1}^{2} \left(s(n-i) + s(n+i) \right)$.

Determine the ROC curve corresponding to a variable α, and determine the best α for the impulse/noise discrimination. How does this method compare with the amplitude threshold method described in section 4.3.3?

4.20 Apply the branch-and-bound method to perform feature selection for the first two classes of the *Cork Stoppers* data.

4.21 Repeat Exercises 4.4 and 4.5 performing sequential feature selection (direct and dynamic).

4.22 Perform a resubstitution and leave-one-out estimation of the classification errors for the three classes of cork stoppers, using the features obtained by dynamic selection. Discuss the reliability of these estimates.

4.23 Compute the 95% confidence interval of the error for the classifier designed in Exercise 4.11, using the standard formula. Perform a partition method evaluation of the classifier, with 10 partitions, obtaining another estimate of the 95% confidence interval of the error.

4.24 Compute the decrease of impurity in the trees shown in Figure 4.41 and Figure 4.45, using the entropy as impurity measure.

4.25 Compute the classification matrix *car* vs. {*mas*, *gla*, *fad*} for the *Breast Tissue* dataset in the tree shown in Figure 4.41. Observe its dependence on the prevalences. Compute the linear discriminant shown in the same figure.

4.26 Using the *CART* approach, find decision trees that discriminate the three classes of the *CTG* dataset, N, S and P, using several initial feature sets that contain the four variability indexes ASTV, ALTV, MSTV, MLTV. Compare search times and classification performances for the several initial feature sets.

5 Neural Networks

In the previous chapters we learned how to design supervised and unsupervised classifiers, which had in common the concept of class or cluster separability, based on a distance measure. Artificial neural networks, or *neural nets* for short, afford a means of classifying data and also use distance measures in a model-free approach, but whereas, previously, class separability was the driving mechanism towards a solution, we now apply another concept, that of minimizing errors between obtained outputs and desired target values. Besides statistical considerations, optimisation techniques play a fundamental role here.

5.1 LMS Adjusted Discriminants

Let us assume that we are searching for a solution in terms of linear discriminants for a c-class classification problem. We are given n labelled patterns and wish to use linear decision functions for their classification. Linear discriminants were already presented in section 2.1; we rewrite here the respective expression 2-2:

$$d(\mathbf{x}) = \mathbf{w}'\,\mathbf{x} + w_0 . \tag{5-1}$$

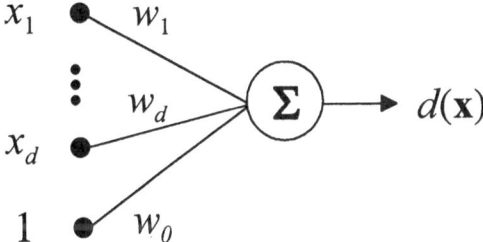

Figure 5.1. Connectionist structure of a linear decision function. Σ is the processing unit.

As we will, in principle, always use bias weights w_0, we will simplify, for the moment, the notation by calling $\mathbf{x}$ the augmented feature vector with an extra feature (bias) of value one, as shown in Figure 5.1. We will also use **w** to denote the whole weight vector, unless we need to refer explicitly to the bias term. This discriminant unit, whose input variables are the features and whose output is the linear function $d(\mathbf{x})$, is also called a *linear network*.

When presenting graphically connectionist structures, such as the one in Figure 5.1, we will use an open circle to represent a processing neuron and a black circle to represent a terminal neuron. In the case of a single output linear network, as shown in Figure 5.1, there is only one processing unit where the contributions from all inputs are summed up.

In general, we will have available c such functions $d_k(\mathbf{x})$ with weight vector $\mathbf{w}_k$, one for each class, therefore for each pattern $\mathbf{x}_i$ we write:

$$d_k(\mathbf{x}_i) = \mathbf{w}_k'\mathbf{x}_i = \sum_{j=0}^{d} w_{k,j} x_{i,j} \ . \tag{5-1a}$$

As in section 4.1.2, the class label assigned to an unknown pattern corresponds to the decision function reaching a maximum for that pattern.

Imagine now that we wanted to adjust the weights of these linear functions in order to approximate some target outputs $t_k(\mathbf{x})$ for each class ω_k. We could do this in the following way:

First, for each feature vector $\mathbf{x}_i$, we compute the deviations of each discriminant output from the target values:

$$\delta_k(\mathbf{x}_i) = d_k(\mathbf{x}_i) - t_k(\mathbf{x}_i) \ ; \tag{5-2}$$

Next, these deviations or *approximation errors*, are squared and summed in order to obtain a total error, E:

$$E = \frac{1}{2} \sum_{k=1}^{c} \sum_{i=1}^{n} \left(d_k(\mathbf{x}_i) - t_k(\mathbf{x}_i) \right)^2 = \frac{1}{2} \sum_{k=1}^{c} \sum_{i=1}^{n} \left(\sum_{j=0}^{d} w_{k,j} x_{i,j} - t_{k,i} \right)^2 \ . \tag{5-2a}$$

In this last formula we simplified the writing by using $t_{k,i}$ instead of $t_k(\mathbf{x}_i)$. We have also included a one half factor whose relevance is merely to ease subsequent derivations. Note that equation (5-2a) can be viewed as the total dissimilarity between output values and the desired target values using a squared Euclidian metric.

Adding the squares of the deviations, as we did in (5-2a), imposes a stronger penalty on the larger ones. Other formulas for E are also possible, for instance using the absolute values of the deviations instead of the squares. However, the sum-of-squares error has the desirable property of easy differentiation and also well-established physical and statistical interpretations. For instance, if our linear network had to approximate voltage values, and the voltage deviations obtained were applied to resistances of the same value, the heat generated by them would be proportional to E. It seems, therefore, appropriate to call E the *error energy*. In order to obtain the best approximation to the target values, corresponding to minimize E, we differentiate it with respect to the weights and equalize to zero:

$$\sum_{i=1}^{n}\sum_{j=0}^{d}(w_{k,j}x_{i,j} - t_{k,i})x_{i,j} = 0; \quad k = 1,\cdots,c .\tag{5-2b}$$

We can write these so-called *normal equations* corresponding to the *least-mean-square* or LMS solution, in a compact form as:

$$\mathbf{X'XW'}= \mathbf{X'T} ,\tag{5-2c}$$

where $\mathbf{X}$ is a $n_x(d+1)$ matrix with the augmented feature vectors, $\mathbf{W}$ is a $c_x(d+1)$ matrix of the weights and $\mathbf{T}$ is a n_xc matrix of the target values. Provided that the square matrix $\mathbf{X'X}$ is non-singular, the weights can be immediately computed as:

$$\mathbf{W'}= (\mathbf{X'X})^{-1}\mathbf{X'T} = \mathbf{X^*T} .\tag{5-3}$$

The matrix $\mathbf{X}^* = (\mathbf{X'X})^{-1}\mathbf{X'}$ is called the *pseudo-inverse* of $\mathbf{X}$ and satisfies the property $\mathbf{X^*X=I}$.

In order to see how the LMS adjustment of discriminants works, let us consider a very simple two-class one-dimensional problem with only two points, one from each class, as shown in Figure 5.2a, where the target values are also indicated. For adequate graphic inspection in the weight space, we will limit the number of weights by restricting the analysis to the discriminant that corresponds to the difference of the linear decision functions:

$$d(x) = d_1(x) - d_2(x) = (w_{11}x + w_{12}) - (w_{21}x + w_{22}) = ax + b .\tag{5-4}$$

Let us compute the pseudo-inverse of $\mathbf{X}$:

$$\mathbf{X}=\begin{bmatrix} -1 & 1 \\ 1 & 1 \end{bmatrix} \Rightarrow \mathbf{X}^* = \left(\begin{bmatrix} -1 & 1 \\ 1 & 1 \end{bmatrix}\begin{bmatrix} -1 & 1 \\ 1 & 1 \end{bmatrix}\right)^{-1}\begin{bmatrix} -1 & 1 \\ 1 & 1 \end{bmatrix}=\begin{bmatrix} -\frac{1}{2} & \frac{1}{2} \\ \frac{1}{2} & \frac{1}{2} \end{bmatrix}.\tag{5-4a}$$

Since our goal now is to adjust one discriminant d, instead of d_1 and d_2, matrix $\mathbf{T}$ has only one column[1] with the respective target values, therefore:

$$\mathbf{W} =\begin{bmatrix} -\frac{1}{2} & \frac{1}{2} \\ \frac{1}{2} & \frac{1}{2} \end{bmatrix}\begin{bmatrix} -1 \\ 1 \end{bmatrix}=\begin{bmatrix} 1 \\ 0 \end{bmatrix} \Rightarrow a = 1; \quad b = 0 .\tag{5-4b}$$

---

[1] Since we are using a single discriminant, $c=1$ in this case.

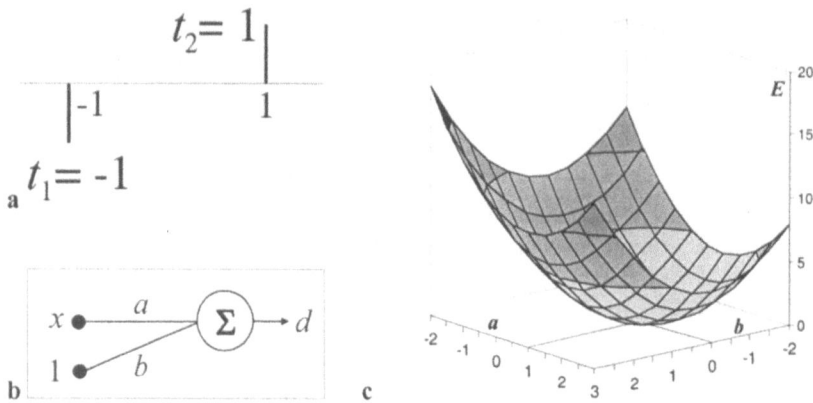

Figure 5.2. Linear discriminant for a two-class one-dimensional situation: (a) Design set; (b) Linear network; (c) Energy surface.

The solution $d(x) = x$ does indeed satisfy the problem. Let us now see what happens in terms of the energy function. Simple calculations show that:

$$E = a^2 + b^2 - 2a + 1 .$$ (5-4c)

The parabolic surface corresponding to E is shown in Figure 5.2c. The minimum of E does indeed occur at the point ($a=1$, $b=0$).

It is interesting to see the role of the bias weights by differentiating (5-2a) in order to the bias weights alone:

$$\frac{\partial E}{\partial w_{k,0}} = \sum_{i=1}^{n} \sum_{j=1}^{d} \left(w_{k,j} x_{i,j} + w_{k,0} - t_{k,i} \right) = 0 ,$$ (5-5)

which, solved for the biases, gives:

$$w_{k,0} = \frac{1}{n} \sum_{i=1}^{n} t_{k,i} - \frac{1}{n} \sum_{i=1}^{n} \sum_{j=1}^{d} w_{k,j} x_{i,j} .$$ (5-5a)

Therefore, the role of the biases for each class is to compensate for the difference between the mean of the target values and the mean of the output values corresponding to the feature vectors alone (without the biases).

Note that by transforming the input variables using non-linear functions, one can obtain more complex decision boundaries than the linear ones. In fact, this corresponds to using the concept of generalized decision functions, presented already in section 2.1.1. Instead of (5-3) we would now have:

$$\mathbf{W'} = \left(\mathbf{Y'Y}\right)^{-1}\mathbf{Y'T} = \mathbf{Y}^{*}\mathbf{T},$$ (5-6)

where $\mathbf{Y}$ is the matrix of the transformed features $y_i = f(x_i)$.

Using generalized decision functions, one can obtain arbitrarily complex decision surfaces at the possible expense of having to work in much higher dimensional spaces, as already pointed out in 2.1.1. Another difficulty is that, in practical applications, when there are several features, it may be quite impossible to figure out the most appropriate transforming functions $f(x_i)$. Also note that nothing is gained by cascading an arbitrary number of linear discriminant units (Figure 5.1), because a linear composition of linear discriminants is itself a linear discriminant. In order to achieve more complex decision surfaces, what we really need is to apply non-linear processing units, as will be done in the following section.

A limitation of the method of minimum energy adjustment is that, in practice, the solution of the normal equations may be difficult or even impossible to obtain, due to $\mathbf{X'X}$ being singular or nearly singular. One can, however, circumvent this limitation by using a *gradient descent* method, provided that E is a differentiable function of the weights, as is verified when using the error energy (5-2a).

In order to apply the gradient descent method we begin with an initial guess of the weight values (e.g. a random choice), and from there on we iteratively update the weights in order to decrease the energy. The maximum decrease of the energy is in the direction along the negative of the gradient, therefore we update the weights on iteration $r+1$ by adding a small amount of the negative of the gradient computed at iteration r:

$$w_{k,j}^{(r+1)} = w_{k,j}^{(r)} - \eta \frac{\partial E}{\partial w_{k,j}}\bigg|_{\mathbf{w}^{(r)}}.$$ (5-7)

The factor η, a small positive constant controlling how fast we move along the negative of the gradient, is called the *learning rate*.

Consider the energy surface represented in Figure 5.2c. Starting at any point at the top of the surface we will move in the direction of the steepest descent of the surface. The choice of the learning rate is critical, since if it is too small we will converge slowly to the minimum, and if it is too big we can get oscillations around the minimum.

The weight updating expressed by equation (5-7) can be performed, one pattern at a time, by computing the derivative of the energy E_i for the current pattern $\mathbf{x}_i$:

$$w_{k,j}^{(r+1)} = w_{k,j}^{(r)} - \eta \frac{\partial E_i}{\partial w_{k,j}}\bigg|_{\mathbf{w}^{(r)}}.$$ (5-7a)

The process of weight adjustment is then repeated many times by cycling through all patterns.

Let us compute the gradient in (5-7a). The energy contribution of each pattern $\mathbf{x}_i$ is computed using equation (5-1a):

$$E_i = \frac{1}{2}\sum_{k=1}^{c}\left(d_k(\mathbf{x}_i) - t_k(\mathbf{x}_i)\right)^2 = \frac{1}{2}\sum_{k=1}^{c}\left(\mathbf{w}_k{}'\mathbf{x}_i - t_k(\mathbf{x}_i)\right)^2 . \tag{5-7b}$$

The gradient is now expressed compactly, using (5-2), as:

$$\frac{\partial E_i}{\partial w_{k,j}} = \left(d_k(\mathbf{x}_i) - t_k(\mathbf{x}_i)\right)x_{i,j} = \delta_k(\mathbf{x}_i)x_{i,j} . \tag{5-7c}$$

Therefore, each weight is updated by summing the following correction:

$$\Delta w_{k,j} = -\eta\delta_k(\mathbf{x}_i)x_{i,j} . \tag{5-7d}$$

For the particular case of two classes we need only to consider one linear decision function. The increment of the weight vector can be then written compactly as:

$$\Delta\mathbf{w} = -\eta(\mathbf{w}'\mathbf{x}_i - t_i)\mathbf{x}_i . \tag{5-7e}$$

This equation shows that the weight vector correction for each pattern depends on the deviation between the discriminant unit output from the target value, multiplied by the corresponding feature vector. If we update the weights by using the total energy function, we just have to sum the derivatives of equation (5-7c) for all patterns, or equivalently add up the increments expressed by equation (5-7d). This mode of operation is called the *batch mode* of gradient descent. An iteration involving the sum of the increments for all patterns is called an *epoch*.

Note that LMS adjustment of discriminants produces approximations to target values whatever they are, be they class labels or not. Therefore, we may as well use this approach in *regression* problems.

As a matter of fact, even a simple device such as an LMS adjusted discriminant can perform very useful tasks, namely in solving regression problems, and we now present such an example of a regression application to signal adaptive filtering. The theory of adaptive filtering owes much to the works of Bernard Widrow concerning adaptive LMS filtering for noise cancelling (see Widrow *et al.*, 1975).

Let us consider an electrocardiographic signal (ECG) with added 50 Hz noise, induced by the main power supply (a common situation in electrocardiography), shown in Figure 5.3. The reader can follow this example using the *ECG 50Hz.xls* file, where this figure, representing 3.4 seconds of a signal sampled at 500 Hz with amplitude in microvolts, is included.

In order to remove the noise from the signal we will design an LMS adjusted discriminant, which will attempt to regress the noise. As the noise has zero mean we will not need any bias weight. The discriminant just has to use adequate inputs in order to approximate the amplitude and the phase angle of the sinusoidal noise. Since there are two parameters to adjust (amplitude and phase), we will then use any two sinusoidal inputs with π/2 phase lag from each other, as represented in Figure 5.4.

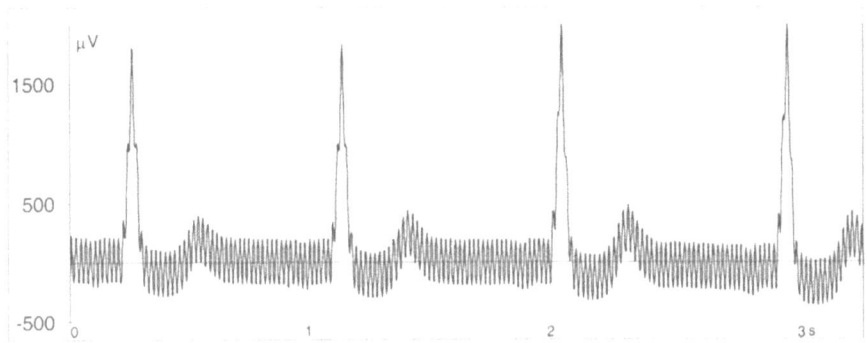

Figure 5.3. Discretized ECG tracing (3.4 seconds) with added 50 Hz noise. Sampling rate is 500 Hz and amplitude is in microvolts. The jagged contour of the signal is due solely to its discrete representation.

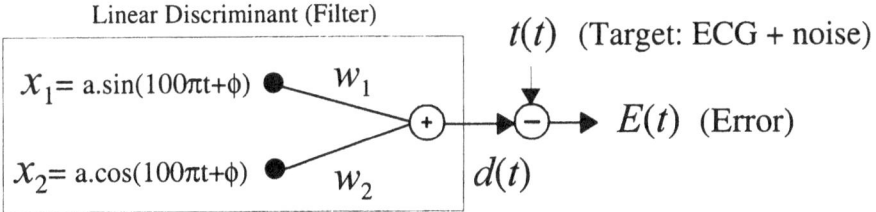

Figure 5.4. Linear discriminant used to regress a 50Hz sinusoid with unknown phase and amplitude.

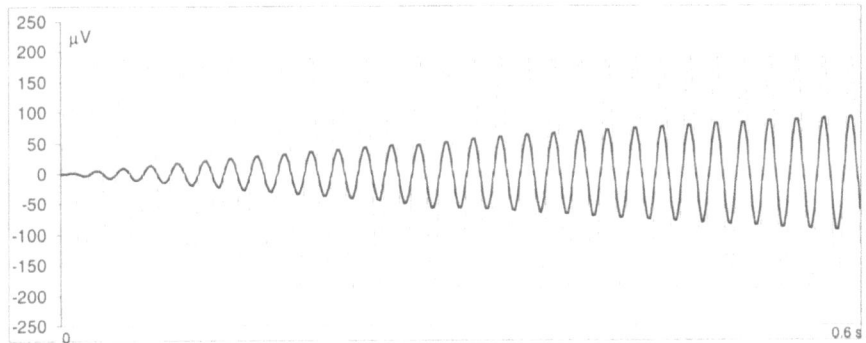

Figure 5.5. Output of the linear discriminant (black) regressing the noise (grey) for a learning rate $\eta=0.002$. Only the first 0.6 seconds are shown.

Note that the amplitude a and phase angle ϕ of the inputs are arbitrary. The weights of the linear discriminant are updated at each incoming signal sample (i.e. pattern-by-pattern) using formula (5-7d), therefore, since the iteration is along time, the gradient descent method corresponds to the following weight adjustment:

$$w_i(t+1) = w_i(t) - \eta E(t) x_i(t).$$ (5-8)

For implementation purposes we can transform this iteration in time into iteration in space as we have done in the *ECG 50Hz.xls* file, where each row represents a new iteration step. Using a suitably low learning rate η the linear discriminant (filter) output will converge to the incoming noise[2], as shown in Figure 5.5. As a result, we will obtain at the error output the filtered ECG shown in Figure 5.6. Note from both figures how the discriminant adjustment progresses until it perfectly matches (regresses) the incoming noise. By varying the learning rate the reader will have the opportunity to appreciate two things:

– Up to a certain point, increasing η will produce faster learning.
– After that, the learning step is so big that the process does not converge, in fact it diverges quickly, producing a saturated output.

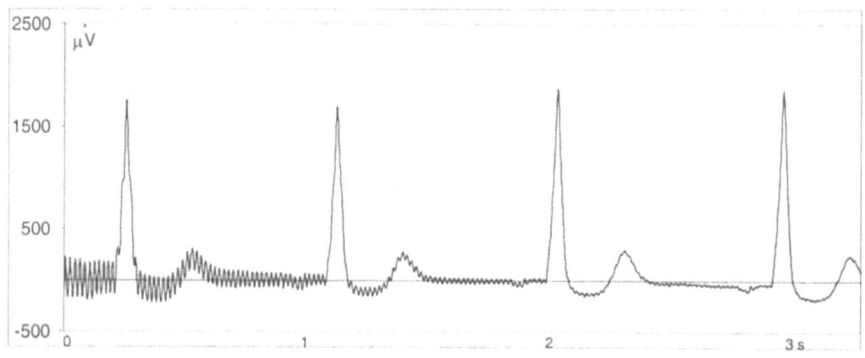

Figure 5.6. Filtered ECG using the LMS adjusted discriminant method with learning rate η=0.002.

The reader can also change the amplitude and phase angle of the discriminant inputs in order to see that their values are immaterial and that the discriminant will make the right approximation whatever value of a and ϕ is used. In fact, the filter will even track slow changes of frequency and phase of the incoming noise signal.

---

[2] The influence of the 50Hz component of the ECG is negligible, since it is uncorrelated with the noise.

5.2 Activation Functions

We have mentioned previously that, in order to obtain more complex discriminants, some type of non-linear function will have to be used as shown in Figure 5.7. The non-linear function f is called an *activation function*. The generalized decision function can now be written as:

$$d(\mathbf{x}) = f(\mathbf{w'}\,\mathbf{x})\,. \qquad (5\text{-}8)$$

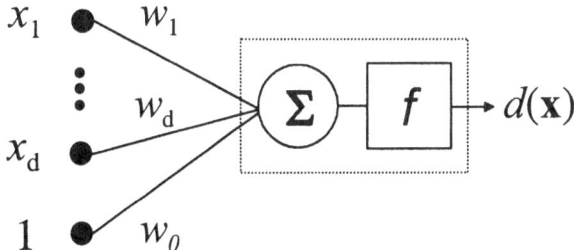

Figure 5.7. Connectionist structure of a generalized decision function. The processing unit (rectangle with dotted line) implements $f(\Sigma)$.

Let us consider the one-dimensional two-class example shown in Figure 5.8a, with three points -1, 0 and 1 and respective target values 1, -1, 1. We now have a class (target value 1) with disconnected regions (points -1 and 1). We try to discriminate between the two classes by using the following parabolic activation function:

$$d(x) = f(ax+b) = (ax+b)^2 - 1\,. \qquad (5\text{-}9a)$$

In order to study the energy function in a simple way, we assume, as in the previous example of Figure 5.2, that the parabolic activation function is directly applied to the linear discriminant, as shown in equation (5-9a). From now on we represent by an open circle the *output neuron* of the discriminant unit, containing both the summation and the activation function, as in Figure 5.8b.

The energy function is symmetric and is partly represented in Figure 5.8c. The rugged aspect of the surface is due solely to the discrete step of 0.5 used for the weights a and b. There are two global minima at $(\sqrt{2},\,0)$ and $(-\sqrt{2},\,0)$, both corresponding to the obvious solution $d(x) = 2x^2-1$, passing exactly by the target points. This solution can be obtained either by solving the normal equations or by using the gradient descent method.

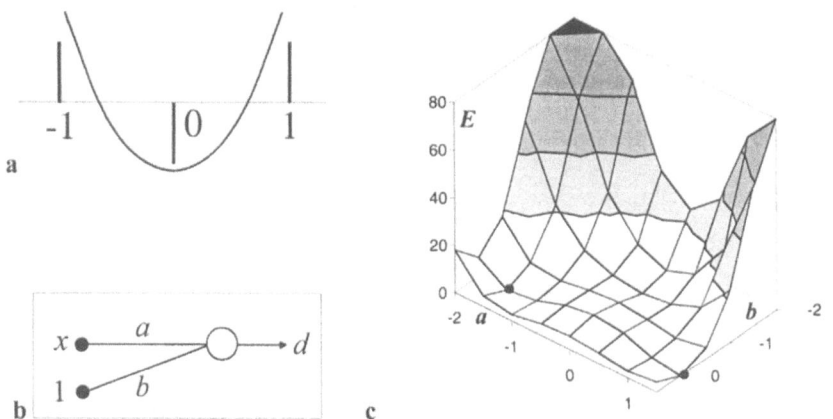

Figure 5.8. Parabolic discriminant for a two-class one-dimensional situation: (a) Design set; (b) Network with parabolic activation function; (c) Energy surface with two global minima.

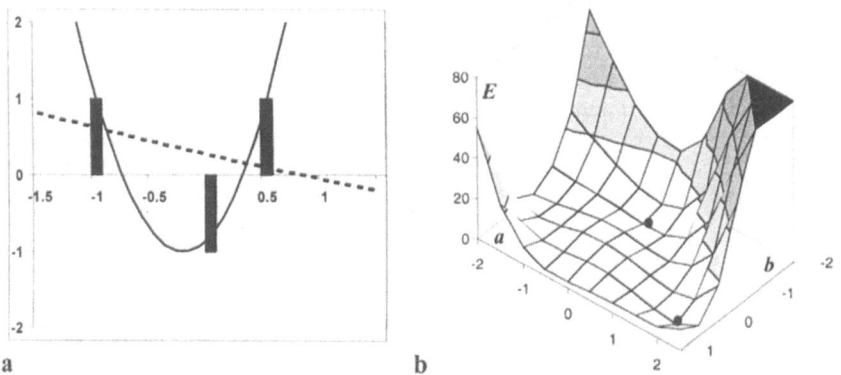

Figure 5.9. Parabolic discriminants for a two-class one-dimensional situation: (a) Discriminants corresponding to the global minima (solid curve) and local minima (dotted curve); (b) Energy surface showing one global and one local minima.

Let us now displace point 1 to the 0.5 position as shown in Figure 5.9a. The energy function has radically changed as shown in Figure 5.9b, where only the part of the function that is of interest is represented. The important aspect is that there are now two global minima, {(1.88, 0.46), (-1.88, -0.46)}, and two local minima, {(0.15, -1.125), (-0.15, 1.125)}.

Corresponding to the global minima we have the parabola represented by a solid line in Figure 5.9a, which fits the data quite well, and has an energy minimum of 0.0466. Corresponding to the local minima is a parabola represented by a dotted line in Figure 5.9a, far off the target points, and with an energy minimum of 2.547. As the normal equations would be laborious to solve, in this case a gradient descent method would be preferred. The problem is that if we start our gradient descent at the point (0,-2), for instance, we would end up in the local minimum, with quite a bad solution. This simple example illustrates, therefore, how drastically different a local minimum solution can be from a global minimum solution, and the need to perform several trials with different starting points when solving an LMS discriminant adjustment using the gradient descent method.

Usually one has no previous knowledge of what kind of activation function is most suitable to the data. This is, in fact, a similar issue to selecting the most suitable transformation function for the input features. There are three popularised activation functions that have been extensively studied and employed in many software products implementing neural nets. These are:

The step function:
$$h(x) = \begin{cases} 1 & \text{if} \quad x \geq 0 \\ -1 & \text{if} \quad x < 0 \end{cases} \qquad (5\text{-}10a)$$

The logistic sigmoid function:
$$sig(x) = \frac{1}{1 + e^{-ax}} \qquad (5\text{-}10b)$$

The hyperbolic tangent function:
$$tanh(x) = \frac{e^{ax} - e^{-ax}}{e^{ax} + e^{-ax}} \qquad (5\text{-}10c)$$

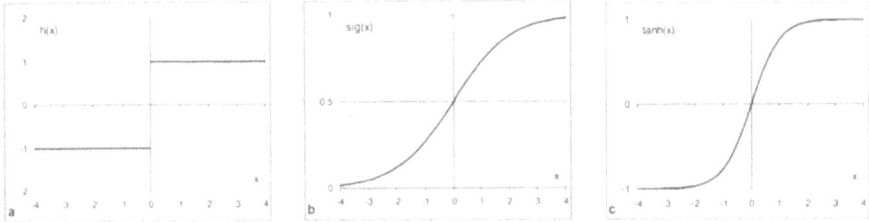

Figure 5.10. Common activation functions: (a) Step; (b) Logistic sigmoid with a=1; (c) Tanh sigmoid with a=1.

These three functions are represented in Figure 5.10. There are variants of these activation functions, depending on the output ranges and scaling factors, without any real practical relevance. The last two are called sigmoidal functions because of their S-shaped appearance. The parameter a governs the sigmoidal slope.

Discriminant units having these activation functions all have outputs in a well-defined range [0, 1] or [-1, 1], which is quite convenient for classification purposes. The step function (also called *hard-limiter* or *threshold function*) is not differentiable in the whole domain. The other activation functions have the advantage of being differentiable in the whole domain with easy derivatives.

Derivative of the logistic sigmoid (with $a=1$):

$$sig'(x) = \frac{e^{-x}}{\left(1+e^{-x}\right)^2} = sig(x)\left(1-sig(x)\right). \tag{5-11a}$$

Derivative of the hyperbolic tangent (with $a=1$):

$$tanh'(x) = \frac{4}{\left(e^x+e^{-x}\right)^2} = \left(1-tanh(x)\right)\left(1+tanh(x)\right). \tag{5-11b}$$

The sigmoidal functions also have the good property that in addition to the limiting aspect of the step function, they provide a linear behaviour near the zero crossing. When approximating target values they are, therefore, considerably versatile.

Compared with the logistic sigmoid, the hyperbolic tangent has the advantage of usually affording a faster convergence. The logistic sigmoid has, however, the relevant advantage that the outputs of the networks using this activation function can be interpreted as posterior probabilities. As a matter of fact, for a two-class Bayesian classifier, we have:

$$P(\omega_1 \mid \mathbf{x}) = \frac{p(\mathbf{x} \mid \omega_1)P(\omega_1)}{p(\mathbf{x} \mid \omega_1)P(\omega_1) + p(\mathbf{x} \mid \omega_2)P(\omega_2)}. \tag{5-12a}$$

We can express this formula in terms of the logistic sigmoid (with $a=1$):

$$P(\omega_1 \mid \mathbf{x}) = sig(t) \quad \text{with} \quad t = \ln\frac{p(\mathbf{x} \mid \omega_1)P(\omega_1)}{p(\mathbf{x} \mid \omega_2)P(\omega_2)}. \tag{5-12b}$$

Assuming normal distributions, with equal covariance for the likelihoods, one readily obtains $t = d(\mathbf{x})$ where $d(\mathbf{x})$ is the linear discriminant depending on the linear decision functions (4.23b) presented in chapter 4. The linear network is therefore mimicking the Bayesian classifier.

5.3 The Perceptron Concept

The network unit depicted in Figure 5.7, with a threshold function $h(x)$ as activation function, was studied by Rosenblatt (1962) who, inspired by the similarity with the physiological structure of the neurons, called it *perceptron*. A similar device was studied by Widrow and Hoff (1960) under the name of *adaline* (ADAptive LINear Element). We will consider, in later sections, cascades of such units that bear some resemblance to networks of physiological neurons, the inputs playing the role of the synapses and the outputs playing the role of the axons. Within this analogy, positive weights are interpreted as reinforcing connections and negative weights as inhibiting connections. It was this analogy that earned the perceptron and its other relatives the name of *artificial neural networks* or simply *neural networks* or *neural nets* for short. However, the reader must not carry the analogy too far, as it is quite coarse, and one should consider the engineering terminology neural networks only as a convenient way of referring to artificial connectionist networks with learning properties.

The perceptron output is given by:

$$d(\mathbf{x}) = h\left(\sum_{j=0}^{d} w_j x_j \right) = h(\mathbf{w}'\mathbf{x}).\tag{5-13}$$

It is of course also possible to use transformed inputs, as already mentioned in the previous section.

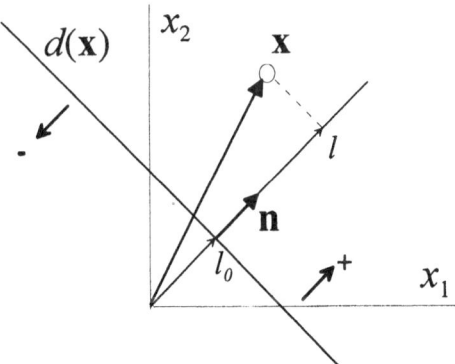

Figure 5.11. Classification of a feature vector **x** using the perceptron rule, based on the distance $l\text{-}l_0$ to the discriminant $d(\mathbf{x})$.

Consider a two-class situation, ω_1 with target value +1 and ω_2 with target value −1. Then, from (5-13) and the definition (5-10a) of the hard-limiting function, we want $\mathbf{w'x}_i > 0$ for patterns $\mathbf{x}_i$ belonging to class ω_1 and $\mathbf{w'x}_i < 0$ for patterns $\mathbf{x}_i$ belonging to class ω_2. These two conditions can be written simply as $\mathbf{w'x}_i t_i > 0$, using the target values. The fact that $\mathbf{w'x}_i t_i$ must be positive for correct classification, suggests the use of the following error function known as the *perceptron criterion*:

$$E(\mathbf{w}) = - \sum_{\mathbf{x}_i \text{ in error}} \mathbf{w'x}_i t_i .$$

(5-14)

Let us look more closely at this error function. Consider the situation with $d = 2$ depicted in Figure 5.11, where the unit length normal to the discriminant, $\mathbf{n}$, points in the positive direction ($d(\mathbf{x}) > 0$), corresponding to class ω_1.

Let us determine the projection distance $l - l_0$ of a feature vector $\mathbf{x}$ onto the positive normal $\mathbf{n}$. The projection of $d(\mathbf{x})$ referred to the origin, l_0, is given by $-w_0/\|\mathbf{n}\|$ [3]. The length l is the projection of $\mathbf{x}$ onto $\mathbf{n}$. Since the components of the normal vector $\mathbf{n}$ to the linear discriminant $d(\mathbf{x})$ are precisely the weights of $d(\mathbf{x})$, $\mathbf{n} = (w_1, w_2)$ [3], we can compute the projection distance $l(\mathbf{x})$ of $\mathbf{x}$ onto the normal of the linear discriminant, as:

$$l(\mathbf{x}) = l - l_0 = \frac{w_1 x_1 + w_2 x_2}{\|\mathbf{n}\|} - \frac{-w_0}{\|\mathbf{n}\|} = \frac{\mathbf{w'x}}{\|\mathbf{n}\|} .$$

(5-15)

This projection $l(\mathbf{x})$ is positive for feature vectors $\mathbf{x}$ lying in the positive half plane and negative otherwise.

Consider now that feature vector $\mathbf{x}$ represented in Figure 5.11 is wrongly classified because it has target value -1. As the target value is negative, the contribution of the pattern to the error (5-14) is a positive value. In the same way, a feature vector lying in the negative half plane, therefore with $l(\mathbf{x}) < 0$, will contribute positively to the error if its target value is $+1$. In general, the contributions of the wrongly classified patterns to the errors are the Euclidian distances to the discriminant.

The perceptron compensates for these errors by applying the following learning rule:

– Pattern correctly classified: do nothing.
– Pattern wrongly classified: add the pattern to the weight vector if the pattern is from class ω_1 ($t_i = +1$) and subtract it if it is from class ω_2 ($t_i = -1$).

Hence, the increment of the weight vector is:

$$\Delta\mathbf{w} = t_i \mathbf{x}_i \quad \text{for wrong } \mathbf{x}_i .$$

(5-16)

---

[3] See expressions (2-2d) relative to the distance of $d(\mathbf{x})$ from the origin and the unitary normal vector pointing into the positive direction.

Let us consider formula (5-7e) for the particular case of $\eta = \frac{1}{2}$ and use the activation step function applied to the linear discriminant:

$$\Delta\mathbf{w} = -\frac{1}{2}\left(h(\mathbf{w'}\,\mathbf{x}_i) - t_i\right)\mathbf{x}_i\,. \tag{5-16a}$$

For correct decisions the output $h(\mathbf{w'x}_i)$ is identical to t_i and no increment is obtained. For wrong decisions the increment obtained is exactly the same as in (5-16). Hence, the perceptron rule is identical to the LMS rule, using the step function and a learning rate $\eta = \frac{1}{2}$.

Note that what the perceptron produces are class labels, therefore it is adequate for *classification* problems. It is interesting to compare how the perceptron performs in the case of the one-dimensional data of Figure 5.2a. In this case the perceptron learning rule can be written:

$$E = \begin{cases} -a+b & \text{if} \quad -a+b \geq 0 \\ -(a+b) & \text{if} \quad a+b < 0 \\ 0 & \text{other cases} \end{cases} \tag{5-17}$$

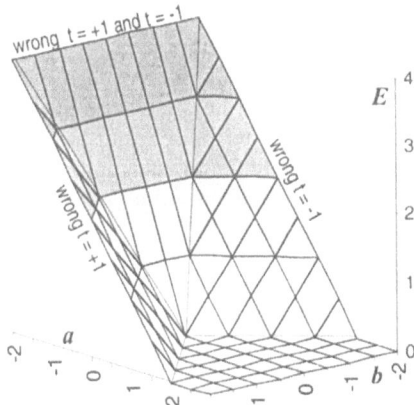

Figure 5.12. Energy surface for the perceptron learning rule in a one-dimensional two-class situation.

Figure 5.12 shows this error surface, exemplifying the piecewise linear nature of the error energy surface for the perceptron learning rule, with jumps whenever a pattern changes from class label.

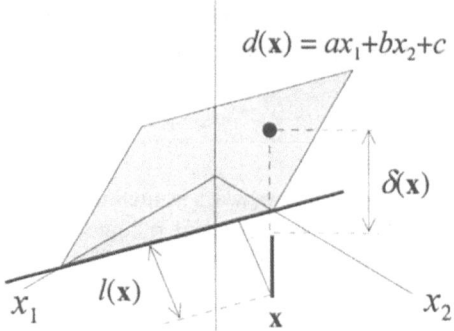

Figure 5.13. Regression error $\delta(\mathbf{x})$ and classification error $E(\mathbf{x})$ with a linear discriminant.

Figure 5.13 illustrates a discriminant function for a two-dimensional problem. The weights have been written a, b and c for simplicity. A feature vector $\mathbf{x}$ is shown with a solid bar representing the target value. For an LMS regression problem, we are interested in minimizing the squared distance $\delta(\mathbf{x})$ to the discriminant function. For a classification problem using the perceptron, we are interested in the distance $l(\mathbf{x})$ to the discriminant surface, i.e., to assess whether or not the pattern is on the "right side of the border".

The simple perceptron learning rule will drive the perceptron into convergence in a finite number of iteration steps if the classes are linearly separable. The reader can find the demonstration of this interesting result in Bishop (1995), for instance. If the classes are not linearly separable, the perceptron learning rule will produce an oscillating discriminant around the borderline patterns.

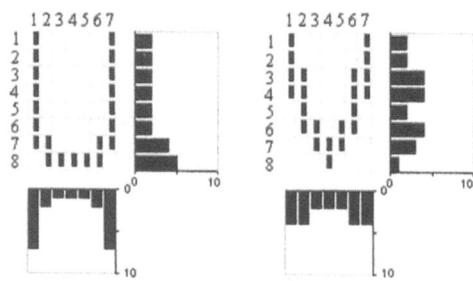

Figure 5.14. Examples of handwritten U and V on a 7x8 grid, with the respective projections.

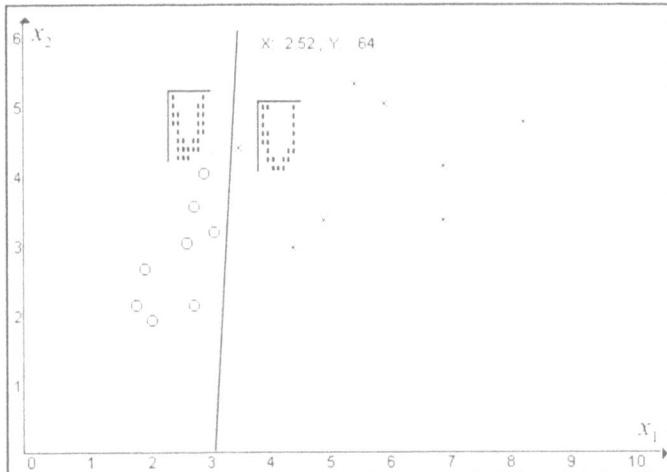

Figure 5.15. Separation of U's (right side) from V's (left side) by a perceptron. Borderline U and V lying near the linear discriminant are also shown.

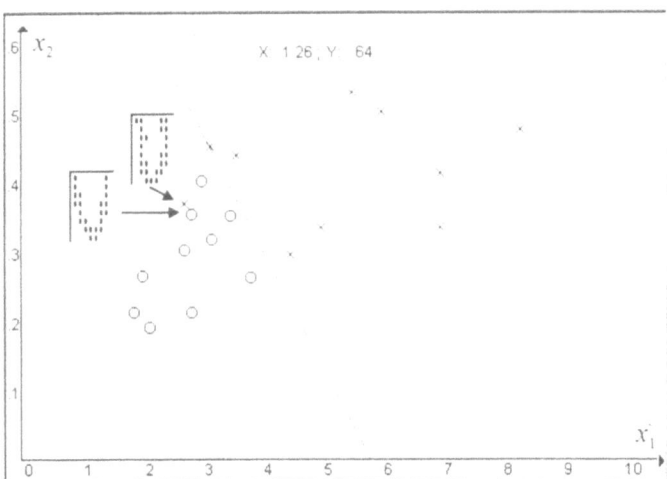

Figure 5.16. Non-separable situation of U's and V's. One of the perceptron's best solutions is shown.

We will illustrate this behaviour using the *Perceptron* program included in the CD (see Appendix B). This program demonstrates the perceptron learning rule for a two-class problem consisting of the discrimination of handwritten U's and V's.

These are written in a 7x8 grid and their images binarised. From the binary images the horizontal (H1 to H8) and vertical (V1 to V7) projections are obtained by counting the dark pixels, as shown in Figure 5.14.

Inspecting these projections for the "prototypes" U and V of Figure 5.14, the following features seem worth trying (other choices are possible):

$$x_1 = (V1+V2+V6+V7) / (V3+V4+V5)$$
$$x_2 = (H7+H8) / (H1+H2+H3+H4+H5+H6)$$

Using a separable set of U's and V's (set 1) the perceptron adjusts a linear discriminant until complete separation, as shown in Figure 5.15. The *Perceptron* program allows learning to be performed in a *pattern-by-pattern* fashion, observing the progress of the discriminant adjustment until convergence.

Using a set of non-separable U's and V's (set 2), the perceptron is unable to converge and oscillates near the border of the U's and V's clusters. Figure 5.16 shows one of the best solutions obtained.

The simple type of decision surfaces that one can achieve with the perceptron is, of course, one of its limitations. Many textbooks illustrate this issue with the classic XOR problem. This consists of separating the two-dimensional patterns shown in Figure 5.17, whose target values correspond to the logical exclusive-or (XOR) of the inputs x_1 and x_2, coding the logical variables as: 1=True, 0=False.

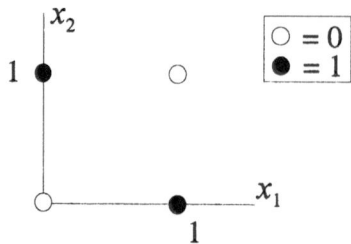

Figure 5.17. The classic XOR problem, often used to illustrate neural classifier performance.

As the two classes of XOR patterns are not linearly separable, it is customary to say that it is not possible to solve this problem with a perceptron. However, we must not forget that we may use transformed features as inputs. For instance, we can use a quadratic transformation of the features. As seen in 2.1.1, we would then need to compute $(d+2)(d+1)/2=6$ new features and use a perceptron with 6 weights:

$$\mathbf{w'x} = w_5 x_1^2 + w_4 x_2^2 + w_3 x_1 x_2 + w_2 x_1 + w_1 x_2 + w_0$$

A little thought shows that by multiplying the original features by 2 and subtracting 1 we convert the original features to the [-1, 1] interval, with the convenient outcome that the product of equal features is now +1, and unequal features −1. Thus, we must have: - $(2x_1 - 1)(2x_2 - 1)$. Therefore, the perceptron with the features and weights of Table 5.1 will solve the XOR problem.

Table 5.1. Features used to solve the XOR problem with a quadratic classifier.

Features	Weights
x_1x_2	-4
x_1	2
x_2	2
bias	-1

For other types of problems requiring complex decision surfaces, such as a generalized version of the U vs. V problem consisting of recognizing all sorts of handwritten characters, one would have to select the appropriate transforming functions of the original features. However, as previously mentioned, this is a difficult selection, with no available rules or guidance except perhaps what a topological analysis of the problem could reveal. Therefore, although the perceptron could in principle solve any classification problem, what we really need is a flexible architecture that can be adapted to any problem. We will see how this is achieved in the following section.

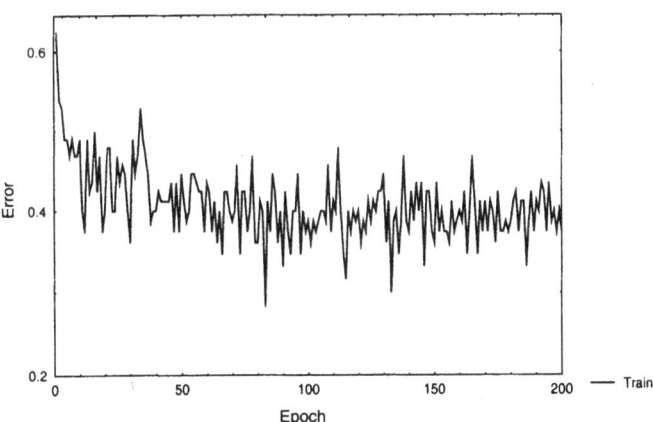

Figure 5.18. Perceptron learning curve for the two-class classification of cork stoppers.

Let us now consider the two-class cork stoppers classification problem, already studied in the previous chapter (features N and PRT10). Using the *Statistica* Neural Networks module we can train a perceptron in order to solve this problem (using a learning rate of 0.5 and a step function as activation function as seen in (5-16a)).

Training the network in batch mode with 200 epochs, we can see in the training error graph of Figure 5.18 (also known as *learning curve*) that the error decreases until stabilizing, always in a jumpy way. The overall classification error is 11%, with 4 misclassifications for class ω_1 and 7 for class ω_2. If we use the logistic function instead of the step function, a smoother convergence and a similar solution is obtained.

When training perceptrons it is customary to scale the inputs, as described in detail in section 5.5.2. The previous solution for the cork stoppers was obtained using a scaling of the inputs to the [0, 1] interval, and computing the following scaled features:

NS = 0.009174xN - 0.1651;   PRT10S = 0.01149xPRT10 - 0.1195.

The perceptron weights computed for these scaled features are:

w_N = - 4.78; w_{PRT10} = 7.68; w_0 = 1.223 (bias).

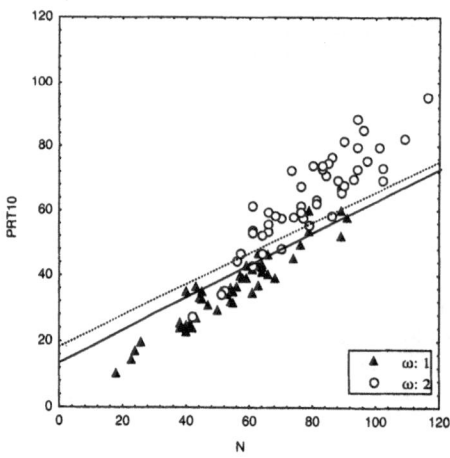

Figure 5.19. Linear discriminants for two classes of cork stoppers. Dotted line: Statistical classifier. Solid line: Perceptron.

Using these weights it is now a simple matter to compute the linear discriminant for the perceptron as:

N - 2xPRT10 - 25.5 = 0.

This linear discriminant is shown in Figure 5.19, with the discriminant derived in section 4.1.3 using a statistical classifier. The similarity is striking. Both discriminants have similar slope. A slight deviation is observed, with the perceptron tending to equalize the misclassifications for both classes.

5.4 Neural Network Types

The neural networks that we have seen in the preceding sections are very simple discriminant devices capable of performing some interesting tasks, as was exemplified. As a matter of fact, with these devices one could in principle succeed in any classification or regression task, provided that one could determine the appropriate transformation functions of the input features, and also the appropriate activation functions. However, this is a difficult task that could also imply, for many problems, having to work in a very high dimensional space. What we need is a generic type of network, which can be easily trained to solve any task. This is achieved by cascading discriminant units, as shown in the *multi-layer perceptron* (MLP) structure of Figure 5.20.

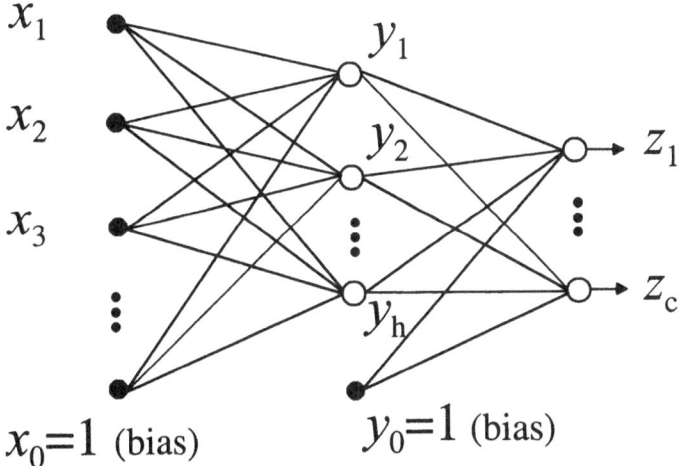

Figure 5.20. Multilayer perceptron structure with input features x_i and output values z_k. An open circle indicates a processing neuron; a solid circle is simply a terminal.

The term multi-layer refers to the existence of several levels or layers of weights in the network. In Figure 5.20 there are two layers of weights: one connecting the input neurons (feature vector **x**) to the so-called *hidden* neurons (hidden-layer vector **y**), and another connecting these to the output neurons (output vector **z**). The previous devices (sections 5.1 and 5.3) with only one layer of weights are also known as *single-layer* networks. Some authors refer to the input level as "input layer", and in this sense the network of Figure 5.20 has three layers instead of two. We prefer, however, to associate the idea of layers with the concept of processing levels, and therefore adopt the above convention. It is customary to denote a neural net by the number of units at each level, from input to output, separated by colons. Thus, a net with 6 inputs, 4 hidden neurons at the first layer and 2 output neurons is denoted a MLP6:4:2 net.

Given an arbitrary neuron with a d-dimensional input vector **s** and output r_j, the computation performed at this neuron is:

$$r_j = f(a_j) = f(\mathbf{w}_j'\mathbf{s}) = f\left(\sum_{i=0}^{d} w_{ji}s_i\right),$$
(5-18)

where w_{ji} denotes the weight corresponding to the connection of the output neuron j to the input neuron i (see Figure 5.21). The function f is any conceivable activation function, namely one of those described in section 5.2. Note, however, that a linear activation function is not of interest for hidden layers, since a composition of linear functions is itself a linear function, and therefore the whole net would be reducible to the single-layer network of Figure 5.1. The quantity a_j is the so-called *neuron activation* or *post-synaptic potential*.

For a multi-layer network it is also possible to have the neurons at each layer performing quite distinct tasks, as we will see in the *radial basis functions* (RBF) and *support vector machine* (SVM) approaches.

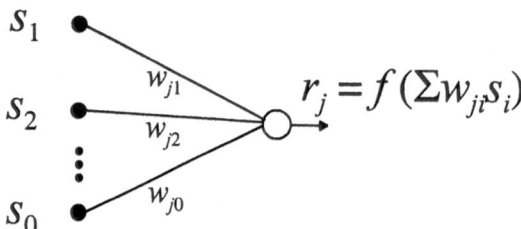

Figure 5.21. A general processing neuron, computing a transformation of the dot product of the weight and input vectors.

Assuming a two-layered network with d-dimensional inputs, h hidden neurons and c outputs, the number of weights, w, that have to be computed, including the biases, is:

$$w = (d+1)h + (h+1)c .$$
(5-19a)

For instance, a two-class six-dimensional problem solved by an MLP6:4:2 involves the computation of 38 weights. The number of these weights, which are the parameters of the neural net, measures its *complexity*. Imagine that we had succeeded in designing an optimal Bayesian linear discriminant for the same two-class six-dimensional problem. The statistical classifier solution demands the computation of two six-dimensional mean vectors plus $d(d+1)/2=21$ elements of the covariance matrix, totalling 33 parameters. Even if the neural net would perfectly mimic the statistical classifier, it represents a more complex and expensive classifier, with more parameters to adjust. Complex classifiers are harder to train adequately and need larger training sets for proper generalization. Whenever possible, a model-based statistical classifier turns out to be simpler than an equivalently performing neural network. Of course, a model-based statistical approach is not always feasible, and the neural network approach is then a sensible choice.

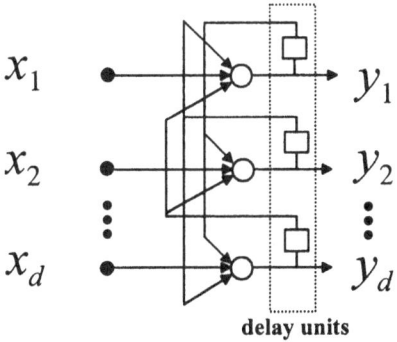

Figure 5.22. A Hopfield network structure with feedback through delay elements.

The MLP network is a *feed-forward* structure, whose only paths are from the inputs to the outputs. It is also possible to have neural net architectures (connectionist structures) with *feedback* paths, connecting outputs to inputs of previous layers through delay elements and without self-feedback, i.e., no neuron output is fed back to its own input. Figure 5.22 shows a *Hopfield* network, an example of such architectures, also called *recurrent* networks, which exhibit non-linear dynamical behaviour with memory properties.

All these types of neural nets are trained in a *supervised* manner, using the pattern classification information of a training set. There are also *unsupervised* types of neural networks, such as the *Kohonen's self organising feature map* (KFM) that we will present in section 5.11.

Table 5.2. Neural net learning rules, with the weight adjustment formulas and examples of networks using the rules.

Rule	Weight adjustment	Network type
Least Mean Square	$\Delta\mathbf{w} = -\eta\left(\mathbf{w'}\,\mathbf{x}_i - t_i\right)\mathbf{x}_i$	MLP
Perceptron	$\Delta\mathbf{w} = -\tfrac{1}{2}\left(h(\mathbf{w'}\,\mathbf{x}) - t_i\right)\mathbf{x}_i$	Perceptron
Hebb	$\Delta w_{ij} = \eta x_{k,i} x_{k,j}$	Hopfield
Winner Takes All	$\Delta w_{ij} = -\eta\left(w_{ij} - x_j\right)$	Kohonen

As there is a large diversity of neural nets, with various architectures and different types of processing neurons, it is no surprise that there are also many types of *learning rules* for the weight adjustment process. Table 5.2 shows some of these learning rules.

The LMS and perceptron learning rules, as previously described, basically consist in the addition of a corrective increment proportional to the value of the wrongly classified pattern and the deviation (error) from the target value.

The Hebb learning rule, one of the earliest and simplest learning rules, is based on the idea of reinforcing the connection weight of two neurons if they are both "on" (+1) at the same time. Using a corrective increment proportional to the multiplication of the respective neuron outputs reinforces the connection weight when the neurons are both "on" or "off" (-1) at the same time.

The winner-takes-all rule is characteristic of a class of networks exhibiting *competition* among the neurons in order to arrive at a decision. In the case of the Kohonen network, the decision is made by determining which neuron best "represents" a certain input pattern. The weight increment reflects the "distance" of the current weight value from the input value.

An introductory taxonomy and description of basic architectures and learning rules can be found in Lippmann (1987). A detailed description of these matters can be found in Fausett (1994).

There is a close resemblance and relation between some neural network approaches and statistical approaches described in the previous chapter, as summarized in Table 5.3. This resemblance will become clear when we present, in the following sections, the neural nets listed on this table.

Table 5.3. Relations between neural net and statistical approaches.

NN approach	MLP	RBF	KFM
Related statistical approach	Bayesian classifier	Parzen window	k-means clustering

5.5 Multi-Layer Perceptrons

In the previous section we presented the feed-forward multi-layer perceptron, whose diagram is shown in Figure 5.20. This type of network is capable of more complex mappings than the single-layer perceptron and, for differentiable activation functions, there exists a powerful algorithm for finding a minimum error solution based on the gradient descent concept, called *error back-propagation*.

Let us first see what kinds of mappings a multi-layer perceptron is capable of, using a constructive argument (Lippman, 1987) for MLPs with activation functions of the threshold type, with outputs 0, 1.

With a single-layer perceptron only one linear discriminant can be implemented, as illustrated in Figure 5.23a for the *MLP Sets* dataset.

Let us now consider the two-layer perceptron of Figure 5.20. Each neuron of the hidden layer implements a linear discriminant. Assuming that the bias of the output neuron, with h hidden neurons, has a value in $]-h, -h+1[$, then the output neuron will produce the value 1 only when all hidden neurons are 1. This corresponds to the intersection (AND operation) of the half-planes produced by the hidden neurons in the 1-value side, as exemplified in Figure 5.23b. We can perform the AND operation in the second layer, upon the discriminants obtained from the first layer, thereby building arbitrarily complex convex regions.

With a three-layer network we can arrange for the first two layers to generate a sufficiently fine grid of hypercubes by using $2d$ hidden units in the first layer for each hypercube (a square in $d=2$ space needs 4 hidden units). Next, we can arrange for the output neuron to perform the reunion (OR operation) of the hypercubes of the second layer neurons using a bias in $]0, 1[$ (e.g. 0.5). The output neuron will "fire" if any of the second layer neurons "fire". In Figure 5.23c we apply this OR operation at the third layer to merge the disjointed clusters. Hence, three-layer networks can generate any arbitrarily complex mapping involving concave or disjointed regions.

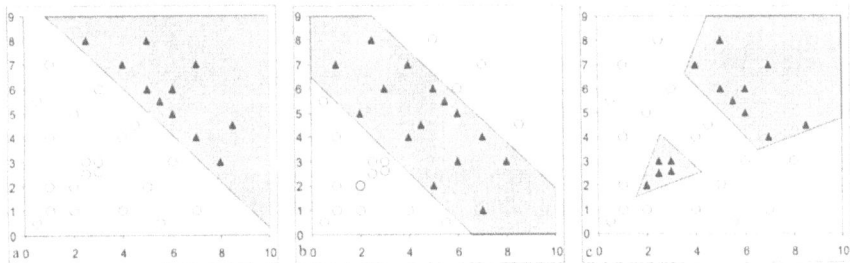

Figure 5.23. Three sets of two class points classifiable by: (a) Single-layer perceptron; (b) Two-layer perceptron; (c) Three-layer perceptron.

Notice that this is a purely constructive argument that justifies why a three-layer network can achieve any arbitrarily complex mapping. It does not mean that MLPs, using any appropriate learning algorithm, will necessarily converge to a solution built with the AND operation at the second layer and the OR operation at the third layer, although, for simple problems they sometimes do (see Exercise 5.7). As a matter of fact, training an MLP2:2:1 with logistic activation functions for the set shown in Figure 5-23b, the first layer weights shown in Table 5.4 were determined. It is a simple matter to confirm that the straight lines implemented by these first layer hidden neurons do indeed correspond to the boundaries of the shaded area in Figure 5.23b, and that for this pattern set the constructive argument is verified.

Although there are decision boundaries that cannot be exactly implemented with two-layer networks, it can be proved that two-layer networks with sigmoidal activation functions can approximate, with arbitrary closeness, any decision boundary (see e.g. Bishop, 1995). Therefore, we will pay more attention to two-layer networks, in particular in what concerns the complexity issue discussed in section 5.6.4.

Table 5.4. Weights obtained for a MLP2:2:1 and dataset of Figure 5.23b.

	Bias	w_1	w_2
Hidden neuron 1	-13.000	9.7278	9.3740
Hidden neuron 2	-8.3262	11.688	10.9780

5.5.1 The Back-Propagation Algorithm

The first and most popular weight adjustment algorithm for the multi-layer perceptron was invented by Rummelhart *et al.* (1986). We will proceed to explain its main steps for a network with two layers, denoting by i, j and k respectively the indices for inputs ($\mathbf{x}$), hidden neurons ($\mathbf{y}$) and output neurons ($\mathbf{z}$).

Let us first rewrite formula (5-2a), concerning the error obtained at an output neuron k, for any input pattern, in a simplified way:

$$E = \frac{1}{2}\left(z_k - t_k\right)^2 , \tag{5-20}$$

where z_k denotes the neuron output.

As seen in (5-18), each neuron of a multi-layer perceptron computes an output that is a function of the dot product of the weight vector and the input vector. We then have for hidden neurons and output neurons:

$$h_j = f(a_j) \equiv f(\mathbf{w}_j{}'\mathbf{x}) ; \tag{5-20a}$$

$$z_k = f(b_k) \equiv f(\mathbf{w}_k{}'\mathbf{y}) . \tag{5-20b}$$

In order to apply the gradient descent concept to the multi-layer perceptron we first have to compute the derivatives of the error as functions of the weights. The derivative of the error as a function of any weight can be written using the chain-rule of partial derivatives, as follows:

$$\frac{\partial E}{\partial w_{ji}} = \frac{\partial E}{\partial a_j}\frac{\partial a_j}{\partial w_{ji}} \; ; \tag{5-21a}$$

$$\frac{\partial E}{\partial w_{kj}} = \frac{\partial E}{\partial b_k}\frac{\partial b_k}{\partial w_{kj}} \; . \tag{5-21b}$$

Note that on the right side of these formulas the first term represents the derivative depending on the activation function, whereas the second term depends only on the dot product, $\mathbf{w}_j'\mathbf{x}$ and $\mathbf{w}_k'\mathbf{y}$, respectively, for the hidden neurons and for the output neurons. The derivatives with respect to w_{ji} and to w_{kj} are simply x_i and h_j, respectively. Therefore, the first term has a decisive contribution to the error and we will denote it as follows:

$$\delta_j = \frac{\partial E}{\partial a_j} \; ; \tag{5-22a}$$

$$\delta_k = \frac{\partial E}{\partial b_k} \; . \tag{5-22b}$$

Let us now compute the error terms δ_j and δ_k. For the output neuron z_k we just have to apply (5-20b) to the error formula, yielding:

$$\delta_k = \frac{\partial E}{\partial b_k} = f'(b_k)\frac{\partial E}{\partial z_k} = f'(b_k)(z_k - t_k) \; . \tag{5-23a}$$

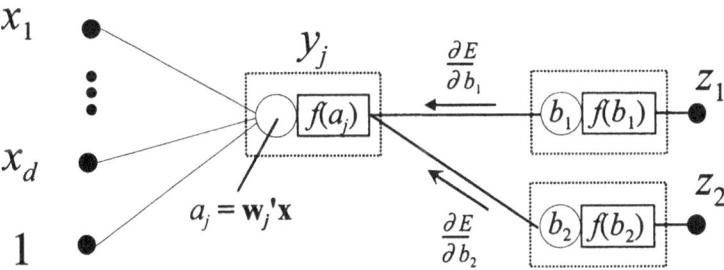

Figure 5.24. A hidden neuron y_j receiving the back-propagated errors from two output neurons.

For a hidden neuron the error term δ_j is more difficult to obtain since it depends on the errors at the output neurons it is connected to, as exemplified in Figure 5.24. For this purpose we express δ_j as a summation of chained derivatives:

$$\delta_j = \frac{\partial E}{\partial a_j} = \sum_{k=1}^{c} \frac{\partial E}{\partial b_k} \frac{\partial b_k}{\partial a_j} . \tag{5-23b}$$

Note that the first term in the summation corresponds to the back-propagated error from an output (δ_k), and the second term reflects the influence of the activation function of the hidden neurons, as well as the weights connecting the hidden neuron to the output neurons. Assuming that all activation functions are equal we can therefore write:

$$\delta_j = f'(a_j) \sum_{k=1}^{c} w_{kj} \delta_k . \tag{5-23c}$$

Notice how the error terms at the output neurons contribute to the error terms at the hidden neurons. This back-propagation of the errors justifies the name of the algorithm.

Using these errors and the gradient descent equations (5-7) we can now write the formulas for updating the weights.

– Weight connecting output neuron k with hidden neuron j:

$$w_{kj}^{(r+1)} = w_{kj}^{(r)} - \eta \delta_k h_j . \tag{5-24a}$$

– Weight connecting hidden neuron j with input neuron i:

$$w_{ji}^{(r+1)} = w_{ji}^{(r)} - \eta \delta_j x_i \tag{5-24b}$$

For more than two layers, the process of error back-propagation generalizes easily using the back-propagation formula (5-23c).

The back-propagation algorithm uses formulas (5-24a) and (5-24b) with initial random weights until the iterative gradient descent process reaches a minimum of the energy function. The error hypersurface of a multi-layer perceptron depends on several weight parameters, and is therefore expected to be quite complex and to possibly have many local minima. Notice that such a simple problem as the one presented in Figure 5.4 already exhibited local minima. Usually many trials have to be performed, with different initial weights and learning factor η, in order to reach the global minimum. Also, for large learning factors, one may obtain divergent behaviour or wild oscillations around the minimum, as previously mentioned in the ECG filter example in section 5.1. As a remedy to this oscillating behaviour it is normal to include a *momentum term* in the weight updating formulas, dependent upon the weight increment in the previous iteration, as follows:

$$w_{kj}^{(r+1)} = w_{kj}^{(r)} - \eta \delta_k h_j + \alpha \Delta w_{kj}^{(r)} \; ; \tag{5-25a}$$

$$w_{ji}^{(r+1)} = w_{ji}^{(r)} - \eta \delta_j y_i + \alpha \Delta w_{ji}^{(r)} . \tag{5-25b}$$

This momentum term, with *momentum factor* α, tends to speed up the network convergence, while at the same time avoiding oscillations. It acts in the same way as the mass of a particle falling on a surface in a viscous medium: away from a minimum the mass of the particle increases the speed along its downward trajectory; near the minimum it dampens the oscillations around it. Similarly the momentum term increases the learning rate in regions of low curvature and decreases it in high curvature regions, therefore reducing oscillations in these regions (for details see Qiang, 1999).

The previous weight updating formulas assume a pattern-by-pattern operation mode. Usually it is more efficient to compute the errors for all the patterns and update the weights using formulas with these total errors. This is the so-called *batch* training, already mentioned in section 5.1. An iteration using all of the available data is called an *epoch*, and the training is conducted by repeating the weight updating process in a sufficiently large number of epochs.

5.5.2 Practical aspects

When training multi-layer perceptrons, and other types of neural nets as well, several practical aspects must be taken into account; these, are described next.

Feature and architecture selection

When designing a neural net, one usually has to perform feature selection in the same way as when designing statistical classifiers. However, the classical search methods are more difficult or cumbersome to apply in the case of neural nets for two reasons: for a given architecture, any configuration of features at the network inputs demands a lengthy training process; for a given configuration of features at the network inputs, the performance of the network depends on the architecture used. Therefore, feature set and architecture work together in a coupled way. Concerning the first issue, we will later present a feature selection method based on genetic algorithms, which is quite fast and often produces quite good results. Regarding the second issue, one may implement searching schemes for the "best" solution in a domain of interesting architectures. This is the approach implemented in *Statistica* under the name of Intelligent Problem Solver (IPS): once we have specified the type of network, the range of features and some constraints on the architecture such as the number of hidden nodes, the IPS will automatically search for the "best" solutions.

Pre-processing

Because of the saturation effect of the most popular activation functions, namely the sigmoidal functions, it is advisable to scale all inputs to a convenient range, otherwise the inputs with higher values will drive the training process, masking the contribution of lower valued inputs. Also, the choice of appropriate initial weights depends on the interval range of the inputs; with weights far away from that range the convergence time can increase significantly.

In general the pre-processing of the inputs consists of performing a linear feature scaling in such a way that all of them occupy the [0, 1] or [-1, 1] interval.

Post-processing

Post-processing operations are related to the application of neural nets for classification purposes. In this situation it is usually convenient to code the outputs as nominal variables, whose values are class labels.

In two-class classification problems one may use a single output, coded as a two-state variable (e.g. -1, +1). When there are more than two classes it is more appropriate to have one output for each class, with one nominal value representing the class decision. For instance, for three classes one would have three outputs with nominal values $\{+1, -1\}$ corresponding to the class decisions $\omega_1=(+1, -1, -1)$, $\omega_2=(-1, +1, -1)$ and $\omega_3=(-1, -1, +1)$. Network output values can be converted to the proper nominal value using thresholds. By setting up appropriate threshold values one can also define reject regions, as done in section 4.2.3. Output thresholding is easily performed using step functions.

Number of hidden neurons

In practical applications one rarely encounters architectures more complex than a two-layer network, which, as we have seen, is capable of producing solutions arbitrarily close to the optimal one. For datasets that are hard to train with two-layer networks, a three-layer solution can be tried, usually with a low number of hidden neurons (2 or 3) in the third layer. Concerning the number of hidden neurons in the first layer, it can be proved (Bishop, 1995) that their role is to perform a dimensional reduction, much in the way of the Fisher discriminant transformation described in section 4.1.4. It is expected, therefore, that their number will be near the number of significant eigenvectors of the data covariance matrix. Bearing this in mind, it must be said that there is no fast guiding rule that will substitute for experimentation.

Learning parameters

As previously seen, the learning rate controls how large the weight adjustment is in each iteration. A large learning rate may lead to faster convergence, but may also cause strong oscillations near the optimal solution, or even divergence. It is normal to choose values below 0.5, and for non-trivial problems it is advisable to use a decreasing learning rate, finishing with a small value after a large number of epochs.

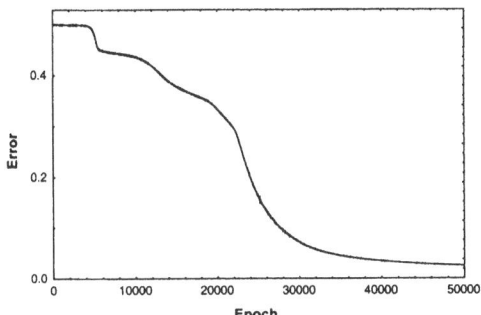

Figure 5.25. Learning curve for the dataset represented in Figure 5.23c. More than 20000 epochs are needed for a definite convergence path.

The momentum factor is chosen in the range [0, 1[, and it is advisable to decrease it during training.

Note that when a class is represented by very few patterns, it may take a long time to train before the optimal solution is reached. This is a consequence of the fact that the error energy will then suffer a small influence from the errors relative to the poorly represented class. This effect is exemplified by the set 3 training of the *MLP Sets* data (Figure 5.23c), as illustrated in Figure 5.25. A convergence to the global minimum, using a MLP2:4:2:1, was observed in one trial only after more that 20000 iterations. For some initial values of the learning parameters no convergence was observed. In such difficult cases it is advisable to use small training factors. In the case of Figure 5.25 a value of 0.02 was used.

Local minima

In order to avoid local minima of the energy function, one can run several training experiments with different specifications for the initial weights and the learning and momentum factors. The number of experiments, r, with different random starting weights, needed to ensure that a network will reach a solution within a desirable lower percentile of all possible experiments is given by (Iyer and Rhinehart, 1999):

$$r = \frac{ln(1-\alpha)}{ln(1-p)},$$

(5-26)

where p is the percentile and α is the confidence level.

For instance, if we want to ensure with confidence $\alpha = 99\%$ that we will reach a solution among the best $p = 20\%$, we will need to perform $r = \ln(1-0.99)/\ln(1-0.2) \approx 20$ experiments.

Besides repeating experiments, there are other techniques that can achieve good results:

- Case shuffling: by shuffling the cases in each epoch, we hope that the network tries alternative descent routes, and avoids getting stuck in a path leading to a local minimum.
- Adding noise: by adding a small amount of random noise to the inputs in each epoch, we hope that a similar effect to case shuffling is achieved, namely the exploration of alternative descent routes. Noise can also provide better generalization of the neural net, preventing it from over-fitting the training set.
- Jogging weights: by adding a small random quantity to the weights it may be possible to avoid a local minimum.

Dimensionality ratio and generalization

If we train a network with arbitrarily complex architecture we may also obtain arbitrarily low errors for the training data, since we are attempting to model exactly the structure of the training data by the neural network. As we have already seen in previous chapters, the real issue is to obtain a solution that performs equally well (on average) in independent test sets. Once more we are confronted with a *dimensionality ratio* issue, here under the form of n/w, n being the total number of patterns in the training set and w the total number of weights to adjust. If w is too small we may obtain a neural net that is under-fitted; if w is too big it may be over-fitted. The criteria for choosing an appropriate dimensionality ratio n/w are not guided by exact formulas as in statistical classification, but rather by some intricate combinatorial considerations about the number of partitions achieved by a neural net, the main results of which will be presented in section 5.6.

It is common practice, in order to avoid over-fitting (except for trivial problems), to reserve a part of the available data for independent *verification* or *validation* purposes during training. At each epoch, the neural net solution is applied to this set and the corresponding graph inspected. When degradation of the validation set error is detected, it is assumed that some over-fitting is present and the training is stopped.

Let us illustrate this aspect with the cork stoppers classification problem for three classes. We divide each available dataset per class into approximately one half of the cases for training, a quarter for validation and another quarter for testing. Next we apply the back-propagation algorithm to an MLP7:5:3 (58 weights), having 7 features (the 10-feature set except NG, PRTG, RAAR) as inputs. The neural network has three nominal outputs corresponding to the three classes. Figure 5.26 shows how the validation error starts degrading after a certain number of epochs, around 500. This means that after this point the neural net is over-fitting the training data and losing the capacity to generalize to other independent sets. We should therefore stop the training around 500 epochs.

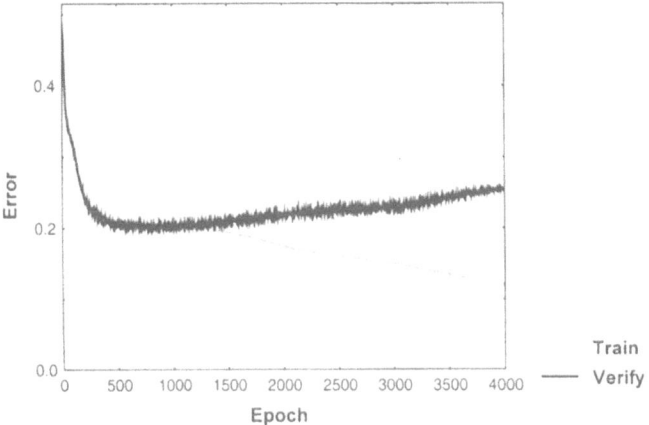

Figure 5.26. Learning curve for the cork stoppers data (3 classes) with a MLP7:5:3. Notice the error degradation for the verification set after approximately 500 epochs.

Choosing the best neural net solution can be quite a tedious job since one has to try several architectures and starting conditions. As previously mentioned, *Statistica* has a helpful IPS tool that allows the user to perform a series of experiments and retain the best solutions, which are displayed at the end in a sorted way. Using this tool it was possible to find an MLP2:2:3 solution with features N and PRT and a much lower number of weights (15), which after training with 200 epochs performed similarly. This is shown in Table 5.5 for the training, verification and test sets. In this and other examples the logistic sigmoid was always used as activation function. Selection of cases for training, validation and test sets is always performed randomly.

Table 5.5. MLP2:2:3 classification matrices of three classes of cork stoppers. True classification along the rows; predicted classification along the columns.

	Training				Validation				Test		
	ω_1	ω_2	ω_3		ω_1	ω_2	ω_3		ω_1	ω_2	ω_3
ω_1	23	2	0	ω_1	12	0	0	ω_1	13	0	0
ω_2	2	20	2	ω_2	1	12	2	ω_2	2	8	1
ω_3	0	0	24	ω_3	0	0	12	ω_3	0	1	13

The training set, validation set and test set errors for this experiment with the MLP2:2:3 are 8.2%, 7.7% and 10.5%, respectively. When conducting an experiment with small datasets and/or low dimensionality ratios, it is advisable not to trust just one run. Instead, several runs should be performed using randomised sets or the partition method explained in section 4.5. When performing ten runs with the cork stoppers data, by randomly shuffling the cases, we obtained different solutions regarding the relative value of the errors, all with small deviations from the previously mentioned results. This is, of course, a good indication that the neural net is not over-fitting the data. Table 5.6 summarizes the results of these ten runs.

Table 5.6. Statistical results of ten randomised runs with the MLP2:2:3.

	Training	Validation	Test
Average error	10.5	9.2	10.3
Standard deviation	2.8	3.4	3.9

From these results we can obtain a better idea of the attainable network performance, and conclude that the overall error should be near 10% with approximately 3% standard deviation.

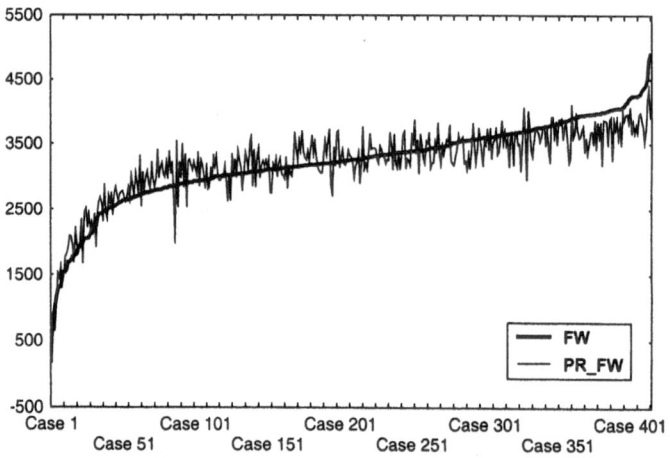

Figure 5.27. Predicted foetal weight (PR_FW) using an MLP3:6:1 trained with the back-propagation algorithm. The FW curve represents the true foetal weight values.

Let us now consider a regression application of multi-layer perceptrons. For this purpose we use the *Foetal Weight* dataset, with the aim of predicting the foetal weight of 414 newborns based on measurements obtained from echographic examination of the foetus. Using *Statistica*'s intelligent problem solver an MLP3:6:1 neural net was found with good performance, using features BPD, AP, FL as inputs. This neural net was trained with the back-propagation algorithm using 100 epochs with learning rate 0.02 and momentum 0.3. In one run the RMS errors (see definition in 5.6.1) obtained were respectively 284.4 g for the training set (207 cases), 275.4 g for the verification set (103 cases) and 289.8 g for the test set (104 cases). High correlations (about 86%) between true and predicted values were found for the three sets.

The proximity of the error figures and correlation values in several runs is an indication of convergence without over or under-fitting and adequacy of the set sizes. The regression solution does indeed perform quite well as shown in Figure 5.27, where the 414 cases are sorted by increasing value.

5.5.3 Time Series

One particularly interesting type of regression problem with multiple practical applications is time series forecasting. In this type of problem one has a sequence of data and wishes to forecast the value of one or more of its variables, some steps ahead. The sequence of data is typically a time series, such as daily weather parameters, daily river flow or share values in the stock exchange market, but can also be any other type of sequence, temporal or not.

Recurrent networks are especially appropriate for this kind of application. A typical problem is the one of estimating the value of one variable z one step ahead, i.e., at time $t+1$, $z(t+1)$, based on its present value and values of other influencing variables $\mathbf{x}(t)$, called *external variables*:

$$z(t+1) = f(z(t), \mathbf{x}(t)), \text{ or equivalently } z(t) = f(z(t-1), \mathbf{x}(t-1)). \tag{5-27}$$

This autoregressive estimation can be performed using a recurrent multi-layer perceptron with a loop feeding back the output z to the input vector, with a one-unit delay. Of course one can also use a k-unit delay, then having a forecast of $z(t + k)$, k steps ahead. It is also possible to have several network outputs fed back to the inputs in multi-variable forecasting.

Recurrent networks are trained in the same way as other networks. However, the feedback loops, as is well known from control theory, may sometimes cause an oscillation effect with rapid divergence of the neural net weights. This divergent behaviour imposes low learning rates and also a limitation on the number of feedback loops. In order to choose the most appropriate neural net for time series forecast, namely which external variables can be of use, it is recommended to first study the normal regression solution, i.e. to regress z based on $\mathbf{x}$.

As a first example of time series forecast we will consider the *Stock Exchange* data (see Appendix A), and set as our task the prediction of firm SONAE share values one day ahead. This type of regression problem was already considered in section 1.2.2 (see Figure 1.5). The time series available covers a period of over one year (June 1, 1999 until August 31, 2000).

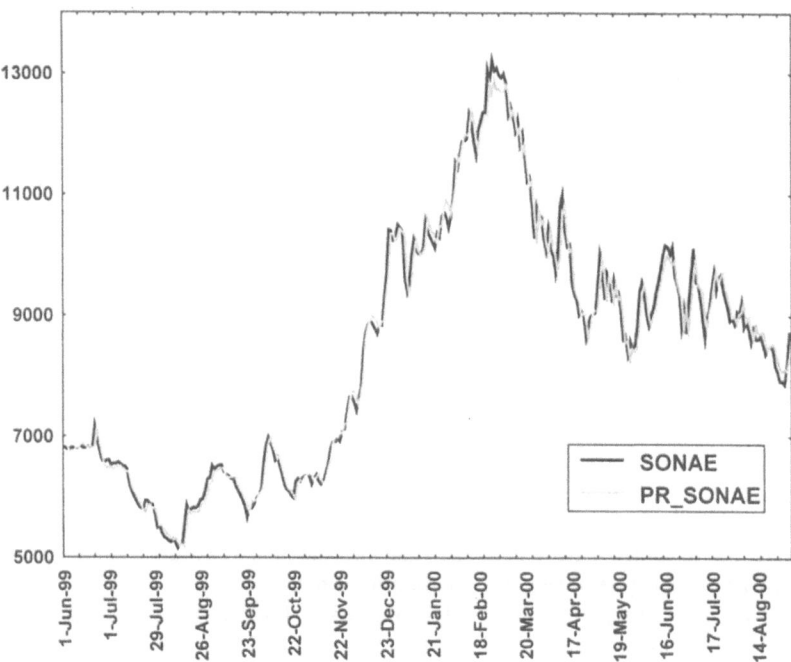

Figure 5.28. Prediction of SONAE share values one day ahead, using a multi-layer perceptron with eight external variables.

Using *Statistica's* intelligent problem solver, an MLP11:4:1 solution was found with good performance when trained with the back-propagation algorithm (correlation over 0.98). This solution used all features except BVL30 and USD. It was found afterwards that it was possible to remove features EURIBOR and BCP with a decrease of the errors. Figure 5.28 shows the predicted value of SONAE shares one day ahead, using a recurrent MLP9:4:1, with eight external variables and SONAE($t - 1$) as extra input. The average RMS error is about 2%. The average absolute deviation is below 39 Escudos, with nearly half of the predictions deviating less than 130 Escudos. Using two steps recurrent inputs it was possible to lower the average RMS error to below 1.5, % with more than half of the cases deviating less than 90 Escudos.

As a second example of time series forecasting we attempt to forecast one day ahead the temperature in Oporto at 12H00, using the *Weather* data covering the period of January 1, 1999 until August 23, 2000. With the help of *Statistica's* intelligent problem solver, an MLP3:3:1 solution was found with features H (relative humidity) and NS (North-South component of the wind) as external variables. Forecast one day ahead was achieved with average RMS error of 8%, and more than half of the cases had absolute deviations between true values and predicted values of the temperature lower than 2° C.

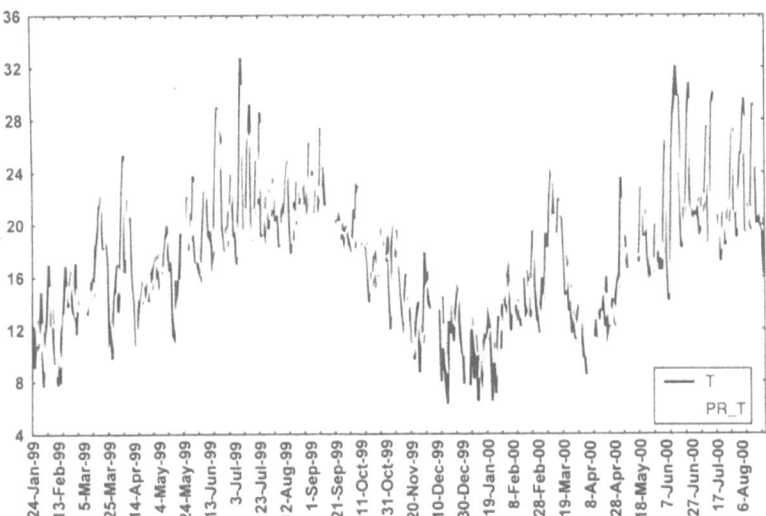

Figure 5.29. Temperature (°C) forecast (Oporto, 12H00), two days ahead, using a multi-layer perceptron with two external variables (relative humidity and North-South wind component).

The following two days ahead prediction of the temperature, $T(t)$, was also tested:

$$T(t) = f\big(T(t-1), T(t-2), \mathbf{x}(t-1), \mathbf{x}(t-2)\big) . \tag{5-28}$$

The multi-layer perceptron implementing this approach achieved, as expected, a better forecast performance with more than half of the cases having absolute deviations lower than 1.5°. This is the solution corresponding to Figure 5.29. Notice that the higher deviations occur when data losses occur; after that the MLP tracks in the incoming data with high performance. Data losses can substantially decrease the prediction performance in time series forecast.

5.6 Performance of Neural Networks

5.6.1 Error Measures

There are several indexes used to evaluate and compare the performance of neural net solutions in classification problems. Most of them are related to the squared error measure defined in (5-2). Considering the individual errors $e_i = z_i - t_i$, of n patterns, the following performance indexes are quite popular:

Error mean:
$$m_e = \frac{1}{n} \sum_{i=1}^{n} e_i \qquad (5\text{-}29a)$$

Absolute error mean:
$$m_{|e|} = \frac{1}{n} \sum_{i=1}^{n} |e_i| \qquad (5\text{-}29b)$$

Relative error:
$$E_{rel} = \frac{1}{n} \sum_{i=1}^{n} |e_i| / |x_i| \qquad (5\text{-}29c)$$

Average squared error:
$$E = \frac{1}{n} \sum_{i=1}^{n} e_i^2 \qquad (5\text{-}29d)$$

Root mean square (RMS) error:
$$E_{RMS} = \sqrt{E} \qquad (5\text{-}29e)$$

Error standard deviation:
$$s_e = \frac{1}{(n-1)} \sqrt{\sum_{i=1}^{n} (e_i - m_e)^2} \qquad (5\text{-}29f)$$

The average squared error is the squared error divided by the number of patterns. Note its relation with formula (5-2a). A problem when comparing neural net classifiers using E and E_{RMS} is the dependence of these indexes on the threshold values of the output activation functions. In some cases it may be advisable to evaluate these indexes only for the misclassified cases, using the threshold value as target value.

The standard deviation of the errors is useful for ranking the solution obtained. In regression problems a good solution should have, besides a high correlation between predicted and true values, a standard deviation of the errors, s_e, at least about an order of magnitude lower than the standard deviation of the target values, s_t, otherwise the regression solution is completely erratic. For instance, for the

Stock Exchange data the standard deviation of the SONAE shares values is 2070 Escudos, whereas for the prediction errors, it is only 224 Escudos.

As a matter of fact, a good ranking index for neural networks comparison is:

$$s_{e/t} = \frac{s_e}{s_t},$$ (5-29f)

This is a normalized index, with value in the [0, 1] interval for all networks, therefore affording more insight when comparing networks. For instance, for the previous *Stock Exchange* figures, $s_{e/t} = 0.11$ represents a good regression solution. Another possibility for comparison of NN solutions is the use of the ROC curve area method, described in section 4.3.3.

Estimation of confidence intervals for neural network errors can be done in a "model-free" approach, as indicated in section 4.5. As seen in that section, confidence intervals obtained by this "model-free" approach can be unrealistically large. More realistic confidence intervals are harder to compute. The respective formulas were derived by Chryssolouris *et al.* (1996) using the so-called Jacobian matrix of the neural network, a matrix whose elements are the derivatives of the network outputs with respect to the inputs.

It is interesting to see the implications of using the squared error criterion for MLP training. For this purpose let us imagine that we have obtained output functions z_k, modelling each class of the input data, such that the target values differ from z_k by an error e_k:

$$t_k(\mathbf{x}_i) = z_k(\mathbf{x}_i) + e_k(\mathbf{x}_i).$$ (5-30)

For a given training set X with n patterns and target set T, assuming that the distributions of the target values conditioned by the patterns $p(t_k(\mathbf{x}_i)|\mathbf{x}_i)$ are independent, we can compute the likelihood of the dataset in a similar way as we did in (4-22):

$$p(X,T) = \sum_{k=1}^{c} \prod_{i=1}^{n} p(t_k(\mathbf{x}_i)|\mathbf{x}_i) p(\mathbf{x}_i).$$ (5-31)

Assuming Gaussian errors with zero mean and equal variance σ, and since the z_k are deterministic, the logarithm of the likelihood is:

$$\ln p(X,T) = \frac{1}{2\sigma^2} \sum_{k=1}^{c} \sum_{i=1}^{n} (t_k(\mathbf{x}_i) - z_k(\mathbf{x}_i))^2 + \text{constant} = \frac{E}{\sigma^2} + \text{constant} ,$$ (5-32)

where E is the error energy expressed as in (5-2a).

We conclude that minimizing the squared error is equivalent to finding out the output functions that maximize the likelihood of the training set. By analysing the relations between E and the data probability distributions, it is also possible to conclude that (see Bishop, 1995):

1. With $n \to \infty$, the error E converges to a minimum corresponding to:

$$z_k(\mathbf{x}) = \int_{T_k} t_k(\mathbf{x}) p(t_k(\mathbf{x})|\mathbf{x}) dt_k(\mathbf{x}) ,$$

(5-33)

where $z_k(\mathbf{x})$ is the regression solution for the training set T_k of target values for the class ω_k. The integral (5-33) is also known as the *conditional average of the target data* and denoted $E[t_k | \mathbf{x}]$.

2. The minimization of E corresponds to the hidden neurons transforming the input data in a way similar to the Fisher discriminant described in section 4.1.4. Therefore, the outputs are obtained as linear combinations in a reduced dimensionality space, obtained by a Fisher discriminant-like transformation.

3. The multi-layer perceptron outputs are the class posterior probabilities for sigmoid activation functions and Gaussian distributions of the patterns (generalization of (5-12b)). Therefore, in this situation we have a neural net solution equivalent to the statistical classification solution. For other types of distributions it is also possible to easily obtain the posterior probabilities.

5.6.2 The Hessian Matrix

The learning capabilities of MLP's, using the minimization of a squared error measure E, depend in many ways on the second order derivatives of E as functions of the weights. These second order derivatives are the elements of the *Hessian matrix* $\mathbf{H}$ of the error:

$$\mathbf{H} = [h_{ij}] \quad \text{with} \quad h_{ij} = \frac{\partial^2 E}{\partial w_i \partial w_j} ,$$

(5-34)

where w_i and w_j are any weights of the network.

The Hessian is a symmetric positive semi-definite matrix, and plays an important role in several optimisation approaches to MLP training, as well as in the convergence process towards a minimum error solution. In order to ascertain this last aspect, let us assume that we had computed the eigenvectors $\mathbf{u}_i$ and eigenvalues λ_i of the Hessian, in a similar way to what we have done for the covariance matrix in section 2.3:

$$\mathbf{H}\mathbf{u}_i = \lambda_i \mathbf{u}_i .$$

(5-35)

Next, we proceed to compute a second order approximation of the error energy function at a point w^*, using Taylor series expansion around that point:

$$E(\mathbf{w}) = E(\mathbf{w}^*) + (\mathbf{w} - \mathbf{w}^*)' \frac{\partial E}{\partial \mathbf{w}} \Big|_{w^*} + \frac{1}{2}(\mathbf{w} - \mathbf{w}^*)' \mathbf{H}(\mathbf{w} - \mathbf{w}^*). \tag{5-36}$$

At a minimum of E the gradient is zero, therefore the linear term vanishes and the approximation becomes:

$$E(\mathbf{w}) = E(\mathbf{w}^*) + \frac{1}{2}(\mathbf{w} - \mathbf{w}^*)' \mathbf{H}(\mathbf{w} - \mathbf{w}^*). \tag{5-37}$$

This approximation has a local gradient given by:

$$\frac{\partial E}{\partial \mathbf{w}} = \mathbf{H}(\mathbf{w} - \mathbf{w}^*). \tag{5-37a}$$

Let us now expand $\mathbf{w} - \mathbf{w}^*$ as a linear combination of the eigenvectors, which, as seen in section 2.3, form an orthonormal basis:

$$\mathbf{w} - \mathbf{w}^* = \sum_{i=1}^{w} \alpha_i \mathbf{u}_i. \tag{5-38}$$

Since the eigenvectors are orthonormal, when multiplying both terms of (5-38) by $\mathbf{u}_i'$ we obtain:

$$\mathbf{u}_i'(\mathbf{w} - \mathbf{w}^*) = \alpha_i, \tag{5-38a}$$

which allows us to interpret the α_i as the distance to the minimum $\mathbf{w}^*$ along the direction $\mathbf{u}_i$.

From (5-38) it is also easy to compute the weight updating as:

$$\Delta \mathbf{w} = \sum_{i=1}^{w} \Delta \alpha_i \mathbf{u}_i. \tag{5-38b}$$

On the other hand, substituting (5-35) and (5-38) in (5-37a), we obtain:

$$\frac{\partial E}{\partial \mathbf{w}} = \sum_{i=1}^{w} \alpha_i \lambda_i \mathbf{u}_i. \tag{5-39}$$

From the gradient descent formula (5-7) we know that

$$\Delta \mathbf{w} = -\eta \frac{\partial E}{\partial \mathbf{w}} \quad \Rightarrow \quad \Delta \alpha_i = -\eta \lambda_i \alpha_i , \tag{5-40}$$

which shows that the learning process in gradient descent depends on the size of the eigenvalues of the Hessian matrix. We can make this more explicit by writing this last equation as:

$$\alpha_i^{(r+1)} = \alpha_i^{(r)} - \eta \lambda_i \alpha_i^{(r)} \quad \Rightarrow \quad \alpha_i^{(r+1)} = \alpha_i^{(r)} \left(1 - \eta \lambda_i \right). \tag{5-41}$$

We conclude that the updating of the weights is directly related to the updating of the distances α_i, and these depend on the $(1 - \eta \lambda_i)$ factors. The distances will decrease only if $|1 - \eta \lambda_i| < 1$; steadily if $1 - \eta \lambda_i$ is positive, with oscillations if negative. In order for the condition $|1 - \eta \lambda_i| < 1$ to be satisfied one must have:

$$\eta < \frac{2}{\lambda_{max}}. \tag{5-42}$$

where λ_{max} is the largest eigenvalue.

On the other hand, the speed of convergence is dominated by the smallest eigenvalue. For the maximum η allowed by formula (5-42), the convergence speed along the eigenvector direction corresponding to the smallest eigenvalue is governed by $(1 - 2\lambda_{min}/\lambda_{max})$.

We have already seen in section 5.1 how the learning rate influences the gradient descent process. Let us illustrate this dependence on the eigenvalues with the example of the error function (5-4c), with two weights denoted a and b for simplicity:

$$E\left(\begin{bmatrix} a \\ b \end{bmatrix} \right) = a^2 + 2b^2 - 2a + 1 . \tag{5-43}$$

The minimum of E occurs at $[1, 0]'$. From Exercise 5.9 it is possible to conclude that $\lambda_{max} = 4$, therefore $\eta < 0.5$ for convergence.

Figure 5.30 shows the horizontal projection of the parabolic surface corresponding to E, with the progress of the gradient descent. If a low learning rate of $\eta = 0.15$ is used, the convergence is slow. For $\eta = 0.45$, near the 0.5 limit, one starts getting oscillations around the minimum, along the vertical line. The reader can use the *Error Energy.xls* file to experiment with other values of η and verify the occurrence of oscillations for $\eta > 0.5$.

The problem of the oscillations is partly solved by using the momentum factor of equations (5-25a) and (5-25b).

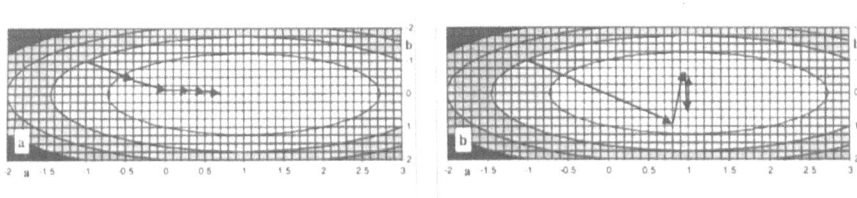

Figure 5.30. Gradient descent in a parabolic error energy. The arrows show the progress of gradient descent starting from the point (-1, -1) and using two different learning factors: (a) $\eta = 0.15$; (b) $\eta = 0.45$.

5.6.3 Bias and Variance in NN Design

When describing the performance of Bayesian classifiers in section 4.5, a trade-off between bias and variance of the error estimates was presented. We saw, namely, that whereas training set error estimates had, on average, zero variance and a bias inversely dependent on the number of training samples, test set error estimates were, on average, unbiased but had a variance inversely dependent on the number of test samples. As a matter of fact, the training and generalization properties of a neural network also exhibit a bias-variance trade-off. This can be understood by decomposing the error energy in bias and variance components, as proposed by Geman *et al.* (1992). We will describe next the main aspects of this issue.

Let us consider the average squared error of a neural network attempting to adjust its outputs $z_k(\mathbf{x}_i)$ to the target values $t_k(\mathbf{x}_i)$ for the input patterns $\mathbf{x}_i$. This, taking into account formulas (5-2a) and (5-29d), is given by:

$$E = \frac{1}{2n} \sum_{k=1}^{c} \sum_{i=1}^{n} \left(z_k\left(\mathbf{x}_i\right) - t_k\left(\mathbf{x}_i\right) \right)^2 . \tag{5-44}$$

If we let the size of the training set grow to infinite, this formula transforms into the integral (see also (5-31)):

$$E = \sum_{k=1}^{c} \int_{X \times T} (z_k - t_k)^2 \, p(t_k \mid \mathbf{x}) p(\mathbf{x}) dt_k d\mathbf{x} , \tag{5-45}$$

with simplified writing of the functions $z_k(\mathbf{x})$, $t_k(\mathbf{x})$.

Adding and subtracting $E[t_k \mid \mathbf{x}]$ to the expression inside parenthesis, the integral can be decomposed into a sum of two terms, as follows:

$$E = \sum_{k=1}^{c} \int_X \left(z_k - E[t_k \mid \mathbf{x}]\right)^2 p(\mathbf{x})d\mathbf{x} + \sum_{k=1}^{c} \int_X \left(E\left[t_k{}^2 \mid \mathbf{x}\right] - E^2[t_k \mid \mathbf{x}]\right)p(\mathbf{x})d\mathbf{x}, \quad (5\text{-}46)$$

with

$$E[t_k \mid \mathbf{x}] \equiv \int t_k \, p(t_k \mid \mathbf{x}) \, dt_k \, ; \qquad (5\text{-}46a)$$

$$E\left[t_k^2 \mid \mathbf{x}\right] \equiv \int t_k^2 \, p(t_k \mid \mathbf{x}) \, dt_k \, . \qquad (5\text{-}46b)$$

We already found the term (5-46a) in (5-33): it represents the conditional regression of the target data. The second term in (5-46) reflects, therefore, the variance in the target data and is totally independent of the network output z_k. It is the first term in (5-46) that is really interesting. The integrand is:

$$\left(z_k - E[t_k \mid \mathbf{x}]\right)^2 . \qquad (5\text{-}47)$$

The optimum output of the network corresponds, of course, to $E[t_k \mid \mathbf{x}]$.

Imagine now that we had many training sets of size n available, and wished to see how the error term, dependent on the network, is influenced by the particular choice of training set. For this purpose let us consider the ensemble average of (5-47), E_D, computed in a potentially infinite number of training sets:

$$E_D\left\{\left(z_k - E[t_k \mid \mathbf{x}]\right)^2\right\}. \qquad (5\text{-}48)$$

The somewhat intricate computation of this ensemble average can be found in Bishop (1995) or Haytkin (1999), where it is shown that it can be expressed as:

$$E_D\left\{\left(z_k - E[t_k \mid \mathbf{x}]\right)^2\right\} = E_D^2\left\{z_k - E[t_k \mid \mathbf{x}]\right\} + E_D\left\{\left(z_k - E_D(z_k)\right)^2\right\}. \qquad (5\text{-}49)$$

- The first term represents the squared average deviation of the network outputs z_k from the optimum solution $E[t_k \mid \mathbf{x}]$. It is therefore called the *bias component of the error*.
- The second term represents the average squared deviation of the output values from their ensemble average $E_D(z_k)$. It is therefore called the *variance component of the error*.

Imagine that we had designed a neural network to regress target values given by the addition of function values $z(\mathbf{x}_i)$ plus a random error term $e(\mathbf{x}_i)$, in a similar way as in (5-30):

$$t(\mathbf{x}_i) = z(\mathbf{x}_i) + e(\mathbf{x}_i). \qquad (5\text{-}50)$$

If the network is complex enough to perfectly fit a given training set, the bias will be zero for that training set at the points x_i, and will also be typically low in the neighbourhood of those points for other training sets; however, the network will show a significant variance, directly related to the variance of the $e(x_i)$. If, at the other extreme, we design a network implementing a very simple function, which will only reproduce the main trend of the target values, then we will obtain a high bias since the implemented function will depart significantly from the target values, but a very low variance since it will be insensitive to the noise term $e(x_i)$.

In general, we will have to make a compromise between using a complex model with a good fit but poor generalization, and a very simple model with good generalization but with significant departure from the desired output. In order to decrease the bias we will have to implement more complex models, but then, in order to decrease the variance, we will have to train the model in larger datasets. For a low size training set a simpler model usually performs better.

The choice of the appropriate model complexity, related to the number of weights, will be discussed in the next section. Experimentally there are several tips that may help to tune the model adequately to the training data, namely:

- *Early stopping.* Use an independent validation set during training and stop the training process when the error of the validation set starts to increase. This technique was already mentioned in 5.5.2.
- *Regularization.* Select a model based not only on its performance but also on its complexity, penalizing models that are highly complex. This regularization technique is applied by *Statistica* in the Intelligent Problem Solver. Another regularization approach is the inclusion in the error formula (5-2a) of an extra term penalizing large weights (*weight regularization*). As a matter of fact, when using sigmoidal activation functions, small weights correspond to the "linear" central part of the functions. Large weights, on the contrary, mean a highly non-linear behaviour, providing high curvature surfaces with a perfect fit of the data. By penalizing the larger weights, the network tends to develop smoother surfaces without over-fitting the data (see Weigend *et al.*, 1991).
- *Training with noise.* By adding a small amount of noise to the input values during training, we are actually forcing the network to learn from several datasets, and therefore decreasing the variance term of the error. The network will improve its generalization capability, as already mentioned in 5.5.2.
- *Network pruning.* After several training experiments inspect the weights and remove those that are very small, and therefore contribute little to the output, and train again the pruned, simpler model. It is also possible to analyse how the error deteriorates by removing each variable (*sensitivity analysis*). If the error before and after variable removal is practically the same, this means that the removed variable has no significant contribution and one can then prune the respective input.

5.6.4 Network Complexity

In order to appropriately solve the bias-variance trade-off described in the preceding section, choosing a sensible network complexity for a given dataset is an important task. Note that the bias-variance trade-off affords the appropriate insight into the dimensionality ratio issue: for adequate training of a complex network with w weights we need to set a lower bound on the needed number n of patterns in order to ensure that the network has generalization capability, yielding reproducible results in independent test sets. Note also that, except for single-layer networks, the number of weights will often be much larger than the dimension d of the pattern vectors.

In statistical classification it is possible to derive formulas describing, for instance, the training set error behaviour of Bayesian normal classifiers with the n/d ratio. The problem is more complicated with neural networks, where no such formulas are available. Instead, it is possible to derive bounds for the n/w ratio. As the modelling capability of a neural network is a function of the discriminants implemented by the neurons, such bounds are essentially based on the combinatorial study of feasible class labels by sets of linear discriminants.

For this purpose, let us first consider the number of linearly separable dichotomies of n points, where a dichotomy is any partition of the n patterns into two disjointed groups. We consider that the n patterns are *regularly distributed* in $\Re^d$, i.e., no subset of $(d+1)$ patterns is contained in a $\Re^d$ hyperpane. For the two-dimensional space, this corresponds to saying that no group of 3 points is co-linear.

It is possible to prove that given n regularly distributed points in $\Re^d$, the number of dichotomies that are linearly separable is given by:

$$
D(n,d) = \begin{cases} 2\sum_{i=0}^{d} C(n-1,i) & , \quad n > d; \\ 2^n & , \quad n \leq d. \end{cases}
\tag{5-51}
$$

When $n=d+1$, both expressions give the same result. The demonstration of this result, known as Cover theorem, can be found in (Cover, 1965).

For $d=2$, the application of (5-51) gives the following results:

- For $n=3$, all the $2^3=8$ dichotomies of the three points are linearly separable;
- For $n=4$, only 14 of the 16 dichotomies are linearly separable;
- For $n=5$, only 22 of the 32 dichotomies are linearly separable.

Using polynomial decision functions is equivalent to using linear discriminants in a higher dimension space, as seen in 2.1.1. Thus, using quadratic decision functions in $d=2$ is equivalent to using linear decision functions in $d-1 = (2+1)(2+2)/2 - 1 = 5$ dimensions. This means that for $n=5$ patterns, all dichotomies would be separable by the quadratic decision functions, since they are linearly separable in the 5-dimension space ($D(5,5) = 32$).

Having seen how the number of possible dichotomies grows with the number of patterns, we now turn to the issue of evaluating the discriminative capability of a given network. We start by analysing the two-class classification case with two-layer perceptrons (i.e., with a single hidden layer) with hard-limiters.

For two-layer perceptrons an interesting result, due to Mirchandani and Cao (1989), is that in $\Re^d$ the maximum number of regions that are linearly separable, with h hidden neurons, $R(h, d)$, is given by:

$$R(h,d) = \sum_{i=0}^{d} C(h,i), \text{ setting } C(h, i) = 0 \text{ for } h < i .$$ (5-52)

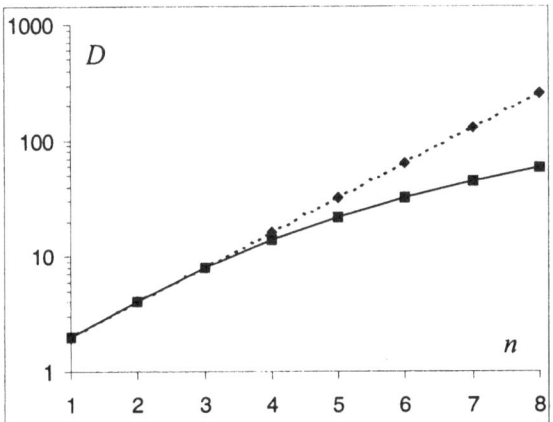

Figure 5.31. Number of total dichotomies (dotted line) and linearly separable regions (solid line), able to be implemented by a perceptron in a two-dimensional space (logarithmic vertical scale).

This formula allows us to set a lower bound to the number of training patterns: $n \geq R(h,d)$, since we need at least one pattern for each trainable region. In particular, the formula yields:

- $R(h, d) = 2^h$ for $h \leq d$;
- $R(h, d) = h+1$ for $d=1$.

In practice, one needs a number of patterns that is significantly greater than $R(h, d)$ in order for the network to be able to generalize. An upper bound on the number of hidden neurons for any single hidden layer MLP is the number of patterns itself (see Huang and Babri, 1998).

Let us analyse in particular the case $d=2$, $h=1$. There are, of course, 2 linearly separable regions by one discriminant, that a single perceptron[4] implements. As confirmation, formula (5-52) gives $R(1,2)=2$. On the other hand, with one discriminant, the maximum number of pattern dichotomies one can have is given by the previous formula (5-51) of $D(n, d)$, represented in Figure 5.31. Notice that up to $n=3$, all 2^n dichotomies are linearly separable. For increasing values of n, the number of dichotomies that can be implemented decreases considerably compared with the number of possible dichotomies.

Let us now increase the number of hidden neurons to $h=2$, for a $d=2$ problem. We then have a maximum of $R(2,2)=4$ linearly separable regions by two discriminants. With regularly distributed $n=4$ patterns, all the possible dichotomies (class labellings) can be implemented with these two discriminants (Figure 5.32a). The same happens for a set of $n=5$ patterns forming a convex hull, as shown in Figure 5.32b. However, for a set of n=6 patterns forming a convex hull, it is not possible to obtain all dichotomies (Figure 5.32c).

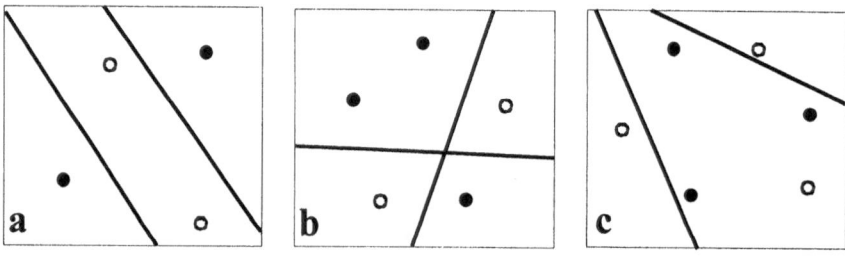

Figure 5.32. Dichotomies for a single layer perceptron with $h=2$: (a) Implemented with three regions, $n=4$; (b) Implemented with four regions, $n=5$; (c) Cannot be implemented with four regions, $n=6$.

Therefore, for $h=2$ hidden neurons we obtain a departure of the number of dichotomies that can be implemented from the number of possible dichotomies, for $n=6$. In general, this behaviour is obtained for any value of h and is related to the important concept of *Vapnik-Chervonenkis dimension*.

Let $G(n)$ be the maximum number of distinct dichotomies implemented by a neural net. This function, called *growth function*, is shown with a solid line in Figure 5.31 for the case MLP:2:1:1. A set of n patterns is said to be *shattered* by the neural net if $G(n) = 2^n$. The Vapnik-Chervonenkis (VC) dimension, d_{VC}, is precisely the largest number of patterns that can be shattered by a neural network. It corresponds, therefore, to the maximum number of training patterns that can be learned without error for all possible class labels. In the case of Figure 5.31, $d_{VC} = 3$. As a matter of fact, for a single perceptron, the number of linearly separable

---

[4] A two-layer MLP with $h=1$ is equivalent to a single perceptron.

dichotomies reaches the value 2^n for a maximum of $n=d+1$ patterns in accordance with formula (5-51). Thus, for this case, $d_{VC}=d+1$.

Below d_{VC} the neural net learns the training set without error and does not generalize. It is only above d_{VC} that the neural net is capable of generalization.

In general, the Vapnik Chervonenkis dimension is, unfortunately, very difficult to determine. Notice that in order to show that the VC dimension of a MLP is at least m, one must simply find some set of m regularly distributed points shattered by the MLP. However, in order to show that the VC dimension of a MLP is at most m, one must show that no set of $m+1$ regularly distributed points is shattered by the MLP. Therefore, in the case of Figure 5.32, a lower d_{VC} bound is 5. As a matter of fact, a lower bound for the VC dimension of a two-class MLP, with hard limiters, is given precisely by the maximum number of linearly separable regions, formula (5-52).

Figure 5.33 shows the values of this lower bound for several values of d and h, obtained with the *PR Size* program (see Appendix B).

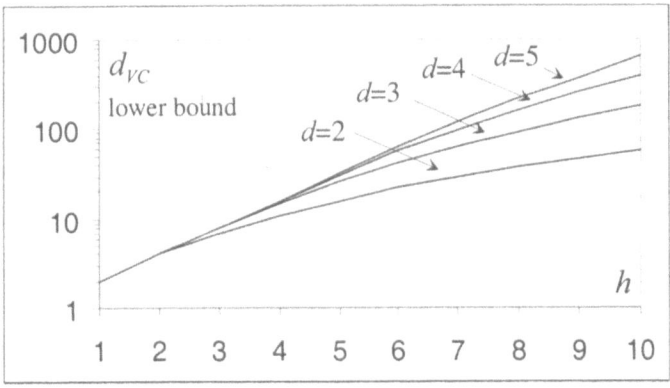

Figure 5.33. Lower bound on the VC dimension for a two-class MLP with hard-limited activation functions (logarithmic vertical scale).

Bounds on the training set size needed for MLP generalization depend on the VC dimension. A lower bound on the number of training samples needed for generalization is due to Blumer *et al.* (1989):

$$n_l = \max\left[\frac{1-Pe}{Pe}\ln\left(\frac{1}{\alpha}\right), d_{VC}\left(1-2(Pe(1-\alpha)+\alpha)\right)\right], \tag{5-53}$$

where Pe is the true error rate of the neural network, and $1-\alpha$ is the confidence level that the design set estimate of the error rate will approximate with arbitrary closeness the true error rate, with an increasing number of patterns. In this formula we may use for d_{VC} the lower bound of formula (5-52).

An upper bound on the sufficient number of patterns for network generalization, is also presented in the same work (Blumer *et al.*, 1989):

$$n_u = \max\left[\frac{4}{Pe}\log_2\left(\frac{2}{\alpha}\right), \frac{8d_{VC}}{Pe}\log_2\left(\frac{13}{Pe}\right)\right]. \tag{5-54}$$

Another, tighter lower bound formula, due to Ehrenfeucht *et al.* (1989) for the special case of $Pe \leq 0.125$ and $\alpha \leq 0.01$, converges asymptotically to the above upper bound, except for a factor of the order of $\log_2(1/Pe)$:

$$n_l = \frac{d_{VC} - 1}{32Pe}. \tag{5-55}$$

The computation of formula (5-54) upper bound presupposes the knowledge of the true VC dimension or at least an upper bound of it. Baum and Haussler (1989) derived an upper bound for the VC dimension of an MLP with u units (hard-limiter neurons) and w weights (including biases), as:

$$d_{VC} \leq 2w\log_2(eu), \tag{5-56}$$

where e is the base of the natural logarithms.

With this result they derived also an upper bound for the sufficient number of patterns achieving generalization for an MLP with $\hat{P}e_d$ (design set error estimate). They proved that such an MLP will have a test set error not worse then $2\hat{P}e_d$ with high probability $1-\alpha$, using:

$$n_u = \frac{w}{\hat{P}e_d}\ln\left(\frac{u}{\hat{P}e_d}\right), \tag{5-56a}$$

with

$$\alpha = 8(2uen_u/w)^w e^{-\hat{P}e_d n_u/16}. \tag{5-56b}$$

The value of α is rather low ($\alpha < 0.005$) even for low values of d and h. A rule of thumb, based on this upper bound, estimates the number of patterns needed for sufficient generalization as w/Pe for complex MLP (high w). This means that for e.g. $Pe = 0.1$, one would need about 10 times more patterns than weights.

With the program *PR Size* (see Appendix B) it is possible to compute the bounds expressed by the formulas (5-53) and (5-56a), for any values of d and h. Figure 5.34 shows these bounds for d=2, 4 and 8. The bounds were computed using $Pe = \hat{P}e_d = 0.05$ and $\alpha = 0.01$.

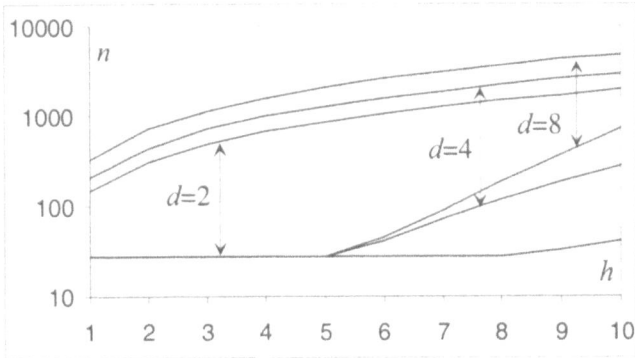

Figure 5.34. Bounds for two-class MLPs with hard-limiters, computed for Pe=0.05 and α=0.01 (logarithmic vertical scale).

The *PR Size* program provides, therefore, the appropriate guidance in the choice of h and n for classification problems with neural networks. For the two-class cork stoppers classification problem described in section 5.3, an MLP2:1 with hard-limiter was used, which for a 95% confidence level of the respective error estimate, corresponds to n_l=27 and n_u=150. The lower bound is satisfied, since we are using 100 patterns. However, we may be somewhat far away from the optimal classifier, since the number of patterns we have available is lower than the estimated sufficient number for generalization, n_u.

When applying these bounds to MLPs one must take into account that these are initially trained with small weights, therefore introducing a bias in favour of solutions with small weights. This, in fact, reduces the effective d_{VC}, favouring smaller training sets. On the other hand, for MLPs with sigmoid activation functions the d_{VC} will be at least as great as formula (5-53) indicates, since a sigmoid unit can approximate a hard-limiter with arbitrary accuracy using sufficiently large weights. Therefore, the lower bound formula (5-55) also applies for networks with sigmoid units. Appropriate formulas for the upper bounds, in this situation, are presented in (Anthony and Bartlett, 1999).

Bounds on the necessary and sufficient number of patterns, needed for learning a regression function, have also been studied by several authors. These bounds depend on a generalized version of the Vapnik-Chervonenkis dimension.

We now present some important concepts on this matter by first defining the *pseudo-shattering* of a set of points $X=\{x_i, x_i \in \Re, i=1, ..., m\}$ by a class of functions F, mapping X into the real numbers set.

We say that X is pseudo-shattered by F if there are m real numbers r_i and 2^m functions of F that achieve all possible "above/below" combinations with respect to the r_i. This is illustrated in Figure 5.35 for a class of linear functions $F = \{ (x, f(x) = ax + b); a, b \in \Re \}$. The points r_i are said to *witness the pseudo-shattering*.

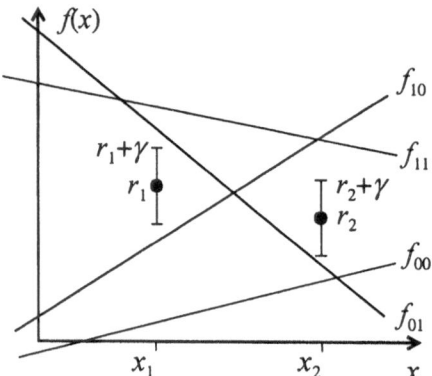

Figure 5.35. The class of functions $F = \{ (x, f(x) = ax + b); a, b \in \Re \}$ pseudo-shatters the set $\{x_1, x_2\}$. The four functions shown achieve all possible "above$\equiv$0/below$\equiv$1" combinations of $\{r_1, r_2\}$.

Notice that the same set X of Figure 5.35 is not pseudo-shattered by the class of functions $G = \{ (x, g(x) = a); a \in \Re \}$.

The pseudo-shattering concept relates to the expressiveness or flexibility that a class of functions must have in order to approximate a set of points. For instance, in the example of Figure 5.35 the class of functions G is not flexible enough to approximate $\{(x_1, r_2), (x_2, r_2)\}$. On the other hand, the class of functions F is not flexible enough in other circumstances (see Exercise 5.14).

The maximum cardinality of a subset of X that is pseudo-shattered by F is called the *pseudo-dimension* of F, and denoted $Pdim(F)$. For the example of Figure 5.35 $Pdim(F)=2$ and $Pdim(G)=1$. Therefore, the pseudo-dimension of a class of functions reflects the expressiveness of the class.

Figure 5.35 shows that the "above/below" combinations of $\{r_1, r_2\}$ are actually achieved with a margin of γ around the points r_i. When it is possible to achieve this separation we say that X is γ-*shattered* by F. The corresponding pseudo-dimension is now called γ-*dimension* or *fat-shattering dimension* and denoted $fat(F,\gamma)$.

A theorem due to Simon (1997) allows the computation of the fat-shattering dimension for all functions mapping $[0, 1]$ into $[0,1]$ and having a total variation of V, as:

$$fat(F,\gamma) = 1 + trunc(V / 2\gamma), \tag{5-57}$$

where the function $trunc(x)$ returns the largest integer less than or equal to x and V is the total function variation:

$$V = \sum_{i=1}^{m-1} |f(x_{i+1}) - f(x_i)|. \tag{5-57a}$$

A lower bound on the number of samples needed for learning a class of functions mapping X into [0,1], with error Pe and confidence level $1-\alpha$, $\alpha < 0.01$, is (Anthony and Bartlett, 1999):

$$n_l \geq \frac{fat(F, Pe/q)-1}{16q}, \quad \text{for any } 0 < q < \frac{1}{4}, \tag{5-58}$$

where q is the quantization level of the function values, i.e., they are computed as $q \cdot trunc(f(x_i)/q)$.

If we use formula (5-57) in (5-58) we obtain the estimated lower bound:

$$n_l = trunc(V/(32Pe)). \tag{5-58a}$$

Let us apply this lower bound to the MLP3:3:1 regressing the temperature T for the *Weather* dataset, with $Pe \approx 0.08$, as analysed in section 5.5.3. The total variation of T(x) is 1573.9 °C, which we refer to the [0,1] interval by dividing by the max(T(x))-min(T(x)) range, obtaining 59.4. Applying formula (5-58a) the estimated lower bound is 23, which is largely exceeded by the number of training samples (378).

5.6.5 Risk Minimization

In the preceding section we saw how to characterize the complexity of a neural network using the Vapnik-Chervonenkis and the fat-shattering dimensions, for classification and regression problems, respectively. We will now proceed to see how the complexity influences the classification or regression risk of a neural network. For this purpose, let us denote $R(\mathbf{w})$ the risk incurred when using a neural network with weight vector $\mathbf{w}$:

$$R(\mathbf{w}) = \int_{XxT} \lambda(t, f(\mathbf{x}, \mathbf{w})) P(\mathbf{x}, t) d\mathbf{x} dt. \tag{5-59}$$

Notice that this is the same formula as (4-20a), section 4.2.1, now applied to a continuous target space T. As we have done in that section we will discuss the simplified situation, without impairing the main conclusions, of zero loss for correct classifications and equal loss for wrong classifications. $R(\mathbf{w})$ will then be, simply, the classifier true error $Pe(\mathbf{w})$. As usual, we do not know the true error but are able to obtain the design set error estimate, $\hat{Pe}_d(\mathbf{w})$, by counting the number of individual errors. An important result due to Vapnik (see Vapnik, 1998) relates these two errors, for any weight vector $\mathbf{w}$ and arbitrarily small quantity ε, as follows:

$$P(|Pe(\mathbf{w}) - \hat{Pe}_d(\mathbf{w})| > \varepsilon) \rightarrow 0 \quad \text{with} \quad n \rightarrow \infty. \tag{5-60}$$

We are therefore guaranteed that, as we use larger training sets, we will obtain an error estimate that comes arbitrarily close to the true error of the classifier, whatever value it may have. This result applies to the general risk functional (5-59) and its *empirical risk* estimation, $\hat{P}e_d(\mathbf{w})$, also known as *empirical error*. The convergence behaviour with increasing n is known as the *principle of empirical error minimization*. We have already applied the ERM principle in the previous chapter, when discussing the application of the Bayes rule for minimum risk.

Usually, we would also like the network (and respective weight vector) that minimizes the empirical error to also minimize the true error. After all, having an excellent estimate of a bad classifier is not of much use! In order to achieve that, the following more restrictive condition, known as *uniform convergence of the errors*, must apply:

$$P\left(\sup_{\mathbf{w}}\left|Pe(\mathbf{w})-\hat{P}e_d(\mathbf{w})\right|>\varepsilon\right)\to 0 \quad \text{with} \quad n\to\infty. \tag{5-61}$$

where sup(x) (supremum of x) of a family of scalar values x, is the smallest scalar larger than any value of the family. What formula (5-61) tells us is that we want to obtain an arbitrarily small deviation of the empirical error from the true error, using the supremum of the deviations for a family of networks. The Vapnik-Chervonenkis dimension allows us to establish the following limit for small values of $Pe(\mathbf{w})$ (Vapnik, 1998):

$$P\left(\sup_{\mathbf{w}}\left|Pe(\mathbf{w})-\hat{P}e_d(\mathbf{w})\right|>\varepsilon\right)<\left(\frac{2en}{d_{VC}}\right)^{d_{VC}}e^{-\varepsilon^2 n/4}. \tag{5-62}$$

Let us denote by $1-\alpha$ the confidence level that we have on a classifier that its error is not deviated from the optimal value more than ε. This corresponds to the so-called *probably approximately correct* (PAC) principle (see e.g. Mitchell, 1997). Then, using formulas (5-62) and (5-61), the following bound holds at the $1-\alpha$ confidence level:

$$Pe(\mathbf{w})\le\hat{P}e_d(\mathbf{w})+\sqrt{\frac{d_{VC}}{n}\ln\left(\frac{2n}{d_{VC}}+1\right)-\frac{1}{n}\ln\left(\frac{\alpha}{n}\right)}. \tag{5-63}$$

In order to study the influence of these terms, let us consider fixed values for α and n and analyse what happens with increasing values of d_{VC}. For an increasing d_{VC} the empirical error will decrease, since the neural network will be better adjusted to the training set up to the limit of having as many hidden neurons as there are patterns. The second term, however, will increase with d_{VC}, representing a structural risk of non-generalization. It works, therefore, as a regularization term that penalizes the network complexity. In general, for any loss function, we will have a guaranteed risk by summing up an empirical risk and a *structural risk* as depicted in Figure 5.36.

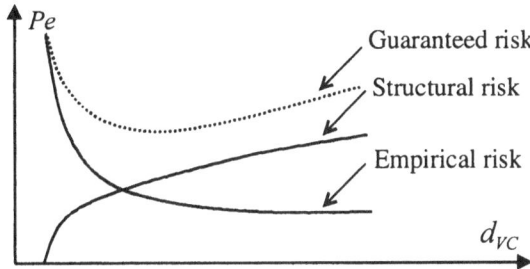

Figure 5.36. Guaranteed risk of a neural network as a sum of empirical and structural risks.

For generalization purposes, we are interested in applying a principle of *structural risk minimization*, SRM. An experimental way of minimizing the structural risk consists of defining a sequence of networks with increasing d_{VC}, by addition of more hidden neurons. For each network the empirical risk is minimized, and one progresses to a more complex machine until reaching a minimum of the guaranteed risk.

5.7 Approximation Methods in NN Training

In section 5.5 we saw how to train MLPs using the back-propagation algorithm, based on a gradient descent technique. Some pitfalls of this technique were explained in that section and in more detail in section 5.6.2, when we analysed the influence of the Hessian matrix on the learning process. There are several alternative algorithms for training MLPs that either attempt to improve the gradient descent technique used in the back-propagation algorithm, or use a completely different approach, not based on the gradient descent method. This last class of algorithms uses ideas and techniques imported from the respectable body of methodologies of multivariate function optimisation. The reader can find a detailed explanation of these techniques in (Fletcher, 1987) and their application to MLPs in (Bishop, 1995). In this section we will present only two of these methods, which are very fast in terms of convergence and do not require the specification of parameters (learning and momentum factor) as in the back-propagation algorithm.

5.7.1 The Conjugate-Gradient Method

The conjugate gradient method uses a *line search* technique, consisting of the determination of the error minimum along a certain line, with an efficient choice of the searching direction on the surface corresponding to the error energy. At each iterative step of this method there are two main tasks to be solved:

1. Find the minimum along the surface line corresponding to a certain search direction.
2. Determine the next search direction as the *conjugate* of the previous one.

Let us illustrate how the method operates with the example of the quadratic function (5-43). At the first iteration ($r=1$), we start with an arbitrary direction $d^{(1)}$ represented by the white arrow in Figure 5.37, with slope -1.2. Next, we determine the minimum of E along this line, which occurs at $\mathbf{w}^* = $ (-1.59, -1.065) (see Exercise 5.20) . Let us compute the gradient at this point:

$$\left.\frac{\partial E}{\partial \mathbf{w}}\right|_{w^*} = \begin{bmatrix} \frac{\partial E}{\partial a} = 2a - 2 \\ \frac{\partial E}{\partial b} = 4b \end{bmatrix}_{w^*} = \begin{bmatrix} -5.18 \\ -4.26 \end{bmatrix}.$$

The gradient, represented with dotted white line in Figure 5.37, has slope 1/1.2, i.e., it is orthogonal to the chosen direction at the minimum point. This is a general property: the gradient projection along the chosen direction and at the minimum point is always zero. If we would choose to move next along the gradient, as in the gradient descent method, we would actually move away from the minimum. Instead, we move along a direction satisfying the following property:

$$d^{(r)}\mathbf{H}d^{(r+1)} = 0, \text{ where } \mathbf{H} \text{ is the Hessian matrix.} \tag{5-64}$$

Directions satisfying this condition are called *conjugate directions*, since they do not interfere with each other. As a matter of fact, along the conjugate direction, represented by the black arrow in Figure 5.37, the component of the gradient parallel to the previous direction (white lines) remains zero, and we are in fact moving along a sequence of minima relative to the previous direction.

Next, we determine again the line minimum, which is in this case the global minimum error, and the process terminates. Otherwise, the previous two steps would have to be repeated until convergence.

In general, for a quadratic error E defined by a wxw matrix $\mathbf{H}$, there are w conjugate directions, which are orthogonal to each other only if $\mathbf{H}=\mathbf{I}$. The conjugate-gradient method guarantees a steadily decreasing error and finds a minimum within at most w iterations. It is, therefore, a very fast method. The only problem is that once a local minimum is reached, it will not move away.

The algorithm for implementing the conjugate-gradient method must solve two main tasks: the determination of the minimum along a line and an efficient method of determining the conjugate directions, using an iterative algorithm that avoids having to compute the Hessian. Details on the algorithm implementation can be found in Haykin (1999).

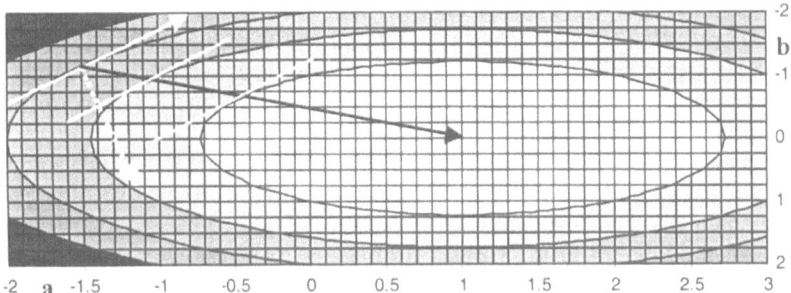

Figure 5.37. Conjugate-gradient descent in a parabolic surface. The black arrow is a conjugate direction of the initial white arrow.

The conjugate gradient method is especially suited for difficult problems with many classes and features. It can then provide a much-improved solution over the back-propagation method.

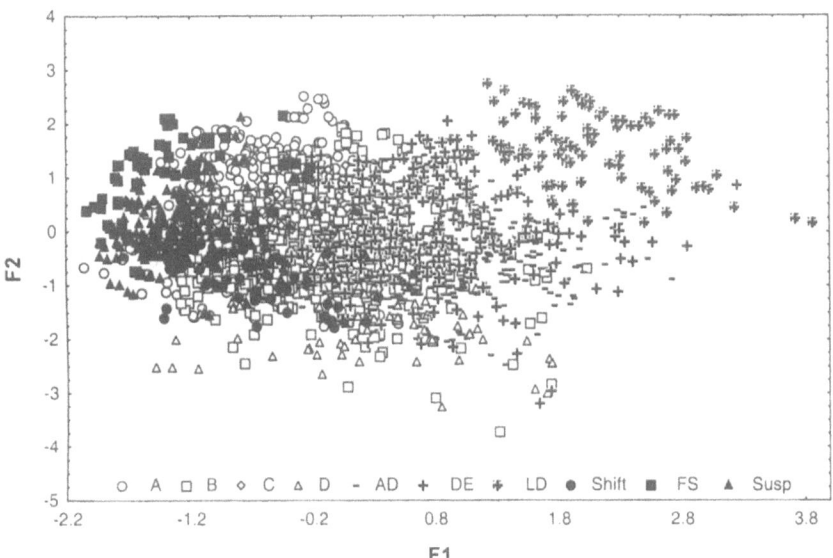

Figure 5.38. Scatter plot of the 10 classes of *CTG* data relative to the two main principal components.

Consider the *CTG* dataset with 10 classes. This constitutes a difficult classification problem, given the proximity and overlap of the classes. By performing Kruskal-Wallis tests and observing box-whiskers plots of the data, it is possible to get some insight about the discriminative capability of the features. It is possible, namely, to discard features that do not contribute to the discrimination (FM, DS, DP, MODE, NZER) and determine the ones that are more discriminative (A, DL, V, MSTV, ALTV, WIDTH, DP, all with Kruskal Wallis H>1000). Factor analysis is also helpful in providing a picture of the extent of class overlap and the main features describing the data (see Exercises 2.12 and 3.8). The difficulty of this problem can be seen in Figure 5.38.

Using the *Statistica* intelligent problem solver, an MLP18:22:10 solution was obtained with good performance. Afterwards, this was trained with the conjugate gradient method and the correct classifications of 90%, 83% and 85.2% were found for the training set (1063 cases), verification set (531 cases) and test set (532 cases), respectively. As a matter of fact, the classification error differences for the three sets were mainly due to class C, represented by few cases in all sets. Without class C patterns the error rates for the three sets were quite similar, making it acceptable to merge the results for the three different sets, in order to obtain an overall classification matrix as shown in Table 5.7.

Table 5.7. Classification matrix of CTG classes, with the conjugate-gradient method. True classifications along the rows; predicted classifications along the columns.

A	B	C	D	SH	AD	DE	LD	FS	SUSP
314	7	36	0	8	3	4	0	2	19
7	544	1	13	2	7	0	0	0	0
4	0	15	0	0	0	0	0	0	0
0	6	0	68	0	0	0	0	0	0
8	8	0	0	55	1	1	0	0	5
1	8	0	0	0	314	12	0	0	0
7	2	1	0	0	7	232	6	0	0
0	1	0	0	0	0	3	101	0	0
4	0	0	0	0	0	0	0	51	16
39	3	0	0	7	0	0	0	16	157
81.77%	93.96%	28.30%	83.95%	76.39%	94.58%	92.06%	94.39%	73.91%	79.70%

Notice the surprisingly high degree of performance (overall error of 87%) obtained with an MLP for this hard classification problem, with the exception of class C. Although the error figures for the training, verification and test sets were quite similar, we must take into account that formula (5-56) for complex MLPs indicates a number of patterns needed for sufficient generalization of approximately w/Pe, which in this case corresponds to 3392 patterns, a higher number of patterns than we have available for training. The previous error figures may be, therefore, somewhat optimistic.

When using the conjugate gradient method in high dimensional feature spaces, it is often found that the algorithm gets stuck in local minima in the early steps of the process. It may be helpful in such cases to use back-propagation in the early steps (e.g. 20 epochs) and conjugate-gradient afterwards.

As an illustration of the conjugate-gradient method applied to a regression task, we used the foetal weight dataset analysed in section 5.5.2, using the same number of epochs and set sizes. Although the algorithm got stuck in local minima in some runs we did obtain, in general, better solutions than with back-propagation. Figure 5.39 shows the result for one of the best runs, with RMS errors of 273 g for the training set, 267 g for the verification set and 287.1 g for the test set.

Notice particularly, in Figure 5.39, a better adjustment in the high foetal weight section.

The foetal weight estimation problem can also be approached as a classification task (see Exercise 5.22).

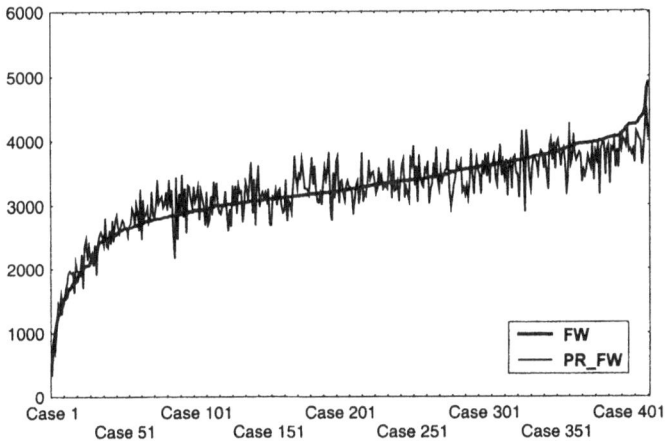

Figure 5.39. Predicted foetal weight (PR_FW) using an MLP3:6:1 trained with the conjugate-gradient algorithm. The FW curve represents the true foetal weight values.

5.7.2 The Levenberg-Marquardt Method

The Levenberg-Marquardt method is also a fast training method, especially designed for a sum-squared error formula as in (5-2a), and single output networks.

In order to understand the main aspects of the method, explained in detail in Bishop (1995), let us rewrite (5-2a) as a squared Euclidian norm of an n-dimensional error vector:

$$E = \sum_{i=1}^{n} e_i^2 = \|\mathbf{e}\|^2 .$$

(5-65)

The error vector $\mathbf{e}$ depends on the weights, and for small deviations of the weights, during the training process, $\mathbf{w}^{(r+1)} - \mathbf{w}^{(r)}$, it can be approximated by a first order Taylor series as:

$$\mathbf{e}\!\left(\mathbf{w}^{(r+1)}\right) = \mathbf{e}\!\left(\mathbf{w}^{(r)}\right) + \mathbf{Z}\!\left(\mathbf{w}^{(r+1)} - \mathbf{w}^{(r)}\right),$$

(5-66)

where $\mathbf{Z}$ is the matrix of the error derivatives:

$$\mathbf{Z} = \left[\frac{\partial e_i}{\partial w_j} \right] .$$

(5-66a)

Substituting (5-64) in (5-63) we get the error approximation:

$$\hat{E} = \left\| \mathbf{e}\!\left(\mathbf{w}^{(r)}\right) + \mathbf{Z}\!\left(\mathbf{w}^{(r+1)} - \mathbf{w}^{(r)}\right) \right\|^2 .$$

(5-67)

Minimizing the error with respect to the new weights, yields:

$$\mathbf{w}^{(r+1)} = \mathbf{w}^{(r)} - \left(\mathbf{Z'Z}\right)^{-1} \mathbf{Z'} \mathbf{e}\!\left(\mathbf{w}^{(r)}\right).$$

(5-68)

The term $(\mathbf{Z'Z})^{-1}\mathbf{Z'}$ is a pseudo-inverse matrix, as in (5-3), and can be computed using the Hessian matrix. This pseudo-inverse matrix governs the step size of the iterative learning process. In order to keep the deviation of the weights sufficiently small so that the Taylor series approximation is valid, the Levenberg-Marquardt algorithm uses instead of (5-67) a modified error formula:

$$\hat{E} = \left\| \mathbf{e}\!\left(\mathbf{w}^{(r)}\right) + \mathbf{Z}\!\left(\mathbf{w}^{(r+1)} - \mathbf{w}^{(r)}\right) \right\|^2 + \lambda \left\| \mathbf{w}^{(r+1)} - \mathbf{w}^{(r)} \right\|^2 .$$

(5-69)

The step size is now governed by $(\mathbf{Z'Z} + \lambda\mathbf{I})^{-1}\mathbf{Z'}$. Far away from a minimum of $\hat{E}$ we will need a large learning step size, therefore a high λ, while still maintaining a small deviation of the weights. In the Levenberg-Marquardt algorithm, an appropriate value of λ is chosen during the training process in order to maintain appropriate learning steps with small deviations of the weights, therefore assuring the linear approximation in (5-68).

A difficulty with the Levenberg-Marquardt algorithm is that the memory required to compute and store the pseudo-inverse matrix is proportional to the square of the number of weights in the network. This restricts its use to small networks.

The Levenberg-Marquardt method was also applied to the foetal weight data set. In several runs it tended to slightly over-fit the training set. Problems with local minima occurred rarely. Figure 5.40 shows one solution with RMS errors of 266.1 g for the training set, 274.4 g for the verification set and 291.7 g for the test set. The performance is only slightly worse than with conjugate gradient.

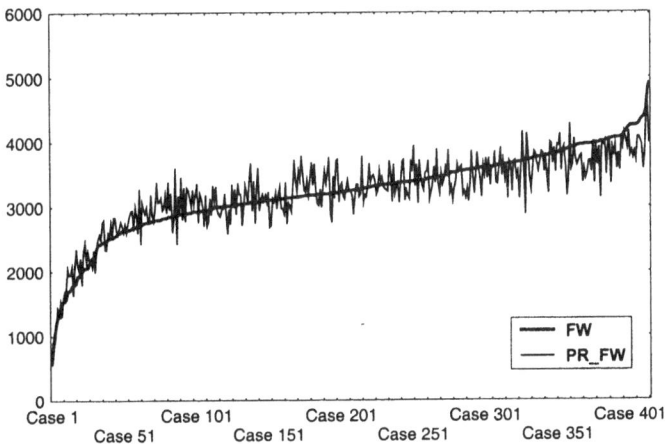

Figure 5.40. Predicted foetal weight (PR_FW) using an MLP3:6:1 trained with the Levenberg-Marquardt algorithm. The FW curve represents the true foetal weight values.

5.8 Genetic Algorithms in NN Training

Genetic algorithms are a class of stochastic optimisation algorithms. They were introduced by Holland (1975) and provide a way of stochastically training MLPs, in addition to many other interesting applications in the Neural Networks field. The key idea is the manipulation of the relevant information, such as neural weights, using rules inspired by the evolution of living beings.

Let us imagine that each weight of a MLP is considered as a *gene* (attribute) of the network device. The whole set of weights (genes) can then be considered as the MLP *chromosome*. To give a concrete example, let us apply this concept to an MLP2:2:1, shown in Figure 5.41.

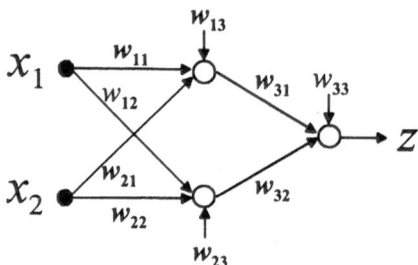

Figure 5.41. An MLP2:2:1 with all its weights plus biases. These are considered chromosome genes.

For this MLP2:2:1 device the chromosome can be expressed by an ordered sequence of the genes, the so-called genotype **g**, such as:

$$\mathbf{g} = \{w_{11}, w_{12}, w_{13}; \ w_{21}, w_{22}, w_{23}; \ w_{31}, w_{32}, w_{33}\}. \tag{5-70}$$

In the representation of **g** we used a semi-colon to separate the weights of individual neurons.

Imagine that we have a *population*, G, of a specified number of such devices (*individuals*) represented by their chromosomes. Each device is characterized by a *fitness factor*, which we may relate in some way with the error achieved with the device. Using the sum of squares error E we can, for instance, define the fitness factor for a device with genotype **g**, as:

$$f(\mathbf{g}) = E_{max} - E(\mathbf{g}), \tag{5-71}$$

where E_{max} is any upper bound of the error.

Inspired by the Darwinian theory of biological evolution, a genetic algorithm generates a new population by repetition of the following two-step process:

1. Select the fittest individuals of the population (the so-called survival of the fittest) for *reproduction*. A common selection process of parent individuals for reproduction is based on the assignment of a probability of selection to an individual, given by the individual's relative fitness:

$$P_{select}(\mathbf{g}) = f(\mathbf{g}) / \sum_{G} f(\mathbf{g}_i). \tag{5-72}$$

This selection rule is also known as *roulette-wheel* selection.

2. Generate a new population based on the selected parent individuals by applying the following operators to the parent chromosomes:

Crossover

Two parent chromosomes may pass unchanged to the next generation or else with a certain probability P_x, called the *crossover rate*, they will generate new chromosomes that result from swapping genes at specific sites or, for real-valued genetics, interpolating the respective gene values. Some interesting crossover types are indicated next for the MLP2:2:1 case, where we simplified the notation by using letters for the weights.

Single crossover:

$$\begin{Bmatrix} a,b,c; & d,e,f; & g,h,i \\ r,s,t; & u,v,w; & x,y,z \end{Bmatrix} \Rightarrow \begin{Bmatrix} r,s,t; & d,e,f; & g,h,i \\ a,b,c; & u,v,w; & x,y,z \end{Bmatrix}. \tag{5-73a}$$

Double crossover:

$$\begin{Bmatrix} a,b,c; & d,e,f; & g,h,i \\ r,s,t; & u,v,w; & x,y,z \end{Bmatrix} \Rightarrow \begin{Bmatrix} r,s,t; & u,v,w; & g,h,i \\ a,b,c; & d,e,f; & x,y,z \end{Bmatrix}. \tag{5-73b}$$

Linear interpolation crossover:

$$\begin{Bmatrix} a,b,c; & d,e,f; & g,h,i \\ r,s,t; & u,v,w; & x,y,z \end{Bmatrix} \Rightarrow \begin{Bmatrix} \dfrac{2a+r}{3}, \dfrac{2b+s}{3}, \dfrac{2c+t}{3}; & \cdots \dfrac{2i+z}{3} \\[2mm] \dfrac{2r+a}{3}, \dfrac{2s+b}{3}, \dfrac{2t+c}{3}; & \cdots \dfrac{2z+i}{3} \end{Bmatrix}. \tag{5-73c}$$

The idea behind crossover is to explore alternative solutions in the weight space, maintaining some good "qualities" of the parent generation. Usually there is also a fixed number of parent chromosomes with high fitness factor that pass unchanged to the next generation, the so-called *elitism*.

Mutation

On the generated chromosomes it is possible to add some mutation effect by adding a small amount of noise, with probability P_m, the *mutation rate*. The possible benefit of adding random noise to the weights during training was already explained in section 5.5.2.

The stopping conditions for the process of generating new populations can be the same as for the MLP trained with back-propagation (see section 5.5.2).

Genetic algorithms rely, therefore, on random crossover and mutations to perform a wide search in the weight space, which hopefully will converge to an optimal solution. The explanation of how a genetically trained MLP will have the ability to reach an optimal solution is essentially based on the *schema theorem*, presented by Holland (1975). Given the insight provided by this theorem, we review here its main ingredients for the case of binary chromosomes. A schema is a *chromosome template*, represented by a sequence using the special symbol * as a representation of any gene value. Consider, for instance, a chromosome with three binary genes. Each possible genetic combination corresponds to a vertex of a 3-dimensional cube. Consider now the schema:

$$H = \{1 * 1\}$$

This schema represents the vertices {101} and {111}, i.e., the cube edge corresponding to a fixed value of 1 for the first and third genes. In general, a schema acts like a hyperplane separating sets of chromosomes.

Let us denote:

- k, *order of schema H*, defined as the number of fixed positions in the schema. The above example has $k=2$. An order of zero corresponds to the full search space.
- $n(\mathbf{g})$, number of instances of $\mathbf{g}$ in the population of chromosomes.
- $n(H) = \sum_{\mathbf{g} \in H} n(\mathbf{g})$, number of schemata in the population of chromosomes.

With this notation we can express, as follows, the average fitness at time t for all sequences in the population that belong to a schema H:

$$f(H,t) = \frac{\sum_{\mathbf{g} \in H} f(\mathbf{g}) n(\mathbf{g})}{n(H,t)},$$
(5-74)

where $n(H, t)$ is the number of schemata at time t.

Using roulette-wheel, the expected number of selections of $\mathbf{g}$ is:

$$E[\mathbf{g}] = f(\mathbf{g}) / \bar{f}(t),$$
(5-75)

where $\bar{f}(t)$ is the average fitness of all chromosomes at time t. Therefore, the number of schemata H at time $t+1$ is:

$$n(H,t+1) = \sum_{\mathbf{g} \in H} n(\mathbf{g}) \frac{f(\mathbf{g})}{\bar{f}(t)} = \frac{n(H,t) f(H,t)}{\bar{f}(t)}.$$
(5-76)

This shows that the number of schemata with above average fitness will increase, while the others, with below average fitness, will decrease. In particular, if $f(H,t) / \bar{f}(t) = a > 1$ then an exponential growth $n(H,t) = n(H,0) a^t$ will be observed.

Let us analyse now the effect of 1-point crossover. For this purpose let us denote by $d(H)$ the *length of a schema*, defined as the distance between the first and last fixed positions of the schema; $d(H) \in [0, m-1]$ for chromosomes with m genes.

Consider the following example of a chromosome with 6 binary genes belonging to two distinct schemas, $H1$ and $H2$:

$$\mathbf{g} = \{1 \quad 0 \quad 0 \quad ; \quad 1 \quad 1 \quad 0\}$$
$$H_1 = \{* \quad 0 \quad 0 \quad ; \quad * \quad * \quad *\}$$
$$H_2 = \{1 \quad * \quad * \quad ; \quad * \quad 1 \quad *\}$$

When crossing $\mathbf{g}$ with another chromosome, there is only a small chance that schema H_2 will survive, unless the other chromosome has genes in the same fixed positions before or after the crossing position. On the contrary, schema H_1 will always survive. As a matter of fact, a little thought shows that a schema survives 1-point crossover if it falls outside its defining length $d(H)$. As there are m-1 different positions for 1-point crossover the probability of survival is:

$$P_s = 1 - \frac{d(H)}{m-1}. \tag{5-77}$$

If crossover is applied with probability P_x the probability of survival is:

$$P_s = 1 - P_x \frac{d(H)}{m-1}. \tag{5-77a}$$

Similar results are obtained for other types of crossover.

Concerning the effect of mutation, a schema is destroyed if mutation is applied to any fixed position. If P_m is the probability of mutation, the chance of a schema surviving is:

$$P_s = (1 - P_m)^k \approx 1 - P_m k, \quad \text{for small } P_m. \tag{5-78}$$

Combining all these effects we have:

$$n(H, t+1) \geq n(H, t) \frac{f(H)}{\bar{f}(t)} \left(1 - P_x \frac{d(H)}{m-1}\right)(1 - kP_m). \tag{5-79}$$

Neglecting a small cross-product term:

$$n(H, t+1) \geq n(H, t) \frac{f(H)}{\bar{f}(t)} \left(1 - P_x \frac{d(H)}{m-1} - kP_m\right). \tag{5-79a}$$

This formula justifies the statement of the Schema theorem that *short, low-order and above average fitness schemata will grow exponentially in subsequent generations.*

The problem with the Schema theorem is that it assumes that important chromosomal information is already present initially, or will appear during crossover and mutation. For a detailed explanation of this issue see, e.g., Vonk *et al.* (1997). As a matter of fact, genetic training of neural networks is also plagued by the local minima problem, and may lead to slow convergence times since important chromosomal information may take a long time before appearing. The advantage of genetic training is that it can be applied to a wide variety of neural architectures, input values and error formulations.

The *Neuro-Genetic* program, included in the book CD (see Appendix B), is a tool for designing neural networks with either genetic or back-propagation algorithms, allowing a comparison of the two approaches. The two-class cork stoppers problem was analysed with the *Neuro-Genetic* for an MLP2:1:1 configuration. Two features were used (N, PRT10) and the cases were equally divided for training and testing (50 cases each). Using an initial population of 10 chromosomes with $P_m=P_x=0.1$, 1-point crossover and elitism, a test error estimate of 10% was achieved, similar to the performance provided by back-propagation.

Genetic algorithms also have other applications, namely for generating and analysing neural nets. An interesting application is the combination of genetic algorithms with the probabilistic neural nets, presented in section 4.3, for performing feature selection quickly. The genetic algorithm then provides a wide search in the feature space. Several datasets analysed in this chapter underwent feature selection using this method. In the many experiments performed it was found that this method of feature selection tends to discard too many features. For instance, for the foetal weight problem, the method only found feature AP as a useful feature, although at least two more features are definitely useful, as shown in sections 5.6 and 5.7.

5.9 Radial Basis Functions

The radial basis functions approach constitutes an alternative feed-forward architecture to the two-layer MLP, for performing classification or regression tasks. It is based on the exact interpolation method of determining a function $h(\mathbf{x})$ that will fit the target values t_i:

$$h(\mathbf{x}_i) = t_i. \tag{5-80}$$

The radial basis functions approach for solving this problem consists of approximating $h(\mathbf{x})$ by a weighted series of a kernel function $\varphi(d)$, which depends on the distance d of a feature vector $\mathbf{x}$ to a prototype vector $\mathbf{x}_i$:

$$h(\mathbf{x}) = \sum_{i=1}^{n} w_i \varphi\left(\|\mathbf{x} - \mathbf{x}_i\|\right). \tag{5-81}$$

Note the striking similarity between this formula and the formula of the generalized decision function (2-4), or the formula of the Parzen window estimate (4-36).

The formula (5-81) can be represented compactly in matrix form:

$$\mathbf{\Phi}\mathbf{w} = \mathbf{t}.$$ (5-82)

For a large class of functions, and assuming that the training set is composed of distinct points, matrix $\mathbf{\Phi}$ is non-singular and the weights needed for an exact interpolation can be computed from:

$$\mathbf{w} = \mathbf{\Phi}^{-1}\mathbf{t}.$$ (5-82a)

The most common kernel function used is the Gaussian function:

$$\varphi_i(\mathbf{x}) = \exp\left(-\frac{\|\mathbf{x} - \mathbf{x}_i\|^2}{2\sigma^2}\right),$$ (5-83)

with σ acting as smoothing parameter.

As we have already seen in previous sections we are not interested in exact interpolation, but rather on an interpolation solution capable of generalization, therefore, some modifications have to be introduced in the exact interpolation method:

- The number of radial basis functions is typically much smaller than n, since they are chosen relative to some centroid patterns, $\mathbf{m}_j$, instead of relative to the training patterns.
- In order to obtain good generalization properties the centroids will have to be adjusted as part of a training process.
- Instead of having a common smooth parameter σ, each basis function can have its own smoothing parameter σ_i, also determined during the network training.
- Bias parameters are included in the summation of the kernel values in order to compensate for the difference between the average value over the basis functions and the average value of the targets.

The radial basis function (RBF) network implements these requisites with the architecture of Figure 5.42.

The weights of the first layer (*radial layer*) of an RBF neural net are used to adjust the centroids $\mathbf{m}_j$ and smoothing factors σ_j used by the kernel functions. Besides a number of ad-hoc methods to choose the centroids (for instance, randomly selected or equally separated in the whole range of the training samples), the centroids can be determined sensibly using the k-means clustering algorithm explained in section 3.5. Next, the smoothing parameters are chosen, for instance, by averaging the distance from a centroid to its k-nearest neighbours. In this way, the smoothing effect is smaller in regions where the pattern distribution is more peaked.

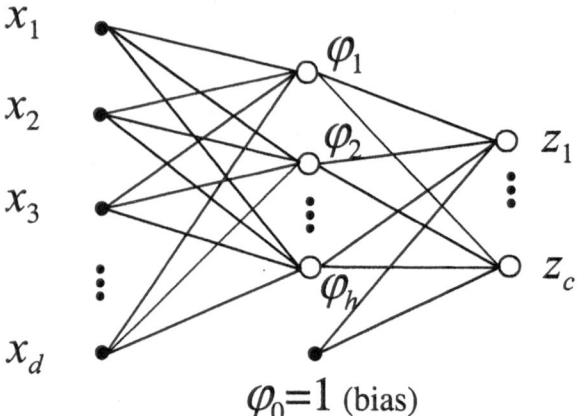

$\varphi_0 = 1$ (bias)

Figure 5.42. Radial basis functions network, with kernel functions φ_i.

The second layer weights are determined using the pseudo-inverse technique described in 5.1.1:

$$\mathbf{W'} = (\mathbf{\Phi'}\mathbf{\Phi})^{-1}\mathbf{\Phi'}\mathbf{T} = \mathbf{\Phi}^*\mathbf{T}.\tag{5-84}$$

Note that formula (5-82a) does not apply, as there are fewer functions than points.

The weights of the two layers of an RBF neural net are, therefore, independently trained, given their different role. As a consequence, RBF nets train much faster in general than equivalent MLP nets.

Instead of using the Euclidian distance in (5-83) it is also possible to use a Mahalanobis distance. It is, however, usually preferred to have more kernels with the Euclidian distance than to have to compute fewer kernels with the Mahalanobis distance, with an additional large number of covariance parameters to estimate.

An important advantage of the RBF approach compared with the MLP approach has been elucidated by Girosi and Poggio (1991). They showed that for an RBF network it is (at least theoretically) possible to find weights that will yield the minimum approximating error of any function. This *best approximation* property does not apply to MLPs.

Further details on RBF properties can be found in Bishop (1995) and Haykin (1999).

Using *Statistica* intelligent problem solver for the foetal weight data, an RBF4:4:1 solution was found with inputs BPD, CP, AP and FL. This solution had RMS errors 287 g, 286.1 g and 305.5 g for training set, validation set and test set, respectively, when trained with Gaussian kernel, k-means centroid adjustment and 6 nearest neighbours for the evaluation of the smoothing factor. Figure 5.43 shows this solution, which performs similarly to the one obtained with the Levenberg-Marquardt algorithm (section 5.7.2).

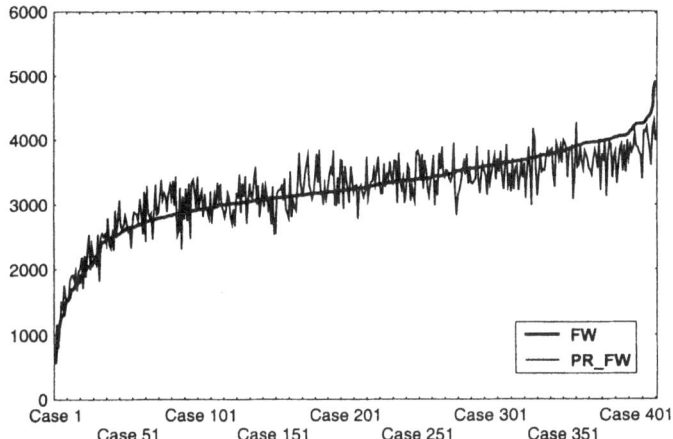

Figure 5.43. Prediction of foetal weight using an RBF4:4:1 network with Gaussian kernel and k-means centroid adjustment (compare with Figure 5.40).

5.10 Support Vector Machines

Support vector machines (SVM) is a distinctive approach to pattern classification and regression, since it tackles the principle of structural risk minimization, described in section 5.6.5, in a special way. As a consequence, support vector machines can provide a good generalization performance independent of the distributions of the patterns.

The central idea of SVM is the adjustment of a discriminating function so that it optimally uses the separability information of the boundary patterns. Let us first assume a linear discriminating function and two linearly separable classes with target values +1 and −1. A discriminating hyperplane will satisfy:

$$\mathbf{w}'\mathbf{x}_i + w_0 \geq 0 \quad \text{if} \quad t_i = +1 ; \tag{5-85a}$$

$$\mathbf{w}'\mathbf{x}_i + w_0 < 0 \quad \text{if} \quad t_i = -1 . \tag{5-85b}$$

or (perceptron rule),

$$t_i\left(\mathbf{w}'\mathbf{x}_i + w_0\right) \geq 1 . \tag{5-85c}$$

Taking into account the hyperplane properties mentioned in section 2.1, the distance of any point $\mathbf{x}_i$ to a hyperplane is precisely $|\mathbf{w}'\mathbf{x}_i + w_0|/\|\mathbf{w}\|$, as shown in Figure 5.44. In particular, the distance to the origin is simply $|w_0|/\|\mathbf{w}\|$.

Given a hyperplane, the distance of the closest pattern to it is called the *margin of separation*. The SVM approach, in its simplest linear version, consists of determining the hyperplane that maximizes the margin of separation, called *optimal hyperplane*.

Imagine that we had found the optimal hyperplane, i.e., the root set of $\mathbf{w'x}+w_0=0$. Concerning the root set, the values of $\mathbf{w}$ and w_0 are obviously not unique, and we may always divide all the weights plus bias by the same scalar factor without changing the hyperplane. Let us assume then that we have scaled $\mathbf{w}$ and w_0 in such a way that the minimum distance of a point to the hyperplane is $1/\|\mathbf{w}\|$, i.e.,

$$\min_{\mathbf{x}_i}\left|\mathbf{w'}\mathbf{x}_i + w_0\right| = 1 . \tag{5-86}$$

A hyperplane satisfying this condition is called a *canonical hyperplane* and the vectors $\mathbf{x}_i$ corresponding to this minimum distance are called *support vectors*. Condition (5-86) can also be written as follows:

$$t_i\left(\mathbf{w'}\mathbf{x}_i + w_0\right)=1 \quad \text{if and only if } \mathbf{x}_i \text{ is a support vector} . \tag{5-87}$$

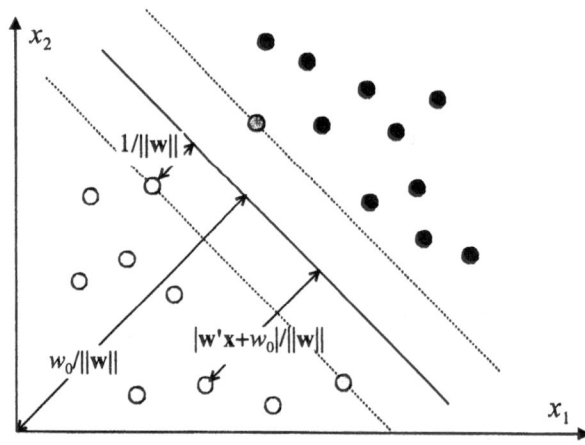

Figure 5.44. Optimal linear discriminant, with margin of separation $2/\|\mathbf{w}\|$ and support vectors (grey coloured circles) from both classes.

It can be shown (Vapnik, 1998) that the Vapnik-Chernovenkis dimension in a d-dimensional space, for a machine using a canonical hyperplane with a margin of separation r, and sample feature vectors within a sphere of radius R, is bounded as follows:

$$d_{VC} \le \min\left(R^2 / r^2, d\right)+1 . \tag{5-88}$$

Hence, when maximizing the separation margin r, we are in fact minimizing the Vapnik-Chervonenkis dimension and, therefore, minimizing the structural risk. As can be seen from expression (5-63), this is particularly beneficial for a small value of n/d_{VC} (say below 20). Also note that the complexity of the SVM approach depends on the number of support vectors used, and is independent of the problem's dimensionality (for more details see e.g. Cherkassky and Mulier, 1998).

For the canonical hyperplane the norm of the weight vector controls the margin of separation. The SVM approach of maximizing the margin of separation (equivalent to minimizing the norm of the weight vector) can be expressed then as the following constrained optimisation problem:

$$\begin{cases} \text{minimize} \quad \Phi(\mathbf{w}) = \frac{1}{2}\|\mathbf{w}\|^2, \\ \text{subject to} \quad t_i(\mathbf{w}'\mathbf{x}_i + w_0) \geq 1, \quad i = 1, \cdots, n. \end{cases} \tag{5-89}$$

Notice that the minimization of the cost function $\Phi(\mathbf{w})$ will assure the minimization of the norm of the weight vector, with the advantage that $\Phi(\mathbf{w})$ being a quadratic function, there is a standard method for solving this so-called *quadratic programming problem*. This standard method is called the *Lagrange multipliers method*, and consists of computing the saddle point of the *Lagrangian function*:

$$J(\mathbf{w}, w_0, \mathbf{a}) = \frac{1}{2}\|\mathbf{w}\|^2 - \sum_{i=1}^{n} \alpha_i (t_i(\mathbf{w}'\mathbf{x}_i + w_0) - 1), \tag{5-90}$$

minimizing the weights plus bias and maximizing the nonnegative *Lagrange multipliers* α_i.

If we differentiate the Lagrangian function with respect to $\mathbf{w}$ and w_0, the following optimality conditions are derived:

$$\mathbf{w} = \sum_{i=1}^{n} \alpha_i t_i \mathbf{x}_i \ ; \tag{5-91}$$

$$\sum_{i=1}^{n} \alpha_i t_i = 0. \tag{5-92}$$

In order to compute the weights all we need now are the values of the Lagrangian multipliers. When we expand the expression of $J(\mathbf{w}, w_0, \alpha)$ and use the results (5-91), an expression depending only on α is obtained:

$$Q(\mathbf{a}) = \sum_{i=1}^{n} \alpha_i - \frac{1}{2} \sum_{i=1}^{n} \sum_{j=1}^{n} \alpha_i \alpha_j t_i t_j \mathbf{x}_i'\mathbf{x}_j. \tag{5-93}$$

The extremal problems (5-89) and (5-93) are known as *primal* and *dual* problems, respectively. The dual problem consists of maximizing $Q(\alpha)$, yielding nonnegative Lagrange multipliers that satisfy condition (5-92). Notice that the solution of (5-93) depends only on the dot products $\mathbf{x}_i'\mathbf{x}_j$. Let us denote by $\tilde{\alpha}_i$ the optimal Lagrangian multipliers. The optimal weight vector is, therefore, from (5-91):

$$\tilde{\mathbf{w}} = \sum_{i=1}^{n} \tilde{\alpha}_i t_i \mathbf{x}_i \ . \tag{5-94}$$

The optimal bias can be derived using the optimal weight vector and condition (5-86), as follows:

$$\tilde{w}_0 = -\frac{1}{2}\tilde{\mathbf{w}}'\left(\mathbf{x}_p + \mathbf{x}_m\right), \tag{5-95}$$

where $\mathbf{x}_p$ and $\mathbf{x}_m$ are any support vectors from the +1 and –1 classes, respectively. Further details concerning this optimisation problem can be found in (Fletcher, 1999), namely a discussion of the so-called *Kuhn-Tucker conditions*, which constrain the Lagrange multipliers, except for the support vectors, to be zero.

Let us see how the Lagrange multipliers method works in a simple example, depicted in Figure 5.45, with two points, $\mathbf{x}_1=[0\ 0]'$ and $\mathbf{x}_2=[1\ 0]'$, for class +1, and two points, $\mathbf{x}_3=[2\ 0]'$ and $\mathbf{x}_4=[0\ 2]'$, for class -1.

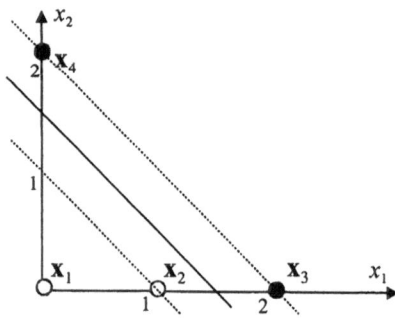

Figure 5.45. An optimal linear discriminant derived by quadratic programming.

We start by solving the dual problem, where the function $Q(\alpha)$ is readily determined from the dot products of the sample vectors:

$$Q(\alpha) = (\alpha_1 + \alpha_2 + \alpha_3 + \alpha_4) - \frac{1}{2}\left(\alpha_2^2 - 4\alpha_2\alpha_3 + 4\alpha_3^2 + 4\alpha_4^2\right). \tag{5-96}$$

Differentiating with respect to the αs and using condition (5-92), the following system of equations is obtained:

$$\begin{cases} \alpha_1 + \alpha_2 - \alpha_3 - \alpha_4 = 0 \\ \alpha_2 - 2\alpha_3 = 1 \\ -2\alpha_2 + 4\alpha_3 = 1 \\ 4\alpha_4 = 1 \end{cases} , \tag{5-97}$$

which has the following solution in nonnegative α's: $\alpha_1=0$; $\alpha_2=1$; $\alpha_3=3/4$; $\alpha_4=1/4$. Applying (5-91), we determine the optimal weight vector:

$$\breve{\mathbf{w}} = + \begin{bmatrix} 1 \\ 0 \end{bmatrix} - \frac{3}{4} \begin{bmatrix} 2 \\ 0 \end{bmatrix} - \frac{1}{4} \begin{bmatrix} 0 \\ 2 \end{bmatrix} = \begin{bmatrix} -1/2 \\ -1/2 \end{bmatrix}. \tag{5-98}$$

Hence, the linear discriminant is a straight line at $-45°$ and the support vectors are the points $\mathbf{x}_2$, $\mathbf{x}_3$ and $\mathbf{x}_4$ (with non-zero Lagrange multipliers), allowing us to determine the optimal bias using points $\mathbf{x}_2$ and $\mathbf{x}_3$:

$$\breve{w}_0 = -\frac{1}{2} \begin{bmatrix} -1/2 & -1/2 \end{bmatrix} \begin{bmatrix} 3 \\ 0 \end{bmatrix} = 3/4. \tag{5-99}$$

The canonical hyperplane is, therefore, $d(\mathbf{x}) = 3 - 2x_1 - 2x_2 = 0$, satisfying condition (5-87) for the support vectors.

Concerning the performance of SVM classifiers in the case of linearly separable classes, the work of Raudy (1997) has shown that the classification error is mainly determined by the dimensionality ratio, and that larger separation margins result, on average, in better generalization.

When the classes are non-separable, the optimal hyperplane must take into account the deviations from the ideal separable situation. In the approach introduced by Cortes and Vapnik (1995), the conditions (5-89) for the determination of the optimal hyperplane are reformulated as:

$$\begin{cases} \text{minimize} \quad \Phi(\mathbf{w}) = \frac{1}{2} \|\mathbf{w}\|^2 + C \sum_{i=1}^{n} \varepsilon_i , \\ \text{subject to} \quad t_i(\mathbf{w}' \mathbf{x}_i + w_0) \geq 1 - \varepsilon_i, \quad i = 1, \cdots, n , \end{cases} \tag{5-100}$$

where the ε_i are nonnegative *slack variables*, penalizing the deviation of a data point from the ideal separable situation.

For a point falling on the right side of the decision region but inside the region of separation, the value of ε_i is smaller than one. This is the situation of point $\mathbf{x}_1$ in Figure 5.46. For a point falling on the wrong side of the decision region a bigger penalty, using $\varepsilon_i > 1$, is applied. This is the situation of the points $\mathbf{x}_2$ and $\mathbf{x}_3$.

The support vectors are now the vectors that satisfy the condition:

$$t_i(\mathbf{w}' \mathbf{x}_i + w_0) = 1 - \varepsilon_i. \tag{5-101}$$

Note that the first condition was reformulated by adding to the cost function $\Phi(\mathbf{w})$ the term:

$$c\sum_{i=1}^{n}\varepsilon_i = C\xi .$$ (5–102)

This term is proportional to the sum of the penalties, ξ, scaled by a parameter C. The minimization of $\Phi(\mathbf{w})$ imposes an inverse influence on C and ξ. For small C the influence of ξ is big, i.e., the solution tends to minimize the errors using a small margin. For large C the influence of ξ in the minimization is small, i.e., there is a large tolerance to misclassification errors with a tendency to use a wide margin. In practice, the value of C has to be chosen experimentally since it may have more than one "optimal" value.

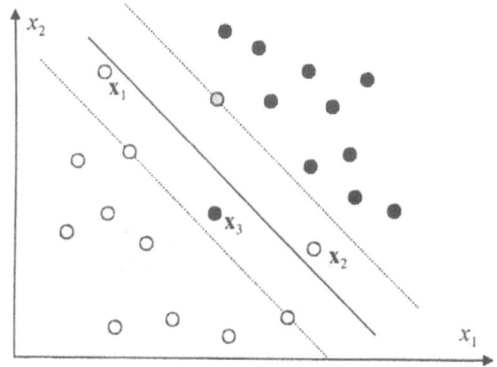

Figure 5.46. Optimal linear discriminant for a non-separable class situation.

The solution of the quadratic programming problem with reformulation (5-100) is obtained in a similar way to the previous linearly separable problem (5-89). In fact, the formulation of the dual problem for determination of the Lagrange multipliers is the same, with the multipliers now satisfying the more restrictive condition:

$$0 \le \alpha_i \le C .$$ (5-103)

Also, formula (5-94) for the weight vector now uses a summation for the support vectors alone:

$$\breve{\mathbf{w}} = \sum_{SVs} \breve{\alpha}_i t_i \mathbf{x}_i .$$ (5-104)

Using the *Support Vector Machine Toolbox* for *Matlab*, developed by S.R. Gunn (Gunn, 1997), several experiments were conducted as explained in the following. Figure 5.47 illustrates the SVM approach for the non-separable situation, exemplifying the influence of the constant C in the separation region, namely for $C=100$ and $C=\infty$ (a very large value of C). In both cases the number of misclassified samples is the same (3 misclassified samples). However, in the first case the margin is smaller, therefore attempting to decrease the value of ξ, with a smaller number of support vectors.

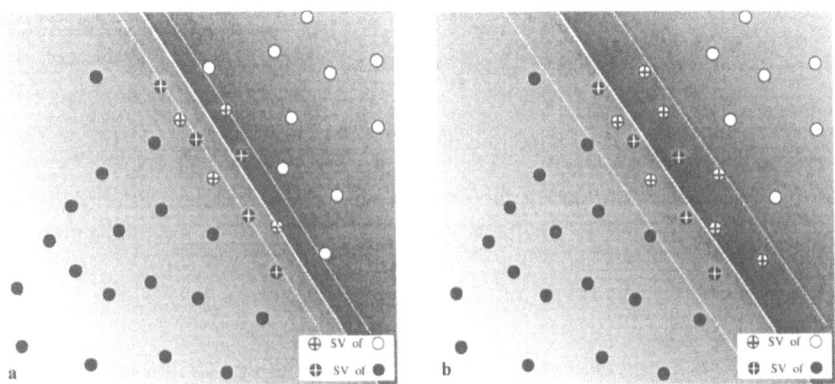

Figure 5.47. SVM linear discrimination of two non-separable classes. (a) $C=100$, with nine support vectors; (b) $C=\infty$, with twelve support vectors.

The SVM approach was also applied to the classification of the first two classes of cork stoppers. Figure 5.48 shows the results obtained for $C=10$. The overall error is 9% (2 misclassified cases of class ω_1 and 7 misclassified cases of class ω_2). The solution is remarkably close to the solution obtained with a perceptron (see Figure 5.19), with somewhat better performance, at least for the training set. Using other values of C similar solutions were obtained, with some variation of the separation margin and the number of support vectors.

Let us now consider the support vector approach for non-linear decision functions. The basic idea is to perform a non-linear mapping into a higher dimension space where the linear approach can be applied. The transformation to a higher dimension, already presented in (2-4), is:

$$d(\mathbf{x}) = w_1 f_1(\mathbf{x}) + \ldots + w_k f_k(\mathbf{x}) + w_0 = \mathbf{w}'\mathbf{y}^*, \tag{5-105}$$

$$\text{with} \quad \mathbf{y}^* = [f_1(\mathbf{x}) \, f_2(\mathbf{x}) \ldots f_k(\mathbf{x}) \, 1]' . \tag{5-105a}$$

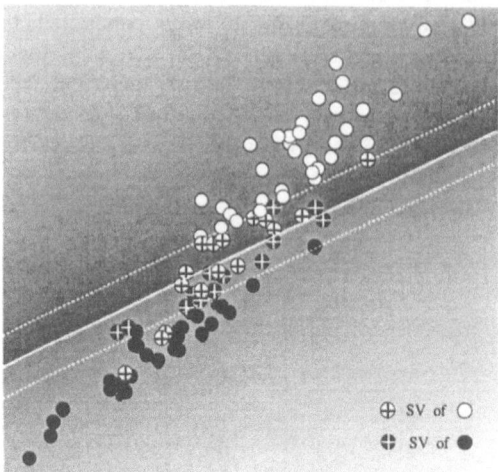

Figure 5.48. SVM solution for the classification of two classes of cork stoppers, using $C=10$. The number of support vectors is 33 (a third of the total number of patterns).

In the transformed feature space we now have the optimal weight vector:

$$\breve{\mathbf{w}} = \sum_{SVs} \breve{\alpha}_i t_i f(\mathbf{x}_i).$$

(5-106)

Using (5-105), the linear decision function in the transformed feature space is:

$$d(\mathbf{x}) = \mathbf{w'}\mathbf{y}^* = \sum_{SVs} \breve{\alpha}_i t_i f(\mathbf{x}_i)' f(\mathbf{x}),$$

(5-107)

or

$$d(\mathbf{x}) = \mathbf{w'}\mathbf{y}^* = \sum_{SVs} \breve{\alpha}_i t_i K(\mathbf{x}_i, \mathbf{x}),$$

(5-107a)

where $K(\mathbf{x}_i, \mathbf{x})$ is known as an *inner-product kernel*, which allows us to express the decision functions in the original feature space.

The kernel $K(\mathbf{x}_i, \mathbf{x})$ will exist, provided some non-stringent conditions are fulfilled (see e.g. Haykin, 1999). In particular, the following kernels can be used:

Polynomial	$K(\mathbf{x}_i, \mathbf{x}) = (\mathbf{x'}\mathbf{x}_i + 1)^p$
Gaussian radial basis function	$K(\mathbf{x}_i, \mathbf{x}) = \exp(-(\mathbf{x}-\mathbf{x}_i)^2/2\sigma^2)$
Exponential radial basis function	$K(\mathbf{x}_i, \mathbf{x}) = \exp(-|\mathbf{x}-\mathbf{x}_i|/2\sigma^2)$
Tanh sigmoid	$K(\mathbf{x}_i, \mathbf{x}) = \tanh(a\mathbf{x'}\mathbf{x}_i + b)$

Notice that the preceding linear approaches can be viewed as particular cases of the kernel approach, using a linear kernel, $K(\mathbf{x}_i,\mathbf{x}) = \mathbf{x}'\mathbf{x}_i$.

The connectionist structure of a generalized support vector machine, using a kernel $K(\mathbf{x}_i,\mathbf{x})$, is similar to the RBF network structure (see Figure 5.42) for a two class problem, with the hidden layer neurons computing the kernels, which are next linearly combined (5-107a) to provide the output .

Figure 5.49 exemplifies an SVM quadratic discrimination, $K(\mathbf{x}_i,\mathbf{x}) = (\mathbf{x}'\mathbf{x}_i+1)^2$, using two different values of C. The influence of C on the margin width and the quadratic shape is evident. Using $C=1000$ for the same data a quadratic solution similar to the $C=\infty$ solution was obtained, with similar margin and misclassified samples, in a clear demonstration that there may be many different "optimal" values for C. The generalization properties of non-linear SVMs are still an open issue.

The Support Vector Machine approach can also be applied to regression problems. A description of this topic can be found in Gunn (1997) and Haykin (1999).

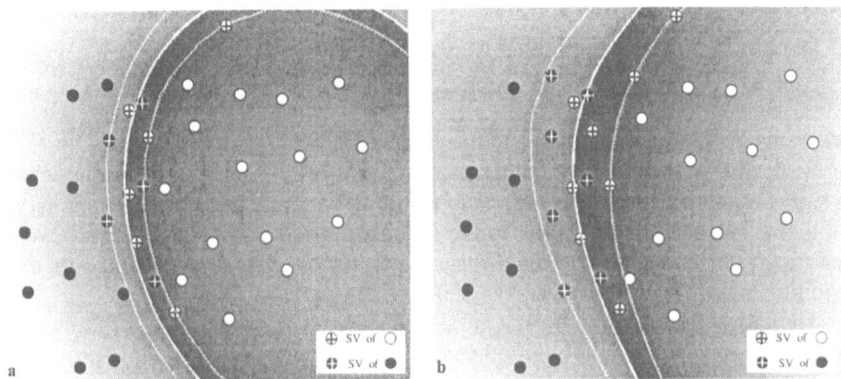

Figure 5.49. SVM quadratic discrimination. (a) C=100, eleven support vectors, 4 misclassified patterns; (b) C=∞, fifteen support vectors, 6 misclassified patterns.

5.11 Kohonen Networks

All the previous neural networks performed supervised classification or regression tasks. Unlike these, *Kohonen's self organising feature map* or Kohonen network for short, constitutes a neural net approach to data clustering. As shown in Figure 5.50, these networks are constituted by just one layer of output neurons, arranged as a two-dimensional grid. The main goal is to iteratively adjust the weights connecting inputs to outputs, such that in the end these reflect the distance relations among input patterns.

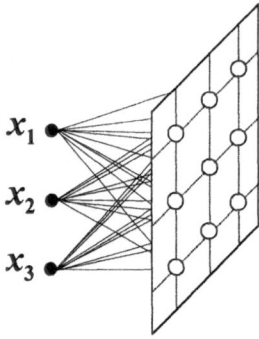

Figure 5.50. Connectionist structure of a Kohonen self organizing map. The output neurons form a two-dimensional grid.

We will denote the output neurons by z_{jk}, the index j denoting the position along the horizontal direction of the grid and the index k along the vertical direction. The distance d_{jk} between an input vector $\mathbf{x}$ and an output neuron z_{jk} is computed as:

$$d_{jk} = \sum_{i=1}^{d} (x_i - w_{jk,i})^2 \,, \tag{5-108}$$

where $w_{kj,i}$ is the weight relative to the connection of input x_i to output z_{jk}.

Basically, the network training consists of adjusting, at any iteration step, the weights of the neuron that is nearest to the input pattern, called the *winning neuron*, so that it becomes more similar to the input pattern, the so called *winner-takes-all* learning rule. At the same time, in the initial iterations, a set of neighbours of the winning neuron have their weights similarly adjusted.

Therefore, the weight adjustment takes place in a neighbourhood of the winning output neuron. The neighbourhood can be large at the beginning of the process and then it decreases as the process progresses. A square or hexagonal grid centred at the winning neuron can be used as neighbourhood, the square grid being more popular. It is normal to use a *radius* measure to define the neighbourhood size; for a square grid the radius is simply the city-block distance to it centre. During the learning process the neurons *compete* in order to arrive at the decision that most resembles a certain input.

The learning algorithm can be described as follows:

1. Initialise the weights, $w_{jk,i}^{(0)}$, with random values in a certain interval, and select the neighbourhood radius, r, and the learning rate, η.
2. Compute d_{jk} for each output neuron and determine the winning neuron (the one with minimum distance).
3. For all neurons in the neighbourhood of the winning neuron, adjust the weights as:

$$w_{jk,i}^{(r+1)} = w_{jk,i}^{(r)} + \eta \left(x_i - w_{jk,i}^{(r)} \right). \tag{5-109}$$

Neurons outside the neighbourhood are not updated. Also, the neighbourhood does not wrap around the borders.

4 Update learning rate and neighbourhood radius (decreasing them).

5. Repeat steps 2 to 4 until the stopping condition (e.g. maximum number of epochs) is reached.

The Kohonen network develops a sort of two-dimensional map, resembling the application of multidimensional scaling techniques. The effect of the neighbourhood is to drag the training cases near their winning prototypes. As the network training progresses, the decrease of neighbourhood radius and learning rate will result in a finer tuning of each neuron to the most similar input pattern. After a sufficient number of epochs the weights will cluster, such that the grid of output neurons constitutes a kind of topological map of the inputs, reflecting the structure of the data, therefore the name of *self-organizing map*. The performance of the mapping is evaluated by an error measure that averages, for all patterns, the distance d_{jk} of each pattern from the winning output neuron.

Table 5.8. Winning frequencies for a Kohonen network trained with the globular data shown in Figure 3.4a.

(a)	$z._1$	$z._2$	$z._3$	(b)	$z._1$	$z._2$	$z._3$
$z_1.$	2	1	1	$z_1.$	5	2	1
$z_2.$	0	5	6	$z_2.$	1	0	3
$z_3.$	1	0	2	$z_3.$	1	1	4

(a) 10 epochs with $\eta = 0.1$, $r=2$.
(b) Convergence situation with $\eta=0.05$, $r=1$.

We now proceed to exemplify the use of a Kohonen mapping, using *Statistica*. We start with the globular data of *Cluster.xls* shown in Figure 3.4a. We use a 3x3 output grid and start with a neighbourhood radius of 2. Training with only 10 epochs and a learning rate of 0.1 we obtain the *winning frequencies*, i.e., the number of patterns for which an output neuron is a winning neuron, shown in Table 5.8. The error (sum of d_{jk}) is then around 0.4. Looking at the local maxima it seems that a cluster centre is forming around z_{23} and possibly another one at z_{11}. With further training using a neighbourhood radius of 1 and a smaller learning rate, we reach the solution shown in Table 5.8 with an error below 0.2, where it is clearly visible that there are now two distinct clusters represented by $\{z_{11}\}$ and $\{z_{33}, z_{23}\}$, separated by zero cases at z_{22} and only isolated borderline cases, e.g. at z_{31} and z_{13}.

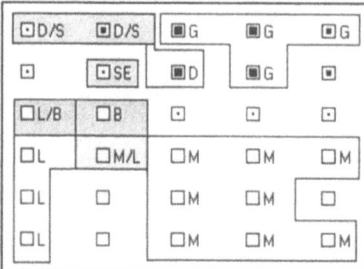

Figure 5.51. Topological map of the rocks dataset, labelled according to the winning neurons for each case: G-granite; D-diorite; S-slate; SE-serpentine; M-marble; L-limestone; B-breccia. Distance measures increase from a full black to a full white neuron. The figured case is the number 1 granite case.

Let us now consider the result of applying Kohonen mapping, with an output grid of 6x5 neurons, to the *Rocks* dataset. Training was performed with 100 epochs starting with an initial neighbourhood radius of 3. Different clustering solutions are obtained depending on the initial weights and small variations of initial and final values of the learning rate. All solutions revealed, however, a similar topology as that exemplified by the topological map of Figure 5.51, where the main categories of rocks are clearly and reasonably identified. In fact, the Kohonen map shows a clear distinction between Si-rich rocks in the upper clusters and Ca-rich rocks in the lower clusters (see also sections 3.4 and 3.5). The other clusters, e.g. M/L, also have a logical interpretation, since they present values for the most relevant features that lie midway between the values of the limiting clusters.

5.12 Hopfield Networks

The Hopfield network is a recurrent neural network with a feedback loop from each output to the inputs of all other units, with no self-feedback, as shown in Figure 5.22. The full analysis of the Hopfield net, with a d-dimensional input vector **x**, requires dynamical considerations that can be found e.g. in Haykin (1999). The main result of the dynamic analysis is the convergence of the net to local minima of the following energy function:

$$E = -\frac{1}{2}\sum_{i=1}^{d}\sum_{\substack{j=1 \\ j \neq i}}^{d} w_{ji} x_i x_j + \sum_{j=1}^{d}\frac{1}{aR_j}\int_0^{x_j} f^{-1}(x)\,dx , \qquad (5\text{-}110)$$

where it is assumed that:

- The inputs x_i (i=1, ..., d) are continuous-valued variables and applied at a given initial instant;
- The weights are symmetric, $w_{ij} = w_{ji}$;
- The activation functions $f(x)$ are sigmoidal functions, identical for all neurons, with parameter a governing the sigmoidal slope (see formulas 5-10b and 5-10c);
- The R_j are non-negative quantities that represent dissipative factors, responsible for energy that is not spent in the "stimulation" of the neurons.

The second term of (5-110) vanishes when $a \rightarrow \infty$, i.e., when the sigmoid converges to the step function. The net then converges to local minima of:

$$E = -\frac{1}{2} \sum_{\substack{i=1 \\ }}^{d} \sum_{\substack{j=1 \\ j \neq i}}^{d} w_{ji} x_i x_j \ . \tag{5-111}$$

A particularly interesting version of the network in this case corresponds to imposing binary valued inputs, e.g. $x_j = \pm 1$, the so-called *discrete Hopfield net*. Suppose that given a matrix $\mathbf{W}$ of weights w_{ij}, with $w_{ii} = 0$ (no self feedback), the output of neuron i, x_i, is computed as:

$$x_i = \text{sgn}\left(\sum_{j=1}^{d} w_{ij} x_j \right), \tag{5-112}$$

where sgn is the *sign function*, identical to the step function 5-10a except that sgn(0)=0. If the linear combination of the inputs yields a positive value, the output is set to +1; if a negative value is obtained, the output is set to –1; for the zero value the output is left unchanged. With this activation function the outputs of the Hopfield neurons will also be binary valued vectors, corresponding to vertices of a d-dimensional hypercube, known as *states*.

The updating can be done in a random serial way - *asynchronous* updating - i.e., each neuron is selected randomly for updating, or in a fully parallel way – *synchronous* updating -, i.e, all the neurons are updated at the same time. When the updating of the outputs is done in an assynchronous way and the matrix $\mathbf{W}$ is symmetric, the net will converge to a *stable state*, with the outputs remaining unchanged with further iterations. The demonstration of this important result can be found e.g. in (Looney, 1997). The stable states of a Hopfield net correspond to minima of the energy function (5-111). If the updating is done in a fully parallel way, the network can either converge to a stable state or oscillate between two states.

The discrete Hopfield net has found interesting applications as a *content-addressed memory* (CAM) device, which allows the retrieval of a previously memorized pattern that most resembles a given input pattern. In this case, the neurons play the role of memories that are able to recall a previously stored prototype pattern. The algorithm for using the Hopfield net as a CAM device is as follows:

1 - Storage phase

Let $\mathbf{z}_k$ be a set of c prototype patterns, with binary-valued features, to be memorized. Assign weights to the net as:

$$w_{ij} = \sum_{k=1}^{c} z_{k,i} z_{k,j} \quad \text{for} \quad j \neq i; \quad w_{ii} = 0; \quad i,j = 1, \cdots, d. \tag{5-113}$$

Note that a symmetric weight matrix is used, therefore only half of the d^2 weights have to be computed.

The weight computation as a product of neuron inputs is known as *Hebb rule* (see Table 5-2). The idea behind this rule is to enhance the "synaptic" link of neurons that are in the same state.

2 - Retrieval phase

2.1 - Let $\mathbf{y}$ be the unknown pattern. At time t=0, initialize the inputs with the unknown pattern:

$$\mathbf{x}^{(0)} = \mathbf{y} . \tag{5-114}$$

2.2 - Iterate until convergence:

$$x_i^{(r+1)} = \text{sgn}\left(\sum_{j=1}^{d} w_{ij} x_j^{(r)} \right). \tag{5-115}$$

The iteration is performed assynchronously, by randomly selecting a neuron from the subset of d neurons not yet selected. The updating of all the d neurons is called a *cycle*. If a stable state has been reached at the end of a cycle, one proceeds to the next step, otherwise a new cycle takes place.

2.3 - The retrieved vector is the one that best matches the network output vector (stable state).

Ideally, the Hopfield net will converge to one of the c vertices of the d-dimensional hypercube, corresponding to the prototypes. In practice, especially for large c, extra stable states will appear, known as *spurious states*. A discussion about the spurious states phenomenon can be found in Haykin (1999). The possible presence of spurious states justifies the need for selecting the prototype vector that best matches the stable state (counting the number of differences in component values, the so-called *Hamming distance*) in the previous step 2.3.

We now exemplify the use of a Hopfield net as a CAM device, using the *Hopfield* program (see Appendix B) with the two-dimensional binary prototype images shown in Figure 5.52.

The *Hopfield* program allows the addition of random noise to the binary images, thereby obtaining "unknown" patterns. It is also possible to create an arbitrary pattern by directly editing the binary grid.

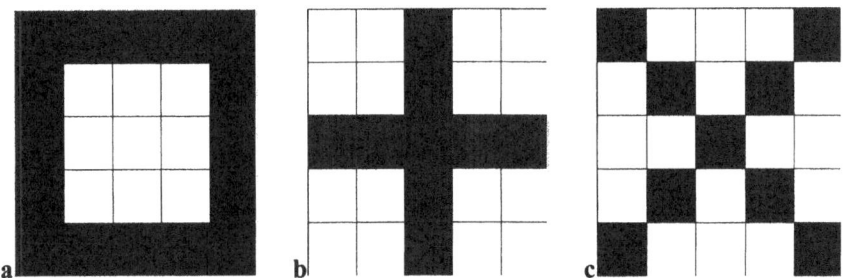

Figure 5.52. Binary image prototypes used in CAM experiments with the *Hopfield* program: (a) "zero"; (b) "plus"; (c) "cross".

Three such "unknown" patterns are shown in Figure 5.53. The first one, Figure 5.53a, corresponds to a "plus" pattern with noise and converges in one cycle to the right prototype.

The second one, Figure 5.53b, corresponds to a "cross" pattern with substantial noise. It can either converge to a cross or to one of the spurious states shown in Figures 5.54a and 5.54b. The type of convergence depends on the random behaviour of the output neuron updating and, therefore, on the particular "trajectory" followed in the space of the d-dimensional hypercube vertices. When the spurious state is the one shown in Figure 5.54a, the matching prototype is the "plus" pattern, therefore corresponding to an incorrect retrieval.

Finally, the "grid" pattern also exhibits convergence to a spurious state. An interesting thing about this pattern is that the Hopfield net will not converge and, instead, will oscillate between two states, the "grid" itself and its complement shown in Figure 5.54c, if the algorithm performs a full parallel updating instead of a random serial updating. The possibility of obtaining oscillations between two states with full parallel updating was previously mentioned.

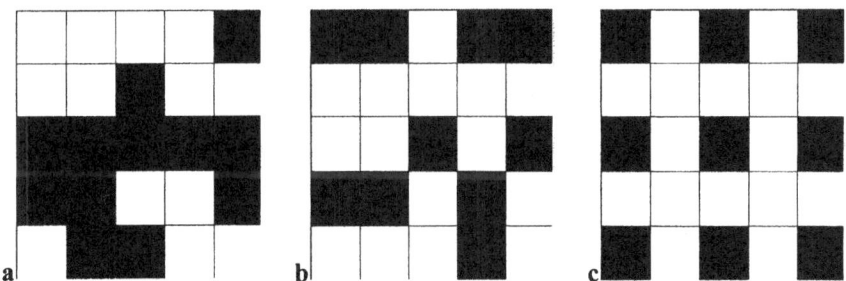

Figure 5.53. Three unknown binary images: (a) "plus" with noise; (b) a highly corrupted "cross"; (c) "grid".

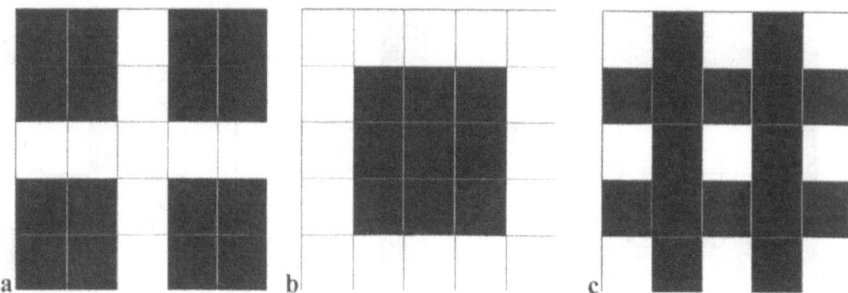

Figure 5.54. Binary images corresponding to spurious states of a Hopfield network trained with the prototypes of Figure 5.52.

Notice that the spurious states shown in Figure 5.54 correspond to the complement of prototype states. Besides the complement, one can obtain spurious states that are a combination of an odd number of prototype patterns or states that are not correlated with any of the prototypes.

Another problem that decreases the efficiency of a Hopfield net, besides the presence of spurious states, is the use of an excessive number of prototypes for the available number of neurons. As a matter of fact, a prototype pattern with moderate noise may converge to an incorrect prototype if it shares many feature values with other prototypes. There is, therefore, an upper limit to the maximum number of patterns that can be memorized and retrieved with practically no errors, the so-called *storage capacity* of the discrete Hopfield net. Formulas and estimates of the storage capacity are presented in (Looney, 1997) and (Haykin, 1999).

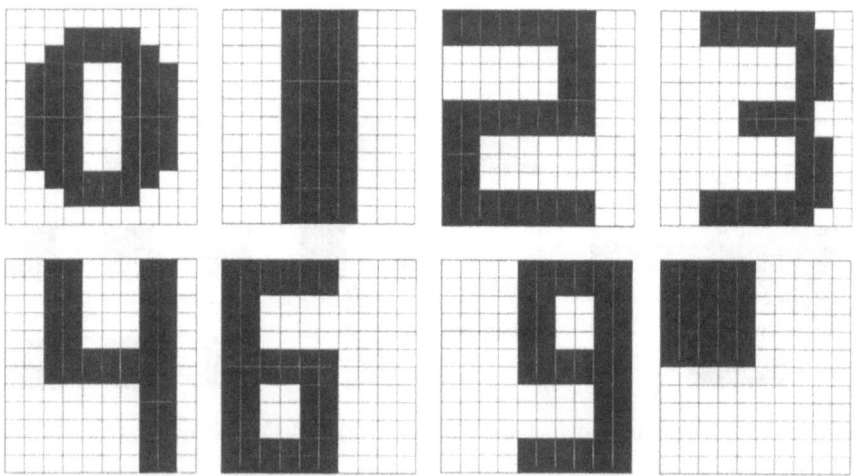

Figure 5.55. Prototype patterns used in CAM experiments with the Hopfield network Lippmann (1987).

In practical applications, a robust estimate of the number of prototype patterns that can be retrieved with a low error rate is $d/10$. For instance, for $c=10$ one must employ a Hopfield net with at least $d=100$ neurons. The prototype patterns must also be carefully chosen, with small correlations among them, in order to obtain the best performance.

Figure 5.55 shows a set of 8 prototype patterns, drawn in a 12x10 grid, presented in the work of Lippmann (1987) and specially designed to produce good performance. Notice that the digit patterns are drawn in such a way that the amount of correlation among them is kept low. The number of classes is also lower than $d/10 = 12$. One obtains, therefore, quite good results even for heavily noise corrupted patterns. An example is shown in Figure 5.56 with a noise corrupted "nine". The network converges to the correct prototype after a few cycles.

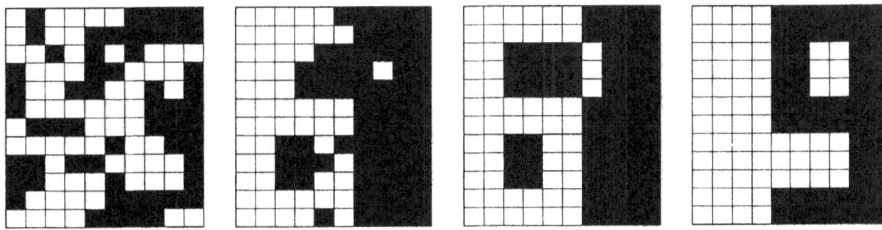

Figure 5.56. A noise corrupted "nine" converges after a few steps (left to right) to the correct prototype.

5.13 Modular Neural Networks

The principle of "divide and conquer", already applied to the decision tree design in section 4.6, can also be applied to obtain improved neural net solutions. Consider the CTG dataset with the difficult 10-class discrimination problem solved with an MLP in section 5.7.1. In this solution a considerable overlap is observed for classes A, FS and SUSP. One could, therefore, consider developing a hierarchical approach for this classification task, starting with a two-class splitting as shown in Figure 5.57.

Let us consider the design of the left side of the tree. Table 5.9 shows the classification matrices that were achieved using neural nets derived by *Statistica*, and trained with the gradient conjugate method. The neural net used for the first level two-class discrimination is an MLP6:7:1, with features LB, AC, MLTV, DL, MEAN and MEDIAN. For the three-class discrimination, at the second level, an MLP9:5:3 with features LB, AC, UC, ASTV, MSTV, ALTV, MEDIAN, MEAN and T was employed. Notice that these neural nets are less complex than the one used in section 5.7.1 and, therefore, substantially easier to train and generalize (see Exercise 5.26).

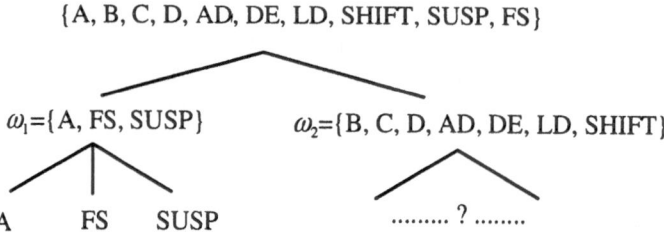

{A, B, C, D, AD, DE, LD, SHIFT, SUSP, FS}

ω_1={A, FS, SUSP} ω_2={B, C, D, AD, DE, LD, SHIFT}

A   FS   SUSP   .... ? ....

Figure 5.57. First levels of a tree classifier for the CTG data, with merged classes A, FS and SUSP.

Looking at Table 5.9 results, we see that in fact some improvement has been made over the previous solution concerning the discrimination of those three classes. In general, the *hierarchical network* approach can achieve better results if the simplified discriminations at the top levels can be solved in a very efficient way. Identification of clusters in the data, factor analysis and multidimensional scaling may be used in order to judge if there are well-separated groups of classes, appropriate for top-level discrimination.

Another motivation to use a modular approach occurs when searching for the "best" neural net solution to a given problem. During the search process one often derives alternative solutions that are discarded. These solutions may use the same inputs with different initial weights, or use alternative input sets. Discarding solutions may not be the most reasonable approach, namely if these solutions can add complementary information to the problem at hand. Instead, we may profit from the complementary characteristics of these nets, and achieve a better performing solution by using an ensemble of neural networks. We can do this by establishing a voting scheme based on the net outputs, as shown in Figure 5.58.

Table 5.9. MLPs classification matrices for the class discriminations shown in Figure 5.57. True classifications along the columns; predicted classifications along the rows.

(a)

	ω_1	ω_2
ω_1	616	82
ω_2	34	1394
P_c	94.77%	94.44%

(b)

	A	FS	SUSP
A	373	1	0
FS	4	59	1
SUSP	7	9	196
P_c	97.14%	85.51%	99.49%
P_{ct}	92.06%	81.04%	94.29%

P_c - Probability of correct classification (training set estimate) at each level.
P_{ct} - Total probability of correct classification (training set estimate for classes A, FS and SUSP).

The voting scheme in these *ensemble networks* can be implemented in a variety of ways, the most common being the *majority vote* (choose the class label that occurs more often at the module outputs), the *max vote* (choose the class label corresponding to the maximum value of the activation function outputs) and the *average vote* (choose the class label corresponding to the highest average value of the activation function outputs of the modules). A detailed discussion about neural network ensembles and voting schemes can be found in (Hansen and Salamon, 1990) and (Kittler *et al.*, 1998), respectively.

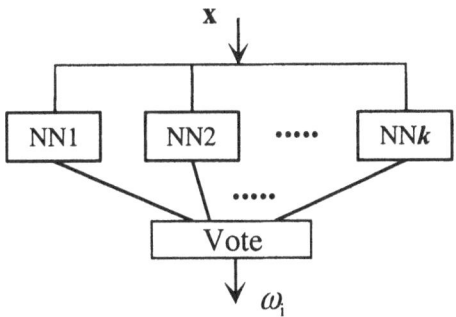

Figure 5.58. An ensemble network with k neural nets and a voting unit.

Table 5.10. Neural net solutions to the three-class cork stoppers problem.

Network	Features	ω_1 errors	ω_2 errors	ω_3 errors	Total errors
MLP2:2:3	N, PRT	2	11	1	14
MLP2:2:3	N, ART	4	10	3	17
MLP3:3:3	N, PRM, ARTG	2	12	1	15
MLP3:3:3	N, PRTG, ARTG	14	4	2	20
MLP3:3:3	RAAR, ARTG, PRTG	6	8	2	16
Majority vote	(ensemble)	3	6	2	11
Averaging	(ensemble)	5	8	2	15

We illustrate this concept using the cork stoppers data example. Instead of using the solution from section 5.6 (Table 5.5), we may choose to build an ensemble network based on neural net solutions with a small number of weights, which were found during the experimentation phase. All these nets were trained with great care in order to achieve the best possible results, which are shown in Table 5.10. Notice that the solutions have distinct qualities, with nets that recognize classes ω_1 and ω_3

very well at the expense of ω_2, a net that recognizes ω_2 well at the expense of ω_1 and finally a net that performs similarly well for all classes.

As shown in Table 5.10, a better solution was achieved with the majority vote scheme than with the first MLP2:2:3 presented in section 5.6. By performing a factor analysis in the feature space of the neural modules, we can obtain representations of the class clusters and draw the boundaries achieved by the neural solutions, as shown in Figure 5.59.

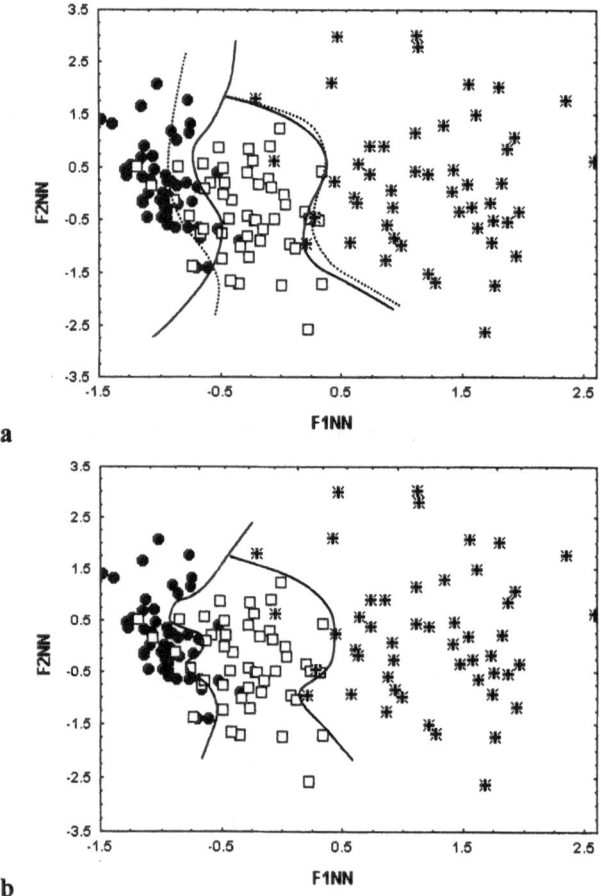

a

b

Figure 5.59. Neural net solutions for the three-class cork stoppers problem (ω_1=●, ω_2=□, ω_3=✳) represented in the space of the two main principal components. (a) MLP2:2:3 with features N, PRT (solid line boundaries) and MLP3:3: with features N, PRTG, ARTG (dotted line boundaries) ; (b) Majority vote of five neural nets (solid line boundaries). Notice how these last boundaries retain the best characteristics of the previous ones.

In general, the idea behind modular neural networks is to profit from what each neural net can do best, so that they co-operate towards the goal of attaining a high classification performance.

The hierarchical and ensemble approaches, although often achieving very good results, use the neural modules in a decoupled way, i.e., there are no mechanisms for guiding the input feature vector to the most adequate module; also, the modules are not trained in a co-operative way, so that each module is tuned to its specialized recognition task taking into account what the other modules are doing. A comparative survey of modular networks with a description of co-operative mechanisms can be found in (Gasser A, Kamel M, 1998).

5.14 Neural Networks in Data Mining

The purpose of data mining and the application of statistical classification in data mining were presented in section 4.7. Neural networks play an important role in data mining, namely the feature selection methods based on genetic algorithms, Kohonen's self organising feature maps and multi-layer perceptrons. These are used for classification or regression tasks, both called *predictive modelling* in data mining jargon. The same requirements on algorithmic performance and evaluation of solutions, presented in section 4.7, are applicable to neural network approaches.

Especially of interest in data mining applications are multi-layer perceptrons solving complex regression/forecast tasks. In order to give a taste of such an application to a typical data mining problem, and to discuss some important issues, we will consider the problem of determining a useful predictive model for the revenue of invested capital using the *Firms* dataset, which contains a table of economic variables for 838 Portuguese firms (year 1995).

In order to build a predictive model for the capital revenue (variable CAPR), defined as the ratio of the net income (NI) over the invested capital (CAP), we may select as variables constituting the search space all those that bear no direct relation with CAPR, namely GI (gross income), CA (capital plus assets), NW (number of workers), P (apparent productivity), GIR (gross income revenue), A/C (assets share) and DEPR (depreciations plus provisions), discarding the variables CAP and NI, which are obviously not of interest here.

Performing feature selection with the genetic algorithm tool yielded variable GIR as the only useful variable. This is a somewhat expected result given that GIR=NI/GI and NI is directly related to CAPR. Running the *Statistica* intelligent problem solver (IPS) for a quick search for an MLP solution, a reasonably performing MLP1:1:1 was found, using variable GIR as input and achieving a 0.765 correlation.

The search time is only about seven seconds on a 733 MHz Pentium. However, with 838 cases we are still far from the typical bulk of a data warehouse! Also, the quick search failed to find any alternative solutions to using GIR, and even failed to see any contribution of the BRANCH variable, which we may rightly suspect of having a definite influence on the results. As a matter of fact, by performing a quick search only for the industrial firms (BRANCH=3, 500 cases), a better

MLP1:3:1 solution using variable GIR is found, with higher correlation and smaller errors, which is shown in Figure 5.60a. By also performing a medium IPS search in the feature space without variable GIR, it was possible to find an alternative MLP3:2:1 solution using variables CA, DEPR and A/C, with much poor correlation (around 0.3). This solution took about 28 seconds to find on the same 733 MHz Pentium. The respective regression result is depicted in Figure 5.60b.

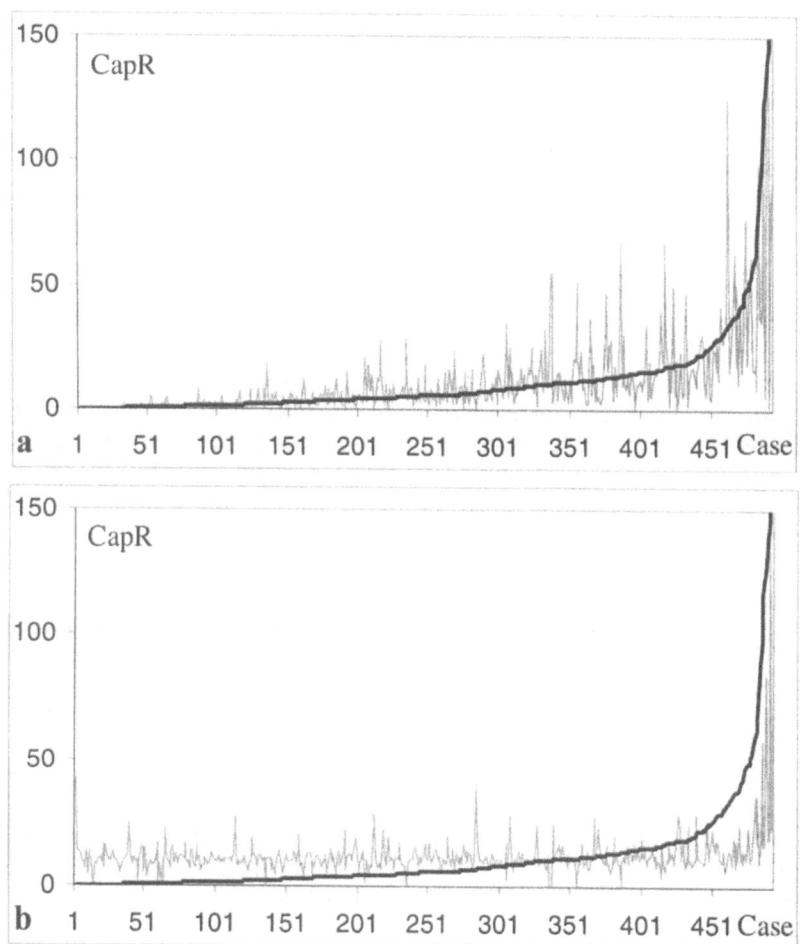

Figure 5.60. Regression (grey line) of the capital revenue (CapR) for 500 industrial firms, sorted (Case) by increasing values of CapR (black line). (a) Using an MLP1:3:1 net with variable GIR as input (correlation ≈ 0.8) ; (b) Using an MLP3:2:1 net with variables CA, DEPR and A/C as inputs (correlation ≈ 0.3).

Summarizing some conclusions of these experiments:

- Quick searches may not yield the solution that performs best (e.g. GIR solution for all values of BRANCH). This obvious conclusion can be dramatically important in data mining applications where "quick search" is a must.
- Quick searches may fail to detect the crucial importance of a variable (BRANCH in the example).
- Solutions that are of interest may require large time-consuming searches. In the example, the {CA, DEPR, A/C} solution could be more interesting from the economical point of view than the solution using GIR.
- Interpretation of the results depends drastically on the solution. In the example, an obvious relationship exists between CapR and GIR because both are ratios with the same numerator, the net income, which is the causal element. A causal inference for the {CA, DEPR, A/C} solution is more problematic, to say the least.

These experiments reflect the difficulties one may face in real data mining applications, especially concerning the usefulness of the mining results.

Bibliography

Anthony M, Bartlett PL (1999) Neural Network Learning: Theoretical Foundations. Cambridge University Press.

Atiya AF, El-Shoura SM, Shaheen SI, El-Sherif MS (1999) A Comparison Between Neural-Network Forecasting Techniques. Case Study: River Flow Forecasting. IEEE Tr Neural Networks, 10:402-409.

Baum EB, Haussler D (1989) What Size Net Gives Valid Generalization? Neural Computation, 1:151-160.

Berson A, Smith SJ (1997) Data Warehousing, Data Mining and OLAP. McGraw Hill Co. Inc.

Bishop CM (1995) Neural Networks for Pattern Recognition. Clarendon Press, Oxford.

Blumer A, Ehrenfeucht A, Haussler D, Warmuth MK (1989) Learnability and the Vapnik-Chernovenkis Dimension. J Ass Comp Machinery, 36:929-965.

Carter MA, Oxley ME (1999) Evaluating the Vapnik-Chervonenkis Dimension of Artificial Neural Networks Using the Poincaré Polynomial. Neural Networks, 12:403-408.

Cherkassky V, Mulier F (1998) Learning from Data, John Wiley & Sons, Inc.

Chryssolouris G, Lee M, Ramsey A (1996) Confidence Interval Prediction for Neural Network Models, IEEE Tr Neural Networks, 7:229-232.

Cortes C, Vapnik V (1995) Support Vector Networks. Machine Learning, 20:273-297.

Cover TM (1965) Geometrical and Statistical Properties of Systems of Linear Inequalities with Application in Pattern Recognition. IEEE Tr Elect Comp, 14:326-334.

Eberhart RC, Dobbins RW (1990) Background and History. In: Eberhart RC, Dobbins RW (eds) Neural Network PC Tools. A Practical Guide. Academic Press, Inc., pp 9-34.

Eberhart RC, Dobbins RW (1990) Implementations. In: Eberhart RC, Dobbins RW (eds) Neural Network PC Tools. A Practical Guide. Academic Press, Inc., pp 35-58.

Eberhart RC, Dobbins RW (1990) Systems Considerations. In: Eberhart RC, Dobbins RW (eds) Neural Network PC Tools. A Practical Guide. Academic Press, Inc., pp 59-77.

Eberhart RC, Dobbins RW (1990) Software Tools. In: Eberhart RC, Dobbins RW (eds) Neural Network PC Tools. A Practical Guide. Academic Press, Inc., pp 81-108.

Eberhart RC, Dobbins RW, Hutton LV (1990) Performance Metrics. In: Eberhart RC, Dobbins RW (eds) Neural Network PC Tools. A Practical Guide. Academic Press, Inc., pp 161-174.

Ehrenfeucht A, Haussler D, Kearns M, Valiant L (1989) A General Lower Bound on the Number of Examples Needed for Learning. Information and Computation, 82:247-261.

Fausset L (1994) Fundamentals of Neural Networks. Prentice Hall Inc., New Jersey.

Fletcher R (2000) Practical Methods of Optimization. J. Wiley & Sons Ltd.

Gasser A, Kamel M (1998) Modular Neural Network Classifiers: A Comparative Study. Journal of Intell. and Robotic Systems, 21:117-129.

Geman S, Bienenstock E, Doursat R (1992) Neural Networks and the Bias/Variance Dilemma. Neural Computation, 4:1-58.

Girosi F, Poggio T (1990) Networks and the Best Approximation Property. Biological Cybernetics, 63:169-176.

Gunn SR (1997) Support Vector Machines for Classification and Regression. Technical Report, Image Speech and Intelligent Systems Research Group, University of Southampton.

Hansen LK, Salamon P (1990) Neural Network Ensembles. IEEE Tr Patt An Mach Intell, 12:993-1001.

Haykin S (1999) Neural Networks. A Comprehensive Foundation. Prentice Hall Inc., New Jersey.

Holland JH (1975) Adaptation in Natural and Artificial Systems. University of Michigan Press, Ann Arbor.

Huang GB, Babri HA (1998) Upper Bounds on the Number of Hidden Neurons in Forward Networks with Arbitrary Bounded Nonlinear Activation Functions. IEEE Tr Neural Networks, 9:224-228.

Iyer MS, Rhinehart RR (1999) A Method to Determine the Required Number of Neural-Network Training Repetitions. IEEE Tr Neural Networks, 10:427-432.

Kearns MJ, Vazirani UV (1997) An Introduction to Computational Learning Theory. The MIT Press.

Kittler J, Hatef M, Duin RPW, Matas J (1998) On Combining Classifiers. IEEE Tr Patt An Mach Intell, 20:226-238.

Lippmann RP (1987) An Introduction to Computing with Neural Networks. IEEE Acc Speech Sig Proc Magazine, 4-22.

Looney CG (1997) Pattern Recognition Using Neural Networks. Oxford University Press.

Mirchandani G, Cao W (1989) On Hidden Neurons for Neural Nets. IEEE Tr Circ Syst, 36: 661-664.

Mitchell TM (1997) Machine Learning. McGraw Hill Book Co., New York.

Nguyen D, Widrow B (1990) Improving the Learning Speed of Two-Layer Neural Networks by Choosing Initial Values of the Adaptive Weights. Proc. 1990 IEEE Int Joint Conf Neural Networks, 3:21-26.

Qian N (1999) On the Momentum Term in Gradient Descent Learning Algorithms. Neural Networks, 2:145-151.

Raudys S (1997) On Dimensionality, Sample Size and Classification Error of Nonparametric Linear Classification Algorithms. IEEE Tr Patt An Mach Intell, 19:667-671.

Rosenblatt F (1962) Principles of Neurodynamics. Spartan Books, Washington DC.

Rumelhart DE, Hinton GE, Williams RJ (1986) Learning Internal Representations by Error Propagation. In: Rumelhart DE, McClelland JL (eds) Parallel Distributed Processing: Explorations in the Microstructure of Cognition, vol.1, chapter 8, MIT Press.

Simon HU (1997) Bounds on the Number of Examples Needed for Learning Functions. SIAM J. of Computing, 26:751-763.

Specht DF (1990) Probabilistic Neural Networks. Neural Networks, 13:109-118.

Specht DF (1991) A Generalized Regression Neural Network. IEEE Tr Neural Networks, 2:568-576.

Vapnik VN (1998) Statistical Learning Theory. Wiley, New York.

Van Rooij AJF, Jain LC, Johnson RP (1996) Neural Network Training Using Genetic Algorithms. World Scientific Co. Pte. Ltd., Singapore.

Vonk E, Jain LC, Johnson RP (1997) Automatic Generation of Neural Network Architecture Using Evolutionary Computation. World Scientific Co. Pte. Ltd., Singapore.

Weigend AS, Rumelhart DE, Huberman BA (1991) Generalization by Weight-Elimination with Application to Forecasting. In: Lippman RP, Moody JE, Touretzky DS (eds) Advances in Neural Information Processing Systems, 3:875-882, Morgan Kaufmann, California.

Widrow B, Glover Jr JR, McCool JM, Kaunitz J, Williams CS, Hearn RH, Zeidler JR, Dong Jr E, Goodlin RC (1975) Adaptive Noise Cancelling: Principles and Applications Proc IEEE, 63:1692-1716.

Widrow B, Hoff Jr M (1960) Adaptive Switching Circuits. In: IRE WESCON Conv. Rec., 4:96-104.

Exercises

5.1 Consider the adaptive noise cancelling application of a linear network, as in the ECG example described in section 5.1. Let $R = E[\mathbf{xx'}]$ represent the auto-correlation matrix of the signal fed at the network inputs.

   a) Compute the error expectation $E[\varepsilon_j]$, noticing that the error for the sample input vector $\mathbf{x}_j$ is $\varepsilon_j = t_j - \mathbf{w'x}_j$. Show that the Hessian matrix of the error energy is equal to R.

   b) Taking into account formula 5-42, prove that an upper bound of the learning factor η, for the 50 Hz noise cancelling example of section 5.1 is $\eta_{max} = 4/(a^2\pi)$, where a is the amplitude of the sinusoidal inputs. Check this upper bound using the *ECG50Hz.xls* file.

   c) The time constant of an exponential approximating the mean-square error learning curve is given by $\tau = w/(4\eta \, \text{tr}(R))$, where $\text{tr}(R)$ is the sum of the eigenvalues of R. Show that for the pure sinusoidal noise cancelling example in section 5.1, the time constant is $\tau = 1/(2\pi a^2 \eta)$.

5.2 Determine the optimal parabolic discriminants for the two-class one-dimensional problems shown in Figure 5.8 and Figure 5.9 by solving the respective normal equations.

5.3 Implement the first two steps of the gradient descent approach for the parabolic discriminant of the two-class one-dimensional problems shown in Figure 5.9, starting at (0, -2) and (3, 1). Verify the convergence towards the local and global minimum, respectively.

5.4 Using equations (5-12), explain why an LMS adjusted discriminant with sigmoid activation function converges to the same solution as the Bayesian classifier. Restrict the analysis to a two-class situation.

5.5 Classify the two-class cork stoppers data with a single perceptron, illustrated in Figure 5.19, using thresholds at the output in order to obtain an appropriate reject region.

5.6 Repeat the single perceptron experiment for the two-class classification of cork stoppers, using activation functions other than hard-limiter. Compare the results and learning curves.

5.7 Design appropriate MLPs for classification of the *MLP* datasets and observe the influence of the learning and momentum parameters on the training:
   a) For the *MLP1* and *MLP2* data, derive the decision boundaries from the weight values and confirm the constructive argument from section 5.5.
   b) What is the structure of a multi-layer perceptron needed for the *MLP3* data, if the constructive argument applies?
   c) Verify, using several training experiments with the structure previously determined, that the constructive argument is not confirmed in the case of the *MLP3* data.

5.8 Change the class labels of the *MLP3* patterns lying in the upper left shaded area of Figure 5.20c and train an MLP2:3:1 classifier. Explain the results obtained.

5.9 Consider that a neural net has an energy function with 2 weights given by (5-4c).
   a) Compute the eigenvectors and eigenvalues of the Hessian.
   b) Compute the value of the learning parameter η_{max}, above which the gradient descent starts to diverge.
   c) Plot the curve showing how the distance to the minimum error evolves, along the direction of the eigenvector corresponding to the minimum eigenvalue, using $\eta = \eta_{max}/2$ and a starting distance of 10.

5.10 Use an MLP approach to classify the three classes of cork stoppers using features *ART, PRM, NG* and *RAAR* (see section 4.2.4). Determine if there are weights with negligible values that can be discarded, and compute the upper bound of the number of training patterns sufficient for training before and after discarding negligible weights.

5.11 Design an MLP that predicts *SONAE* share values (*StockExchange* dataset) two-days ahead, using the same external inputs as in the solution illustrated in Figure 5.28. Compare the results obtained with those relative to one-day ahead prediction, using the ranking index (5-29f).

5.12 Repeat the previous exercise, using the *Weather* dataset.

5.13 Estimate the lower bound of the number of samples necessary for training the MLP prediction one-day ahead of the SONAE share values, described in section 5.5.3.

5.14 Consider a set of three points $X=\{x_i, x_i \in \Re, i=1, 2, 3\}$.
  a) Show that X is not pseudo-shattered by the class of linear functions F (see Figure 5.35).
  b) Show that X is pseudo-shattered by the class of quadratic functions $Q=\{ (x, f(x) = ax^2 + b); a, b \in \Re \}$.

5.15 Using an MLP approach, determine which shares of the *StockExchange* dataset are best predicted one-day ahead, using features *LISBOR* and *USD*.

5.16 Design an RBF classifier for the three classes of cork stoppers, using features *ART*, *PRM*, *NG* and *RAAR*. Compare the solution obtained with the one derived in Exercise 5.7, using ROC curve analysis.

5.17 Train the MLP18:22:10 classifier for the *CTG* data, described in section 5.7.1, with the back-propagation algorithm. Compare the results with those shown in Table 5.7. What is the lower bound of the number of training samples needed for training and the VC dimension, assuming hard-limiting activation functions?

5.18 Design an MLP classifier for the *CTG* data for the three classes *N*, *S* and *P* with a reduced feature set. Use the conjugate-gradient method for training.

5.19 Train the MLP classifier from the previous exercise with the genetic algorithm approach (use the *NeuroGenetic* program). Compare the solution obtained with the one from the previous exercise, regarding classification performance and convergence time.

5.20 Determine the progress of the conjugate-gradient method for the error surfaces shown in Figures 5-8b and 5-9b by determining the successive minima and gradients at those points.

5.21 Design a two-layer MLP for classification of the *Rocks* data into three classes: granites, limestones and marbles. Use features *SiO2*, *CaO* and *RMCS*, and perform the training with the conjugate-gradient and genetic algorithm methods.

5.22 Foetal weight estimation is also clinically relevant when approached as a classification task. Design an MLP classifier for the foetal weight dataset, considering the classes corresponding to the following weight intervals (in grams):
  a) ω_1=below 1000; ω_2=[1000, 1500[; ω_3=[1500, 3000[; ω_4=[3000, 4500[; ω_5=above 4500.
  b) ω_1=below 2000 (too low); ω_2=[2000, 4000]; ω_3=above 4000.

5.23 Design an RBF network with Gaussian kernel for the same *Rocks* data classification as in the previous exercise. Compare both solutions, using scatter plots with the class boundaries determined by the classifiers.

5.24 Determine the optimal SVM hyperplane for a data set as in the example of Figure 5.44, the only difference being that point x_3 is now $x_3=(0,1)$.

5.25 Design an SVM for classification of the Rocks data into two classes: granites vs. limestones+marbles. Use features *SiO2*, *CaO* and determine experimentally the kernel with best generalization.

5.26 Design a Kohonen network for the *CorkStoppers* dataset. Compare the solution obtained with the supervised classification and with the cluster solution from Exercise 3.7.

5.27 Consider the hierarchical classification of the CTG data, shown in Figure 5.57. Estimate the bounds for proper learning of the respective MLP6:7:1 and MLP9:5:3 used in the hierarchy.

5.28 Design a majority vote ensemble of MLPs for classifying the *Rocks* data into the following classes: granite, diorite, slate, marble and limestone.

5.29 Determine useful predictor variables of the pathologic+suspect classes of the CTG dataset, using probabilistic neural nets with a genetic algorithm. With these predictors derive MLP, RBF and SVM solutions for the CTG classification task normal vs. abnormal. Compare the solutions and assess their generalization capability.

5.30 A Hopfield net is applied for the retrieval of binary images using an array of 10x10 neurons. Five classes of simple geometric shapes are used and the network must retrieve the prototype that best matches an input image. When applying the network, it was found that it produced much better results when the images occupied the whole 10x10 array than when they occupied only half of it. Explain why.

5.31 Consider the binary images shown in Figure 5.52. Use the *Hopfield* program in the random serial and full parallel mode with noise corrupted versions of the prototypes and explain the results obtained, namely for the two-state oscillations in the full parallel mode.

5.32 Consider the eight digit images shown in Figure 5.55, used as prototypes in a Hopfield network.
  a)   Explain how the spurious state shown in Figure 5.56 is formed.
  b)   Perform experiments of prototype retrieval using noise corrupted images of the several digits, and determine which pattern is found more often when an incorrect retrieval is made. Explain why.

6 Structural Pattern Recognition

In the preceding chapters several methodologies of pattern classification and regression were presented, all based on a numerical similarity measure. Structural pattern recognition has a completely different approach, as briefly mentioned in section 1.4. Its main concern is the structure of a pattern, i.e., how a pattern can be described and interpreted as an organization of simple sub-patterns, usually designated as *pattern primitives*.

Structural pattern recognition has two main classes of methods: syntactic analysis and structural matching methods. Syntactic analysis methods are based on the use of formal language theory. Structural matching methods use specific techniques based on mathematical relations among the primitives.

Error bounds and generalization capability of structural recognition methods are problem-dependent. The performance of a syntactic analyser or of a structural matching method has to be assessed in a test set of patterns in the usual way.

Structural pattern recognition is often used in combination with statistical classification and/or neural network methods in hybrid approaches in order to achieve complex pattern recognition tasks, namely in applications of two-dimensional and three-dimensional object recognition.

6.1 Pattern Primitives

As the first step to describing and analysing pattern structures, they are decomposed into simple and well-defined elements, called *primitives*. The choice of primitives depends on the application, and can be of varied nature (see the bibliography section). In the following, we limit our discussion to methods of primitive extraction that can be applied to a large class of situations and are, therefore, quite popular.

6.1.1 Signal Primitives

Usually signals are decomposed into line segments or other simple curves. A *piecewise linear approximation* of a signal is by far the most popular method of signal decomposition. Suppose that we have a signal $s(x)$ that we want to approximate by a piecewise linear function $h(x)$ with d segments h_i. The approximation error is:

$$E = \sum_{i=1}^{d} \sum_{x_j \in h_i} \left\| s(x_j) - h_i(x_j) \right\|, \qquad (6\text{-}1)$$

where an appropriate norm, usually the Chebychev norm or the Euclidian norm, is used to evaluate the deviations of $s(x_j)$ from $h_i(x_j)$.

A piecewise linear approximation of this kind is implemented in the *SigParse* program using the following simple algorithm:

1. Specify a maximum error, E_{max}, for every line segment.
2. Start the approximation search with the first signal sample x_1, which initiates the first line segment, $i=1$.
3. Set the number of signal samples to regress, $k=1$.
4. Generate a line regressing k signal samples, from x_i to x_{i+k-1}.
5. Evaluate E for the regressing line. If E is smaller than E_{max}, increase k and go to 4, otherwise start a new line segment, increase i, and go to 3.

Figure 6.1 shows a piecewise linear approximation obtained with *SigParse* for an electrocardiographic (ECG) signal. The original signal has 702 samples. The approximation using the Chebychev norm with $E_{max} = 17$ μV (in a 682 μV pp. ECG) has only 21 segments.

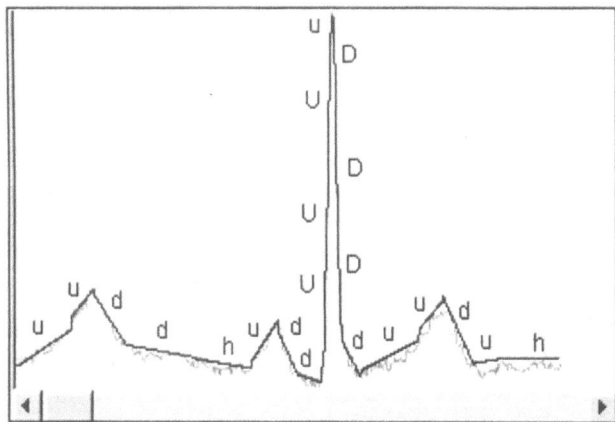

Figure 6.1. Piecewise linear approximation (black) of an ECG signal (grey). The line segments are labelled according to specified slope thresholds.

Sometimes it may be desirable to minimize the number of line segments by a careful adjustment of the segment ends, guaranteeing that an error norm is not exceeded, as described in Pavlidis (1973). In this case, the whole signal must be known beforehand, whereas the previous algorithm can also be used in real time signal processing.

After the signal is decomposed into line segments, one can label these according to a specific rule. For instance, one may use the information on the slope of each segment to set slope thresholds in order to obtain the labels h, u, d, U, D mentioned in section 1.2.3. In that section we defined an h primitive as a line segment with zero slope; usually it is more convenient to set two slope thresholds, Δ_1 and Δ_2, used for the segment labelling as u or d and as U or D, respectively, therefore defining h as any segment with slope below Δ_1. This was done for the ECG signal shown in Figure 6.1 with $\Delta_1=0.1$ and $\Delta_2=5$. We will use this labelling approach in the following examples.

6.1.2 Image Primitives

Image primitives can be obtained through the application of a large variety of image analysis techniques, such as image segmentation, edge detection, contour following and medial axis transformation, described in detail in many textbooks on the subject (e.g., Duda and Hart, 1973 and Rosenfeld and Kak, 1982). In the following we describe some popular ways of deriving image primitives.

Chain Code and Templates

Chain code (*Freeman chain code*) constitutes an easy way of encoding a two-dimensional curve, represented in a rectangular grid with sufficient resolution. It consists of following the curve from a specified starting point and, for each line segment, connecting the grid points that fall closest to the curve. The grid point connections are then coded according to a set of octal primitives, as shown in Figure 6.2.

This technique is usually applied to binary images when one wants to encode the silhouette of an object by contour tracking, as shown in Figure 6.2, where the string starting at the highest vertical point and following the contour in the clockwise direction is: $\mathbf{x} = 6007656454324221002$.

Chain coding of binary images is easy to implement and often provides a very good description. The difficulty with this technique is that, for an accurate enough representation, it may need a very fine grid, then generating very long strings. An alternative is to use template images, which are then considered the primitives. Classic templates are also shown in Figure 6.2. Starting from the highest vertical grid cell that is not empty, one can follow the contour in a clockwise direction, selecting the template that best corresponds with the current contour cell, obtaining in this case the string $\mathbf{x} = 482611999\ 337741812$.

The use of templates for primitive description of binary images is applied in many image recognition tasks, for instance, in some implementations of character recognition and in fingerprint identification.

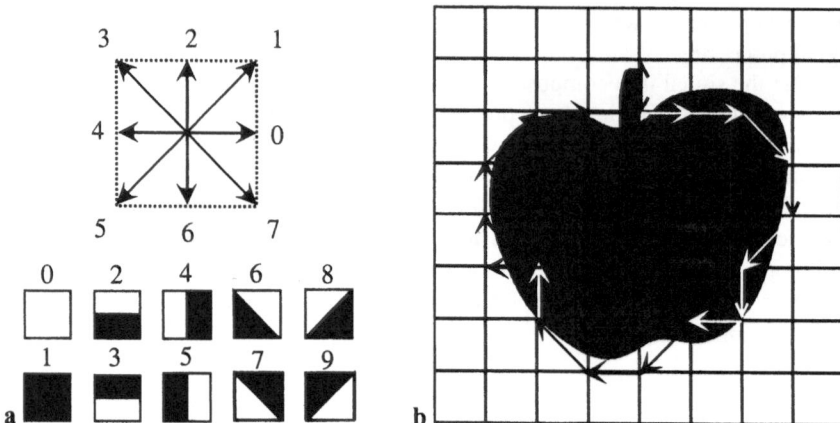

Figure 6.2. (a) Octal primitives (top) and templates (bottom); (b) Binary image with contour line segments according to the octal primitives.

Curve segments

Images described by curve segments, particularly line segments, can be obtained by applying edge detectors to them, as shown in Figure 6.3. They are usually called *shape primitives* or *image silhouette primitives*. In some applications, instead of image silhouettes, one may be interested in obtaining a skelotonised description of an image, by applying thinning or medial axis transformation to a binary image. An application of this technique can be found in character recognition (see e.g., Di Baja, 1996).

After obtaining the curve segment description, one may label the segments in a similar way to what we have done for line primitives of signals, or extract other descriptions from the curve segments (perimeter, curvature, slope of the segment linking the ends, etc.).

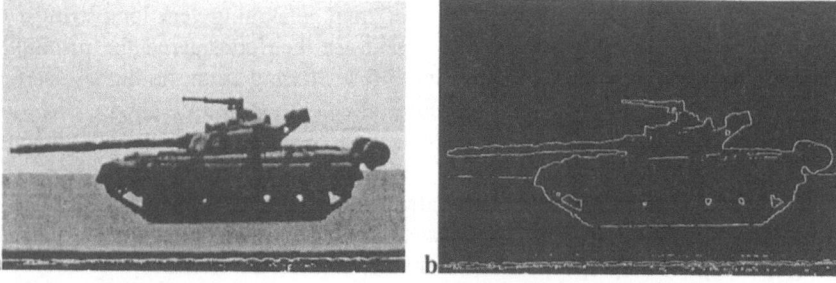

Figure 6.3. (a) Image of a tank (toy model); (b) Image contours detected by an edge detection algorithm.

A particularly useful description can be obtained from line segments derived by the application of the *Hough transform*, a transformation that maps a straight line $y = ax+b = \rho \cos\theta$ into a point in the (a, b) plane or the (ρ, θ) plane. The straight line Hough transform can also be applied to the description of arbitrary curves. Details on how to use this technique can be found in Pao and Li (1992).

Regions

The segmentation of an image into distinct regions is often used as a means of obtaining structural descriptions of images, e.g., based on proximity relations of region centroids and using labels related to the image properties of the regions such as perimeter, area, colour, light intensity and texture. This approach is used, for instance, in image registration applications, such as the structural matching of satellite images (see e.g., Ton and Jain, 1989), which we discuss in section 6.4.2.

Region primitives such as centroids and corners can also be obtained from binary images by using morphologic operators (see e.g., Shapiro, 1988).

6.2 Structural Representations

The representation of a pattern in terms of its constituent elements can be done in many ways. Here we will describe the most common ways of structural representation.

6.2.1 Strings

A *string* is an ordered sequence of symbols, each symbol representing a primitive. We denote by S the set of all possible strings that can be built with the elements of a symbol set T. A string $\mathbf{x}$ is then a sequence of symbols of T represented as:

$$\mathbf{x} = a_1 a_2 ... a_m, \quad a_i \in T . \tag{6-2}$$

The number of symbols, m, is the *string length*, denoted $|\mathbf{x}|$. The string with no symbols, $m=0$, is called the *null string* and denoted λ.

We define the *concatenation* of strings $\mathbf{x} = a_1 a_2 ... a_m$ and $\mathbf{y} = b_1 b_2 ... b_n$ with m symbols and n symbols, respectively, and denote this operation as $\mathbf{x} + \mathbf{y}$, yielding the string with $m+n$ symbols:

$$\mathbf{z} = \mathbf{x} + \mathbf{y} = a_1 a_2 ... a_m \, b_1 b_2 ... b_n . \tag{6-3}$$

Note that the null string is the neutral element for the concatenation:

$$\mathbf{x} + \lambda = \lambda + \mathbf{x} = \mathbf{x} . \tag{6-3a}$$

Strings are useful for representing concatenated structures, for instance, segment joining in signal descriptions. Even in some apparently complex relations of primitives, describing 2D and 3D structures, it is still possible to use strings, as we will see in section 6.3.4.

Sometimes the ordered sequence of primitives expressed by a string does not contain enough information to achieve pattern discrimination. For instance, when analysing signals, such as electrocardiograms or heart rate tracings, not all peaks described by strings such as $\mathbf{x} = ud$ or $\mathbf{x} = du$ are relevant, i.e., meet the requirements necessary for attributing them to a certain class of waves. Extra conditions often have to be imposed on the duration and amplitude of the peaks. We deal with this requirement through the formalism of *attributed strings*, i.e., strings that have an associated *attribute vector*:

$$\mathbf{a}(\mathbf{x})=[a_1 \ a_2 \ldots \ a_k]' \in \Re^k \ . \tag{6-4}$$

For waveforms described by line segments the attribute vector usually has two elements, namely duration and height of each segment. In some cases there are categorical attributes (e.g., colour), and the attribute vector will contain labels (e.g., red). In the case of strings with single labels, we will refer to them as *labelled strings*.

6.2.2 Graphs

A graph G is an ordered pair:

$$G = \{N, R\}, \tag{6-5}$$

where N, the *node set*, is a set of nodes, and R, the *edge set*, is a set of binary relations defined in NxN.

The elements of R represent arcs (or edges) connecting nodes of N. An arc of G is denoted (a, b) with $a, b \in N$.

A directed graph, or *digraph*, is a graph where each arc has a direction, emanating from a node and incident onto either another node or the same node. An arc from a digraph, represented by the pair (a, b), means that a is the emanating node and b is the incident node. Generally, in a digraph, (a, b) will mean a different relation than (b, a).

The number of nodes b, such that $(a, b) \in G$, i.e., the number of emanating arcs from a, is the *out-degree* of node a. The number of nodes a, such that $(a, b) \in G$, i.e., the number of arcs incident in b, is the *in-degree* of node b.

Graphs are a very flexible way of expressing relations among primitives. As there are attributed and labelled strings, we can similarly have attributed or labelled graphs. Figure 6.4 illustrates the use of digraphs in character recognition. At the left side of the figure, primitives and relations describing capital letters are indicated. At the right side of the figure, two examples are shown of digraphs using these primitives and relations, for the letters "R" and "E".

Primitives

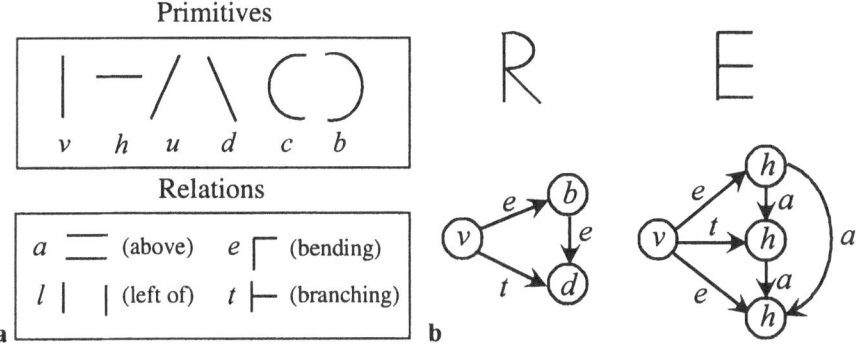

Relations

a ⎯	(above)	e ⎾	(bending)
l ⎢ ⎢	(left of)	t ⊢	(branching)

a

b

Figure 6.4. Primitives and relations used to describe capital letters (a) and labelled digraphs for the letters R and E (b).

6.2.3 Trees

A tree is an undirected graph with no closed loops (*acyclic graph*) and with a special node, the *root node*, with in-degree of zero and every other node with out-degree ≥ 1, except the terminal or *leaf nodes*, which have out-degree zero.

Trees provide a useful representation of hierarchical structures, namely when such structures have a recursive nature. Notice that we have already used trees for hierarchical classifiers in previous chapters.

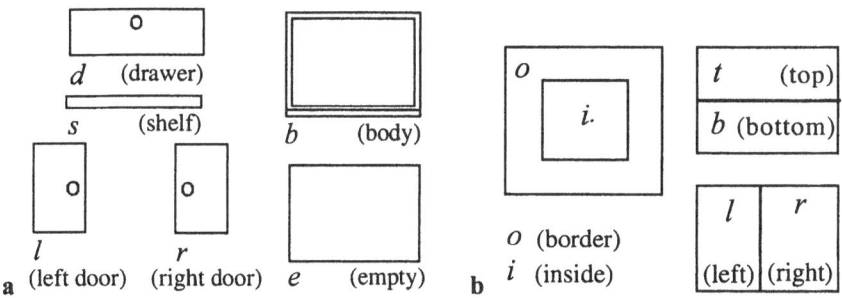

Figure 6.5. Primitives (a) and relations (b) used to describe furniture, as in Figure 6.6.

As an illustration of trees used for the description of hierarchical structures, we consider the task of recognizing pieces of furniture, based on the set of primitives and the set of relations shown in Figure 6.5. Each relation is applied hierarchically. For instance, we can apply the relations "left"-"right" to any sub-pattern previously labelled as "bottom". Figure 6.6 shows how a tree using these primitives and relations can represent a cupboard. This method has been used in several applications, namely in character recognition (e.g., Tai and Liu, 1990; Chen and Lee, 1996).

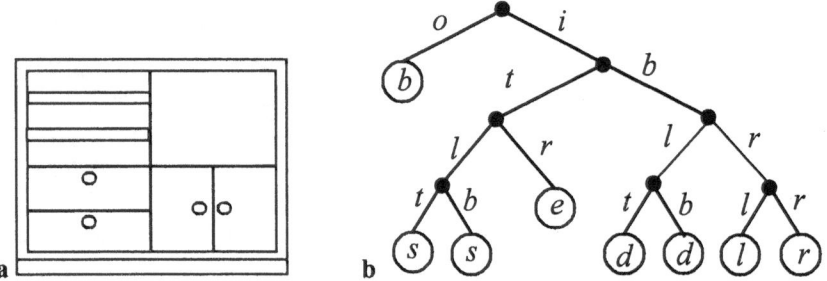

Figure 6.6. A cupboard (a) and its description tree (b) using the primitives and relations of Figure 6.5.

6.3 Syntactic Analysis

Syntactic analysis is the approach to structural pattern recognition based on the theory of formal languages. In the literature, this approach is generally called *Syntactic Pattern Recognition*. The use of grammars to describe patterns is advantageous, given the well-developed body of knowledge in this area and the standardized way one can apply the same approach in many different circumstances.

The disadvantages of the syntactic approach relate to the lack of sufficient representational capability for complex patterns, and also the difficulty in automating inference and learning procedures, which means that in general one first has to devise the appropriate grammar for the problem at hand.

6.3.1 String Grammars

The theory of formal languages allows us to apply structure rules to strings of pattern primitives in a similar way as we apply grammar rules to words in a natural language.

We proceed to define a formal string grammar as a quadruple $G = (T, N, P, S)$:

1. T is a set of symbols, called *terminal symbols*, corresponding in the case of the patterns to the set of primitives, also called *pattern alphabet*.
   The set of strings built with the elements of T is usually denoted T^+:

$$T^+ = \{a_1 a_2 \cdots a_n; a_i \in T, n \geq 1\}. \tag{6-6a}$$

A formal language L is a subset of $T^+ \cup \{\lambda\}$, constituted by strings obeying certain rules.

2. N is a set of *class symbols*, also called *non-terminal symbols*, i.e., symbols that denote classes of elements of T. For instance, when describing natural languages, we would use non-terminal symbols to denote the classes of words that are "nouns", "adjectives", "verbs", etc.
   The sets T and N are disjointed and their union, $V = T \cup N$, constitutes the language vocabulary.

3. P is a set of syntactic rules, known as *production rules*, used to generate the strings. Each rule is represented as:

$$\alpha \mapsto \beta, \qquad \text{with} \qquad \alpha \in V^+, \ \beta \in V^+ \cup \{\lambda\}. \tag{6-6b}$$

The production rule $\alpha \mapsto \beta$, read "α produces β", means that any occurrence of α in a string can be substituted by β.

4. S is a special *parent class symbol*, also called *starting symbol*, used to start the generation of any string with the rules of P.

Let us apply the above definitions to a waveform recognition example, by considering signal waveform descriptions where a waveform is built with only three primitives: horizontal segments, h; upward segments, u; downward segments, d. Hence, the pattern alphabet is, in this case, $T = \{h, u, d\}$.
We now consider the following classes of strings of T:

P^+ : upward peak;
P^- : downward peak;
H : horizontal plateau.

Hence, $N = \{P^+, P^-, H\}$.
We can now define a production rule for an upward peak as:

$$P^+ \mapsto ud . \tag{6-7a}$$

Another production rule for the same class could be:

$$P^+ \mapsto uP^+d . \tag{6-7b}$$

As this last rule is a recursive rule, we are in fact describing upward peaks as an arbitrary number of u primitives followed by the same number of d primitives. We can write the previous rules (6-7a) and (6-7b) compactly as:

$$P^+ \mapsto u\left(P^+ \mid \lambda\right) d \,.$$

(6-7c)

The symbol | denotes an exclusive "or" choice and the parentheses allow a kind of factorisation, meaning that P^+ can be substituted with $u\,P^+\,d$ or with $u\lambda d$, which is in fact ud.

Consider now that our waveform grammar has the following set of productions:

$$P = \begin{cases} S \mapsto (P^+ \mid P^- \mid H)(S \mid \lambda), \quad P^+ \mapsto u(P^+ \mid \lambda)\, d, \\ P^- \mapsto d(P^- \mid \lambda)\, u, \quad H \mapsto h(H \mid \lambda) \end{cases}.$$

(6-7d)

The starting symbol S stands for "any waveform obtainable with the rules of P".

The set P determines a language $L(G)$ (or simply L) of waveforms, which is a subset of all possible waveforms of $T^+ \cup \{\lambda\}$. Consider the waveform of Figure 6.7a, represented by the pattern string $\mathbf{x} = hhuuddh$. Is it an element of L (describable by P)? In order to answer this question, we have to see if it is possible to generate $\mathbf{x}$ using the rules of P starting from S:

$$S \mapsto HS \mapsto HP^+S \mapsto HP^+H \mapsto hHuP^+dh \mapsto hhuuddh \,.$$

(6-7e)

We have indeed been able to generate $\mathbf{x}$ with the rules of P, or, in the jargon of formal language theory, we were able to *parse* $\mathbf{x}$.

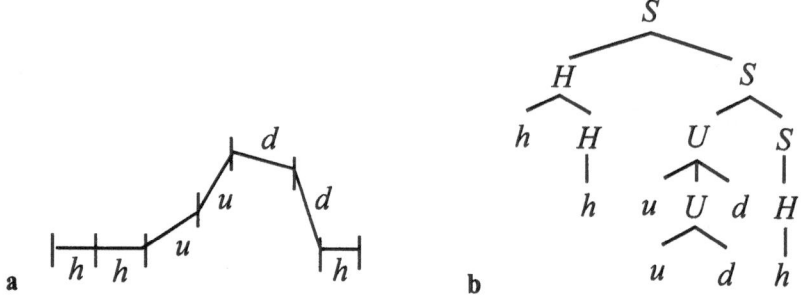

Figure 6.7. A signal wave (a) represented by the string $\mathbf{x} = hhuuddh$ and its top-down parsing tree (b).

The chain of rules (6-7e) generating $\mathbf{x}$ is called a *derivation* of $\mathbf{x}$. The application of rules for obtaining this derivation is called *top-down parsing*, since we started from the initial symbol S and went down until the terminal symbols, as shown in the *parsing tree* of Figure 6.7b. It is also possible to start from the string applying the rules in reverse order as a *bottom-up parsing* chain:

$$hhuuddh \mapsto hHuP^+dh \mapsto HP^+H \mapsto HP^+S \mapsto HS \mapsto S \ . \qquad (6\text{-}7f)$$

Since we were able to reach the starting symbol, we have confirmed that **x** belongs to L generated by P, i.e., the grammar G recognizes **x**, or $\mathbf{x} \in L(G)$.

Let us now consider the pattern string **y** = *hhuudh*. It is easy to see that **y** does not belong to $L(G)$, since no parsing is possible in this case. We see, therefore, that the task of determining whether or not a pattern belongs to a given class is reduced to seeing whether or not it can be parsed with the grammar rules. The reader may find it interesting to change the rule set P in order to recognize string **y**, and other strings as well.

Let us now modify the rules of P^+ and P^- as follows:

$$P = \begin{cases} S \mapsto (P^+ \mid P^- \mid H)(S \mid \lambda), & P^+ \mapsto u(S \mid \lambda)d, \\ P^- \mapsto d(S \mid \lambda)u, & H \mapsto h(H \mid \lambda) \end{cases}. \qquad (6\text{-}7g)$$

Consider the string **x** = *udud*. It can de derived in two ways:

$$S \mapsto P^+S \mapsto udS \mapsto udP^+ \mapsto udud \ . \qquad (6\text{-}7h)$$
$$S \mapsto P^+ \mapsto uSd \mapsto uP^-d \mapsto udud \quad . \qquad (6\text{-}7i)$$

When a grammar admits more than one derivation for the same string we call it an *ambiguous* grammar. In general, there is a different semantic value for each derivation. In the present example, we may interpret *udud* as a sequence of two positive peaks or as a positive peak with a negative peak in the middle.

String grammars can be generalized to apply to more complex structures such as trees and graphs.

6.3.2 Picture Description Language

Grammar strings that use concatenation as the only operation have a limited representational capability, namely when relations among two-dimensional or three-dimensional objects have to be represented. One way to cope with this limitation is to use higher dimensional grammars such as tree or graph grammars. This approach has met limited success in practical applications, given the inherent difficulty of dealing with such grammars, namely in what concerns the building of efficient parsers. Another way is to incorporate operations that are more complex than concatenation into the grammar. This is the approach of the *picture description language*, PDL, which provides an adequate representation of two-dimensional patterns.

In PDL each primitive has two attaching points, *tail* and *head*, where it can be linked to other primitives. The set of terminals includes four binary operators and one unary operator that can be used to join primitives as shown in Table 6.1.

Table 6.1. PDL operators and their meaning.

Operator	Meaning	Geometric interpretation
$a+b$	$head(a+b)=head(b)$ $tail(a+b)=tail(a)$	
$a\text{-}b$	$head(a)$ linked to $head(b)$ $head(a\text{-}b)=head(b)$ $tail(a\text{-}b)=tail(a)$	
$a\times b$	$tail(a)$ linked to $tail(b)$ $head(a\times b)=head(b)$ $tail(a\times b)=tail(b)$	
$a*b$	$head(a)$ linked to $head(b)$ and $tail(a)$ linked to $tail(b)$ $head(a*b)=head(a)$ $tail(a*b)=tail(a)$	
$\sim a$	$head(\sim a)=tail(a)$ $tail(\sim a)=head(a)$	

It can be shown that any digraph with labelled edges can be represented by a PDL expression. Therefore, any pattern that can be represented by a digraph can also be described by a PDL expression. As an example, let us look back to the digraphs of Figure 6.4 and describe them with PDL strings, denoting **r** for the letter "R" and **e** for the letter "E", respectively, using the new version of the primitives shown in Figure 6.8:

$$\mathbf{r} = (v + (\sim b)) + (\sim d); \tag{6-8a}$$
$$\mathbf{e} = (v \times h) + ((v \times h) + h). \tag{6-8b}$$

Note that the strings now incorporate the PDL operator symbols and the parentheses as terminals. Note also that, in general, more than one representation is possible. For instance, the following are also valid expressions:

$$\mathbf{r} = d + (b + (\sim v)); \tag{6-9a}$$
$$\mathbf{e} = (\sim h) + ((v - (\sim h)) + (v - (\sim h))). \tag{6-9b}$$

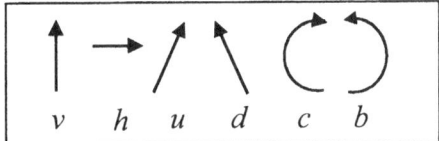

Figure 6.8. Primitives for character description using picture description language.

String grammars are easily generalized to PDL descriptions. We will show this by presenting the string grammar that describes the characters "P", "R", "F" and "E":

$G = \{T, N, P, S\}$;
$T = \{v, h, d, b, \sim, +, -, (,)\}$;
$N = \{S, P, R, F, E, LEFTCORNER\}$;
$P = \{\ S \mapsto (P \mid R \mid F \mid E),\ \ R \mapsto d + P,\ \ P \mapsto b + (\sim v),$
$\qquad LEFTCORNER \mapsto v - (\sim h),\ \ F \mapsto LEFTCORNER + LEFTCORNER$
$\qquad E \mapsto (\sim h) + F\ \}$.

Shape descriptions can also be generated using other types of features, namely line segments derived by chain coding, as explained in section 6.1.2. A variant of this method, using appropriate concatenation rules, is described in the work of Nishida (1996) and applied to structural analysis of curve deformation.

6.3.3 Grammar Types

The string grammar defined in section 6.3.1 states the production rules in the most general way, constituting what is called an *unrestricted grammar*. By imposing restrictions on the production rules of this grammar, it is possible to define other types of grammars, as listed in Table 6.2.

Table 6.2. Chomsky's hierarchy of grammar types.

Type	Name	Production rules
G0	Unrestricted	$\alpha \mapsto \beta$, with $\alpha \in V^+, \beta \in V^+ \cup \{\lambda\}$
G1	Context-sensitive	$\alpha \mapsto \beta$, with $\alpha, \beta \in V^+$ and $\lvert \alpha \rvert \leq \lvert \beta \rvert$
G2	Context-free	$\alpha \mapsto \beta$, with $\alpha \in N, \beta \in V^+$
G3	Regular	$\alpha \mapsto a\beta \mid a \mid \lambda$, with $\alpha, \beta \in N, a \in T$

The following relations exist for these four types of grammars: $G0 \supset G1 \supset G2 \supset G3$. This is called the Chomsky' hierarchy, named after Noam Chomsky whose contribution to the formal language theory was capital.

The representational power of a grammar decreases as we go from a type $G0$ grammar to a type $G3$ grammar.

Production rules of a type $G1$ grammar can also be written:

$$\alpha_1 \alpha \alpha_2 \mapsto \alpha_1 \beta \alpha_2, \quad \text{with} \quad \alpha \in N, \quad \beta \in V^+, \quad \alpha_1, \alpha_2 \in V^+ \cup \{\lambda\}. \tag{6-10}$$

Therefore, α substitutes β in the context of α_1 and α_2. This justifies the context-sensitive name given to this type of grammars (see also Exercise 6.2). For a context-free grammar, the substitution of α by β is independent of the context in which α appears. Since these grammars allow self-embedded productions of the type $\alpha \mapsto \beta_1 \beta \beta_2$, they can generate arbitrarily long sequences of terminals by iteration of the same rule. Regular grammars are a special case of context-free grammars that allow very simple representation and parsing, as will be explained in the following section.

As we saw in the previous section, the task of assessing a pattern structural class is equivalent to seeing whether it can be parsed by a suitable parser, which applies the grammar's rules. Parser building for $G0$ and $G1$ grammars can be a very hard task. Fortunately, structural recognition problems can often be solved using $G2$ and $G3$ grammars, which allow a broad range of string expressiveness. For these grammars there is a bulk of knowledge about parser building. As a matter of fact, there are commercialised and free-ware parsers that can, in principle, be applied to syntactic pattern recognition. The reader may also obtain information on how to build a parser for $G2$ grammars in (Schalkoff, 1992).

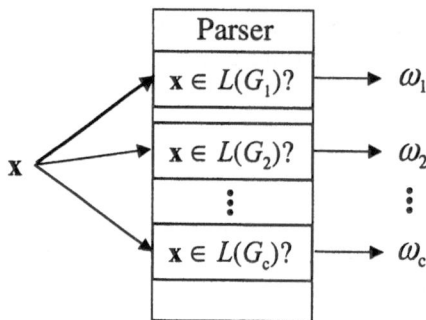

Figure 6.9. Block diagram of a syntactic pattern classifier. $L(G_i)$ are the class languages.

Figure 6.9 represents the block diagram of a syntactic recogniser, having the primitive string as input and class labels together with the syntactic derivations obtained by the parser as outputs. A language $L(G_i)$ represents the set of all strings corresponding to class ω_i. For the example in the previous section the languages would correspond to the sub-grammars producing the derivations for the characters "P", "R", "F" and "E".

Notice that, when parsing a string, one of the following three situations may occur:

- The string belongs to only one of the class languages. This is the desirable situation.
- The string belongs to more than one of the class languages. This is an ambiguous "borderline" string, reminiscent of feature vectors that lie in a reject region.
- The string does not belong to any of the class languages. This is also a reject or a "don't care" situation. For instance, when parsing strings of signal primitives, we may encounter in the tail of a parsed signal wave a sequence of primitives that are not parsed, corresponding to a "don't care" situation.

6.3.4 Finite-State Automata

A broad variety of syntactic recognition tasks can be achieved with the simple $G3$ grammars referred to previously. Fortunately for these grammars the parsing task is quite simple to implement, using a device known as a *finite-state automaton*.

We define a finite-state automaton (or *finite-state machine*) as a quintuple $M=\{T, Q, \delta, q_0, F\}$:

- T is a symbol set (corresponding to the set of primitives);
- Q is a set of states of the machine;
- δ is a function mapping from $Q \times T$ into subsets of Q;
- $q_0 \in Q$ is the initial machine state;
- $F \subseteq Q$ is the set of final states.

A finite-state automaton can be represented as a labelled digraph, known as *state-diagram*, with arcs representing state transitions. Let us exemplify this with:

$T = \{h, u, d\}$
$Q = \{S, U+, D+, U-, D-, F\}; \quad q_0 \equiv S$

$\delta(S, h)=S;$	$\delta(S, u)=U+;$	$\delta(S, d)=D-;$
$\delta(U+, h)=S;$	$\delta(U+, u)=U+;$	$\delta(U+, d)=D+;$
$\delta(D+, h)=F;$	$\delta(D+, u)=F;$	$\delta(D+, d)=D+;$
$\delta(D-, h)=S;$	$\delta(D-, u)=U-;$	$\delta(D-, d)=D-;$
$\delta(U-, h)=F;$	$\delta(U-, u)=U-;$	$\delta(U-, d)=F;$

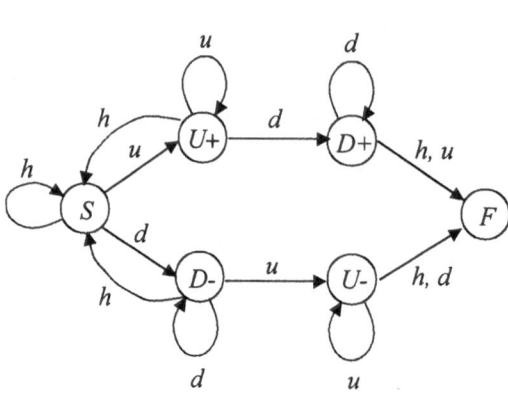

Present State	Input Symbol	Next State
S	h	S
S	u	U+
S	d	D-
U+	h	S
U+	u	U+
U+	d	D+
D+	h	F
D+	u	F
D+	d	D+
D-	h	S
D-	u	U-
D-	d	D-
U-	h	F
U-	u	U-
U-	d	F

Figure 6.10. Finite-state automaton represented by its state-diagram, with corresponding state-transition table. The automaton recognizes waveform peaks without horizontal plateaus.

Figure 6.10 shows the state-diagram corresponding to this finite-state automaton, together with the *state-transition table*, which is a convenient way of representing the mapping δ.

Assuming that the symbols of T represent the signal primitives mentioned already in section 6.3.1, it is clear that this finite-state automaton recognizes any positive or negative peaks that do not include any horizontal plateaus.

A string is said to be *accepted* by M if starting with the initial state we can use the successive string symbols to progress in the state-diagram until a final state. The set of all strings *accepted* by M, denoted $A(M)$, is formally defined as:

$$A(M) = \{\mathbf{x};\ \delta(q_0, \mathbf{x}) \in F\}. \tag{6-11}$$

For any regular grammar $G = \{T, N, P, S\}$, it can be proved that there is a finite-state automaton M such that $A(M) = L(G)$ and vice-versa. The finite-state automaton M uses the set of terminals T, and is implemented as follows:

- $Q = N \cup \{A\}$;
- $q_0 = S$;
- A production $\alpha \mapsto a\beta$ corresponds to $\delta(\alpha, a) = \beta$;
- A production $\alpha \mapsto a$ corresponds to $\delta(\alpha, a) = F$;
- If P contains the production $S \mapsto \lambda$ then $F = \{S, A\}$ else $F = \{A\}$.

Specifying a grammar that corresponds to a finite-state machine is now an easy task, by simply reversing the above rules.

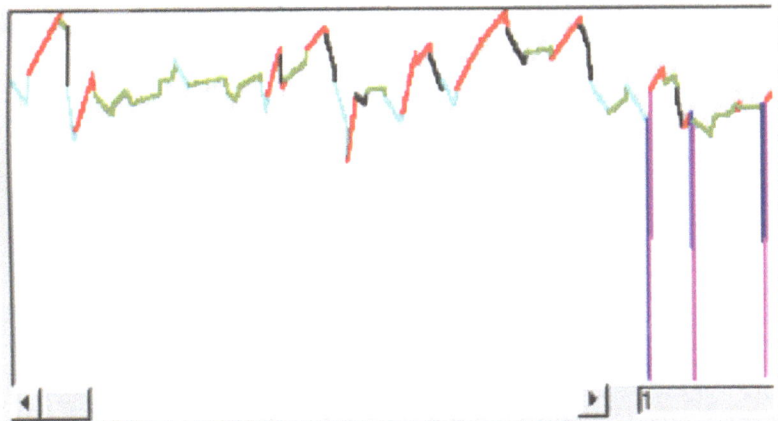

Figure 6.11. FHR signal parsing after approximation by line segments. Line segments are labelled as: h=green; u=red; d=cyan; U=magenta; D=blue. Final states are represented in black. The original signal (in the background) is in grey.

We see therefore that a finite-state machine constitutes a parser for a regular grammar. As a matter of fact, given the expressiveness of a state-diagram, one usually goes directly to the specification of the state-diagram or the state-transition table, omitting the specification of the grammar.

The *SigParse* program allows one to specify a state-transition table for recognizing regular string grammars. We exemplify its use by considering foetal heart rate (FHR) signals, such as the one depicted in Figure 6.11.

Imagine that we want to detect the presence of downward spikes (class *DSPIKE*) in such signals. We start by performing a line segment approximation using the Chebychev norm with a tolerance E_{max}=3, and use slope thresholds of 0.3 and 20 for the segment labelling. These are colour-coded as shown in Figure 6.11. Next, we use the following simple set of rules for the recognition of *DSPIKE* strings:

$$\{DSPIKE \mapsto DA; \quad A \mapsto hB; \quad A \mapsto U; \quad B \mapsto U\}. \tag{6-12a}$$

For the detection of accelerations (class *ACEL*), the set of rules is somewhat more elaborate:

$$\{ACEL \mapsto uA; \quad A \mapsto d; \quad A \mapsto uA; \quad A \mapsto hB; \quad B \mapsto uA; \quad B \mapsto d\}. \tag{6-12b}$$

This corresponds to the finite-state machine of Figure 6.12.

Events detected as "accelerations" by this machine may not qualify as true accelerations in the clinical sense. They only qualify as accelerations if they satisfy a set of conditions on the minimum duration and minimum amplitude. For instance, in Figure 6.11 the second and fourth events do not satisfy such conditions, although they parse as "accelerations". We will see in the following how to take into account primitive attributes.

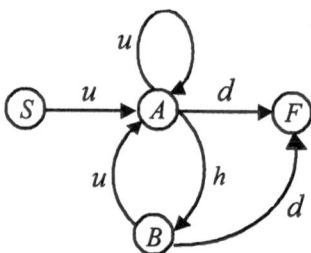

Figure 6.12. State-diagram of a finite-state automaton for the recognition of FHR accelerations.

6.3.5 Attributed Grammars

Until now, we have only considered grammars for string descriptions alone. However, as seen in the previous example of FHR acceleration detection, the qualitative information provided by a string may not be enough for correct recognition. In the mentioned example, if we want to detect "true" accelerations, we will have to appropriately use the information on the length and slope of the segments. In other applications other information may have to be used, such as angle orientation of line segments, textural information or surface orientation. For this purpose, we will have to deal with attributed strings and use an *attributed grammar*, with the same definition as before, plus the addition of *semantic rules*. A pair "syntactic rule - semantic rule" for a regular grammar is:

$$\alpha \mapsto b; \quad \mathbf{a}(\alpha) = f(\mathbf{a}(b)), \tag{6-13}$$

where $\mathbf{a}(\alpha)$ is the attribute vector of the non-terminal α computed in terms of the attribute vector of the terminal b.

An attribute vector can be interpreted as a feature vector. When parsing a string with attributed grammars, one may assume that the production rules for each symbol make its attribute dependent either on the left or on the right side of the productions. For instance, in top-down parsing, attribute values for each symbol are inherited from each right side symbol. We exemplify this for the first production rule of the FHR acceleration rules (6-12b):

$$l(ACEL) = l(u) + l(A); \quad t(ACEL) = t(u) + t(A), \tag{6-14}$$

where l is the length attribute and t is height of the upper segment end.

The height attribute is computed from the length and slope for the u primitives, and may be set to zero for h and d. When a wave event is correctly parsed as an acceleration, the values of $l(ACEL)$ and $t(ACEL)$ are compared with pre-specified thresholds in order to arrive at a final decision.

Attributed strings can be used for shape categorization of object silhouettes described by line segments, using as attributes the length and the angle of the segments. Details on this application can be found in the works of You and Fu (1979) and Stenstrom (1988).

6.3.6 Stochastic Grammars

Stochastic grammars provide a good example of combining structural and statistical approaches and applying them to pattern recognition problems. Stochastic grammars are particularly useful in situations where the same pattern can be interpreted as belonging to more than one class, therefore having the possibility of being generated by alternative grammars.

A *stochastic grammar* is a grammar whose production rules have probabilities associated with them, such that for every symbol α_i producing symbols β_j there are probabilities P_{ij} satisfying:

$$P_{ij} : \alpha_i \overset{P_{ij}}{\mapsto} \beta_j \quad (\text{or } \alpha_i \mapsto \beta_j), \quad \text{with} \quad 0 < P_{ij} \le 1, \quad \sum_{j=1}^{n_i} P_{ij} = 1. \tag{6-15}$$

Therefore, the probabilities associated with the same left side symbol of a production add up to one.

The probability of $\mathbf{x} \in L(G)$, $P(\mathbf{x} \mid G)$, is computed as:

1. If $\mathbf{x} \in L(G)$ is unambiguous and has a derivation with k rules, each with probability P_j, then:

$$P(\mathbf{x} \mid G) = \prod_{j=1}^{k} P_j . \tag{6-16a}$$

2. If $\mathbf{x} \in L(G)$ is ambiguous and has l different derivations with probabilities $P_i(\mathbf{x} \mid G)$, then:

$$P(\mathbf{x} \mid G) = \sum_{i=1}^{l} P_i(\mathbf{x} \mid G). \tag{6-16b}$$

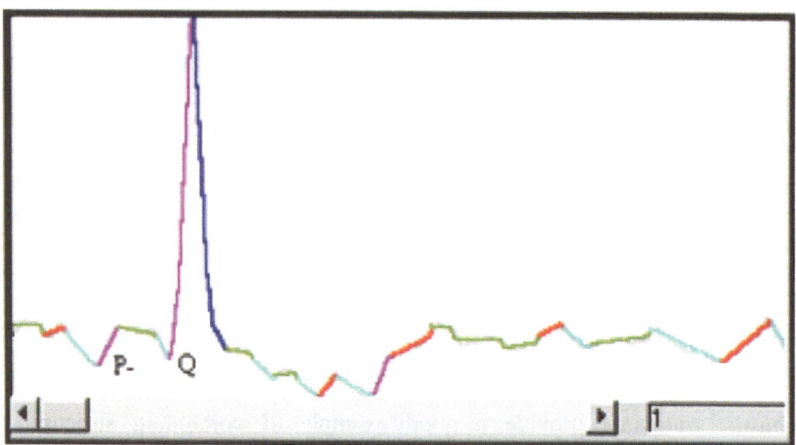

Figure 6.13. An ECG signal, zoomed 4x, described by a piecewise approximation using Chebychev norm with tolerance 20, with segments labelled using slope thresholds of 5 and 22. Colour coding as in Figure 6.11.

As an example, let us consider the distinction between negative P waves and Q waves in an electrocardiographic signal, as shown in Figure 6.13. A brief description of these waves can be found in section 1.3. P waves can be positive and/or negative. Q waves, by definition, are negative. Figure 6.13 shows a negative P wave, described by the string *dU*, followed by a Q wave, described by the same string.

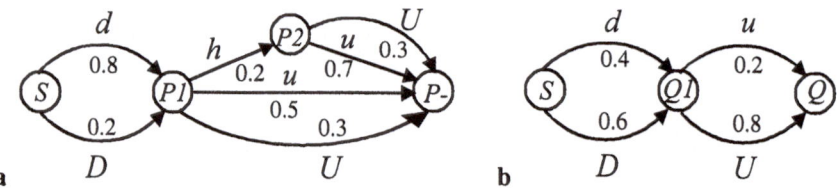

Figure 6.14. State-diagrams of finite-state automata for the recognition of negative P waves (a) and Q waves (b).

The state-diagrams of finite-state automata recognizing negative P waves and Q waves are shown in Figure 6.14. Each arc in these diagrams is labelled with the corresponding transition probability. Notice that rule (6-15) is satisfied. Notice also that the state transition probabilities reflect the fact that a negative P wave is usually less peaked than a Q wave.

The string dU, corresponding to either the first negative P wave or the following Q wave in Figure 6.13, can be parsed by both grammars corresponding to the state-diagrams of Figure 6.14.

The probabilities of generating this string are:

P- grammar: $P(\mathbf{x} \mid P\text{-}) = 0.8 \times 0.3 = 0.24;$
Q grammar: $P(\mathbf{x} \mid Q) = 0.4 \times 0.8 = 0.32.$

When a string can be accepted by multiple grammars we apply the Bayes rule, used already in statistical classification, in order to arrive at a decision. For this purpose, assume that $\mathbf{x}$ can be produced by c grammars G_i with probabilities $P(\mathbf{x} \mid G_i)$. Assume further, that the prior probabilities for the productions are $P(G_i)$. Application of the Bayes rule corresponds to choosing the grammar that maximizes $P(G_i \mid \mathbf{x})$, or equivalently:

Decide $\mathbf{x} \in L(G_k)$ if $P(G_k) P(\mathbf{x} \mid G_k) = \max \{P(G_i) P(\mathbf{x} \mid G_i), i=1,...,c\}.$ (6-17)

In the case of the electrocardiographic signals, the distinction between negative P waves and Q waves is usually a simple task, based on the presence of a peaked R wave after the Q wave. However, there exist less frequent situations where Q waves can appear isolated and there are also rare rhythmic pathologies, characterized by multiple P waves, which may superimpose over the QRS sequence. The signal shown in Figure 6.13 corresponds precisely to such a pathology. Supposing that in this case the prior probabilities are:

$P(P\text{-}) = 0.6; \; P(Q) = 0.4 ,$

we obtain:

P- grammar: $P(P\text{-})P(\mathbf{x} \mid P\text{-}) = 0.144;$
Q grammar: $P(Q)P(\mathbf{x} \mid Q) = 0.128;$

and would decide then for the presence of a negative P wave, although the distinction is somewhat borderline.

In the case of "typical" negative P and Q waves there is a clear distinction:

Typical negative P wave, with string du:

P- grammar: $P(P\text{-})P(\mathbf{x} \mid P\text{-}) = 0.336;$
Q grammar: $P(Q)P(\mathbf{x} \mid Q) = 0.032.$

Typical Q wave, with string DU:

P- grammar: $P(P\text{-})P(\mathbf{x} \mid P\text{-}) = 0.036;$
Q grammar: $P(Q)P(\mathbf{x} \mid Q) = 0.192.$

For the situation shown in Figure 6.13, with string dU, one would probably consider the application of further criteria for discriminating negative P waves from Q waves before making any definite decision.

6.3.7 Grammatical Inference

Until now the grammar rules were supposed to be known beforehand. Grammatical inference is the learning process that extracts from a training set of classified examples the grammatical rules that are able to syntactically describe those examples. It is therefore a concept-driven approach, which bears some resemblance to the supervised classification methods. Instead of parameter learning we are here interested in rule learning.

Many algorithms have been proposed for grammatical inference; a good survey on these is given in (Miclet, 1990). Particular simple and efficient methods have been devised. for inferring regular grammars. One of these methods, called the *successor method*, starts by building a state diagram with a node corresponding to each different production symbol, and then merges the nodes that have the same successors. Let us imagine that we were given the following set of examples of FHR accelerations: $T = \{ud, uhd, uud, uuhuud, uhud\}$. From these examples we start listing all the successors of each symbol in T:

State S – Successors of λ in T: $\{u\}$
State q_u – Successors of u in T: $\{u, h, d\}$
State q_h – Successors of h in T: $\{u, d\}$
State q_d – Successors of d in T: $\varnothing$

With this information we can now build the finite-state automaton of Figure 6.15, where each node corresponds to a symbol, and the arcs are labelled in correspondence with the successors of the symbol. As a matter of fact, the automaton of Figure 6.15 is the same as the one shown in Figure 6.12, with $q_d = F$.

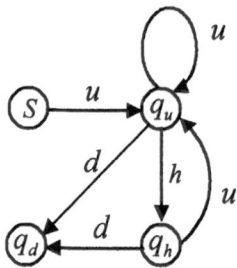

Figure 6.15. Finite-state diagram of an example-inferred automaton for FHR accelerations.

Imagine now that the training set T also contained the example *uhhud*. In this case, the successors of h contain h itself, therefore, the state diagram shown in Figure 6.16a represents the corresponding automaton.

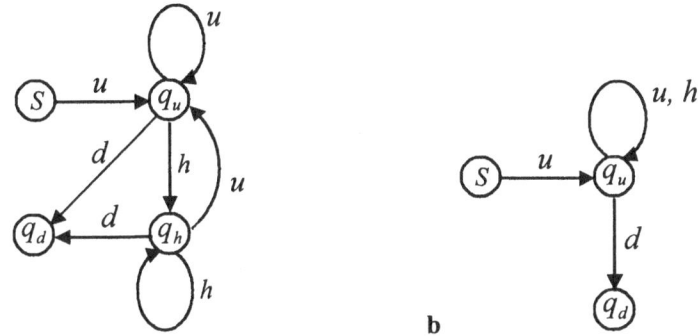

a   **b**

Figure 6.16. A modified finite-state diagram for FHR accelerations (a) and its minimized version (b).

Since states q_u and q_h now have the same successors, they can be merged, leading to the minimized automaton shown in Figure 6.16b. The rules for building the initial state diagram based on successors of symbols and the rules for merging states are easily put into algorithmic form. Once the minimized state diagram is obtained the inferred grammar can be derived by the following inverse rules from section 6.3.4:

- $N = Q$;
- $S = q_0$;
- $A \mapsto aB$ if $\delta(A,a) = B$ with $A, B \in Q$, $a \in T$;
- $A \mapsto a$ if $\delta(A,a) = C \in F \subseteq Q$.

6.4 Structural Matching

The key idea in structural matching is to determine the similarity between an unknown pattern and some prototype pattern by using a similarity measure adequate for the structural representations of the patterns.

6.4.1 String Matching

String matching is based on a similarity measure between two strings **x** and **y** with n and m symbols, respectively, and is defined in terms of the number of elementary edit operations that are required to transform the string **x** into the string **y**. The most common edit operations are:

1. Substitution of a symbol a in **x** by a symbol b in **y**;
2. Insertion of a symbol a in **y**;
3. Deletion of a symbol a in **x**.

We denote these operations as follows:

1. $a \rightarrow b$;   (6-18a)
2. $\lambda \rightarrow a$;   (6-18b)
3. $a \rightarrow \lambda$;   (6-18c)

where λ represents the null string.

Consider, for example, $T = \{h, d, u\}$, **x** = *duuh* and **y** = *hdhuh*. String **x** can be transformed into **y** as follows:

– insert h in **x**: *hduuh*;
– substitute u in **x** by h in **y**: *hdhuh*.

Another alternative is:

– substitute d in **x** by h in **y**: *huuh*;
– insert d in **x**: *hduuh*;
– substitute u in **x** by h in **y**: *hdhuh*.

In order to define a matching distance between **x** and **y**, we start by associating costs with the edit operations: $c(e_i)$, where e_i is any one of the edit operations. Next, we compute the total cost of a sequence, s, of k edit operations that transforms **x** into **y**, as:

$$c(s) = \sum_{i=1}^{k} c(e_i).$$ (6-19)

The dissimilarity distance between **x** and **y** is defined as the minimum cost of all sequences of edit operations that transform **x** into **y**:

$$d(\mathbf{x}, \mathbf{y}) = \min\{c(s), s \text{ transforms } \mathbf{x} \text{ into } \mathbf{y}\}.$$ (6-20)

An algorithm for computing this so-called *Levenshtein distance* is based on the enumeration in matrix form of the computation of all sequences of edit operations that transform **x** into **y**.

First, a matrix $D(i, j)$ with $(n+1)$ by $(m+1)$ elements is built, as shown in Figure 6.17. In this matrix, any path from $D(0, 0)$ to $D(n, m)$ represents a sequence of edit operations transforming **x** into **y**. The top row of the matrix is labelled with the **y** symbols, and the first column with the symbols of **x**, with the seed element $D(0, 0)$ = 0 representing a situation where no edit operations have been performed. From this seed element, the algorithm proceeds to fill up the matrix by examining the following three predecessors of $D(i, j)$ (see Figure 6.17):

1. $D(i, j\text{-}1)$: Progressing from $D(i, j\text{-}1)$ to $D(i, j)$ means the insertion of the corresponding top symbol of **y** into **x**, with a cost of $D1 = D(i, j\text{-}1) + c(\lambda \rightarrow a)$.
2. $D(i\text{-}1, j)$: Progressing from $D(i\text{-}1, j)$ to $D(i,j)$ means the deletion of the corresponding left symbol of **x**, with a cost of $D2 = D(i\text{-}1,j) + c(a \rightarrow \lambda)$.
3. $D(i\text{-}1, j\text{-}1)$: Progressing from $D(i\text{-}1, j\text{-}1)$ to $D(i, j)$ means the substitution of the corresponding left symbol of **x** by the corresponding top symbol of **y**, with a cost of $D3 = D(i\text{-}1, j\text{-}1) + c(a \rightarrow b)$. If both symbols are equal, the cost of this operation is zero.

The minimum of $D1$, $D2$ and $D3$ is assigned to $D(i, j)$.

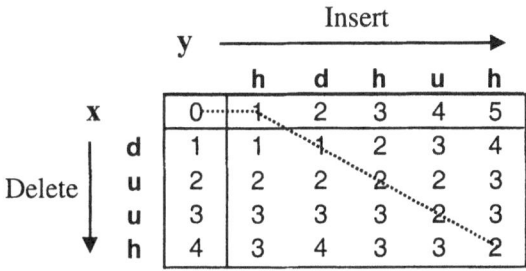

Figure 6.17. Computation of the Levenshtein distance between **x** and **y**, using unitary costs for all elementary edit operations. The dotted line corresponds to the minimum cost path.

Let us use Figure 6.17 to exemplify this procedure, assuming, for simplicity, unitary costs for all edit operations. Applying rules 1 and 2 immediately fills up the top row and left column. Now consider $D(1, 1)$. It can be reached from $D(0, 0)$, $D(0, 1)$ and $D(1, 0)$, adding a cost of one to any of these transitions. If we now consider $D(3, 4)$, we find a minimum cost for the substitution, since both symbols are equal, therefore we obtain $D(3, 4) = D(2, 3)$.

As shown in Figure 6.17 the minimum cost of transforming **x** into **y** is 2, representing the two previously mentioned edit operations as the first alternative to transforming **x** into **y**. The path corresponding to this sequence of operations is also shown in Figure 6.17.

In order for the Levenshtein distance to have the properties of a metric, the following non-stringent conditions must be satisfied:

1. $c(a \rightarrow b) \geq 0$ for any a, b;
2. $c(a \rightarrow b) = 0$ if and only if $a = b$;
3. $c(a \rightarrow b) \leq c(\lambda \rightarrow b) + c(a \rightarrow \lambda)$ for any a, b;
4. $c(a \rightarrow b) = c(b \rightarrow a)$ for any a, b.

In practice, even if these conditions are not satisfied, we still use $d(\mathbf{x}, \mathbf{y})$ as the distance between $\mathbf{x}$ and $\mathbf{y}$. In order to classify patterns described by strings, we can now use the k-nearest neighbour classification approach, described in section 4.3.2, for assigning patterns to classes, given a training set of patterns.

The basic algorithm for computing the Levenshtein distance can be modified in order to cope with a variety of aspects, such as context dependent costs or string attributes (see Bunke, 1990b, for details). Let us consider this last aspect, of matching strings $\mathbf{x}$ and $\mathbf{y}$ with d-dimensional attribute vectors $\mathbf{a}$ and $\mathbf{b}$, respectively. We define a new dissimilarity distance between $\mathbf{x}$ and $\mathbf{y}$ in the following way:

$$d_m(\mathbf{x}, \mathbf{y}) = d_s(\mathbf{x}, \mathbf{y}) + d_a(\mathbf{x}, \mathbf{y}), \tag{6-21}$$

where $d_s(\mathbf{x}, \mathbf{y})$ is the previous dissimilarity distance and $d_a(\mathbf{x}, \mathbf{y})$ is the dissimilarity distance relative to the attributes.

This distance takes account of the attribute differences for the different symbols as:

$$d_a(x, y) = \sum_{r,s} \sum_{i=1}^{d} w_i |x_{ri} - y_{si}|, \tag{6-21a}$$

where $|x_{ri} - y_{si}|$ takes account of attribute differences for homologous attributes and w_i is a suitably chosen weight.

The summation is taken for all x_r symbols that substitute different y_s symbols. As a matter of fact, this rule can be implemented by inserting an attribute cost into steps 1-3 of the basic algorithm. A particular implementation of this procedure for line segment primitives with length, l, and orientation angle, α attributes, is:

$$c(\lambda \rightarrow a) = I_a + (l_a/m); \tag{6-22a}$$
$$c(a \rightarrow \lambda) = D_a + (l_a/n); \tag{6-22b}$$
$$c(a \rightarrow b) = f(\alpha_a, \alpha_b) + |l_a/n - l_b/m|. \tag{6-22c}$$

where I_a and D_a are the usual insertion and deletion costs. The length attribute is divided by the string length, for the purpose of normalization. Function f takes care of the difference in angular attributes.

Let us see how this applies to the very simple situation shown in Figure 6.18, where the only line segments used are horizontal and vertical. Instead of taking into account an orientation attribute, we use a PDL approach so that the 3 symbols u, h, d with length attribute are used. As the only structural operator used is +, we can neglect it when computing distances.

From the results shown in Figure 6.18, obtained with the algorithm implemented in the *String Match.xls* file, some difficulties of this approach are visible. For instance, the dissimilarity between the prototype and shape (b) is only smaller than the dissimilarity corresponding to shapes (c) or (d) when the substitution cost is sufficiently high compared with the insertion cost. In practical applications, some tuning of elementary costs may therefore be necessary in order to obtain the best results.

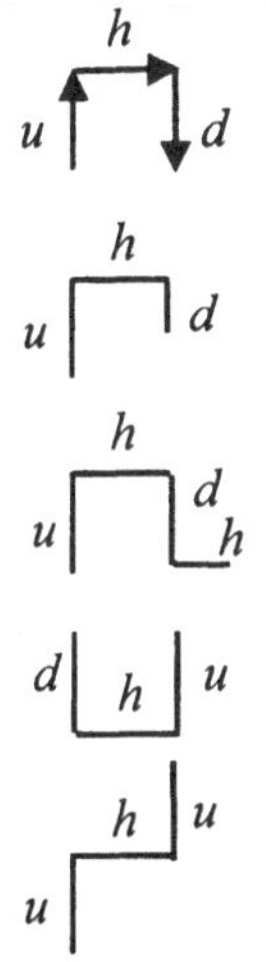

Prototype u		$c_i = 1$ $c_d = 1$ $c_s = \frac{1}{2}$	$c_i = 1$ $c_d = 1$ $c_s = 1$	$c_i = 1$ $c_d = 1$ $c_s = 2$	$c_i = \frac{1}{2}$ $c_d = 1$ $c_s = 3$
(a)		0	0	0	0
(b)		1.3	1.3	1.3	1.3
(c)		1	2	4	3.3
(d)		0.5	1	2	2.2

Figure 6.18. Levenshtein distance between a prototype pattern and each of four patterns, (a) to (d). Edit costs are shown at the top.

Despite the difficulties of string matching, this technique can often achieve surprisingly good results in pattern recognition applications. The basic idea consists of obtaining the matching score of an unknown pattern relative to the prototypes, choosing the classification corresponding to the closest prototype. Of course, a generalization of this principle using k-nearest neighbour classification is also possible.

We now illustrate the application of string matching with the recognition of toy models of tanks (*Tanks* dataset). Figure 6.19 shows profile views of three tank prototypes. Figure 6.20 shows one of the prototypes seen at variable distance and orientation, corresponding to the unknown pattern we wish to classify.

String matching is performed using the Levenshtein distance algorithm (*String Match.xls*) with the following modifications: first, because all primitives are attributed line segments, we do not have in this case different string symbols, and a substitution cost is always computed according to (6-21c); second, we now have to deal with an angular attribute measured in $[-180°, 180°]$. We choose a dissimilarity function $f(\alpha_a, \alpha_b)$, which yields a zero cost for angular differences of $0°$ or $360°$ and positive increasing cost for other angular differences, up to a maximum of one for line segments lying in opposite directions. The following function satisfies this requirement:

$$f(\alpha_a, \alpha_b) = 1 - ||\alpha_a - \alpha_b| - 180|/180. \qquad (6\text{-}23)$$

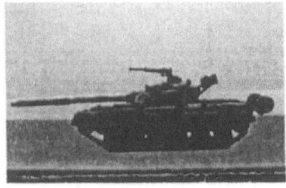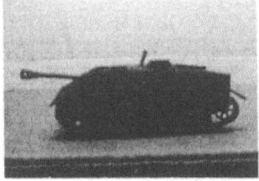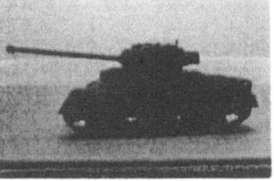

Figure 6.19. Three prototype tanks (toy models), labelled T1, T2 and T3, from left to right.

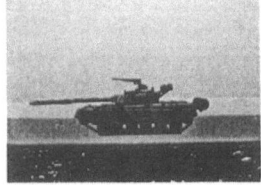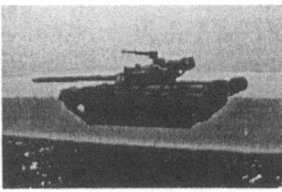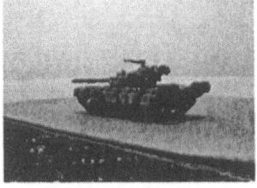

Figure 6.20. Three views of prototype T1 taken at variable distance and perspective angle, labelled T11, T12 and T13, from left to right.

The matching scores between prototypes T1 vs. T2 and T1 vs. T3 are 59 and 57, respectively. Table 6.3 shows the matching scores obtained for each of the "unknown" patterns vs. the prototypes. In all cases, the unknown pattern is correctly classified. It is clear, however, that the discrimination degrades with increasing perspective angle.

Table 6.3. Matching scores between an "unknown" tank and each prototype. The minimum always occurs for the prototype T1.

T11:T1	26		T12:T1	30		T13:T1	41
T11:T2	59		T12:T2	51		T13:T2	55
T11:T3	56		T12:T3	48		T13:T3	48

Improvement of the basic algorithm in order to achieve flexible structural matching, while coping with the issues of scale and orientation changes, as well as contour gaps provoked by occluding objects, is described in the work of Gdalyahu and Weinshall (1999).

The basic ideas of string matching (minimization of a cost function dependent on edit operations) can be generalized and applied to tree or graph matching.

6.4.2 Probabilistic Relaxation Matching

The string matching procedure described in the previous section, performs a sequence of edit operations in order to obtain a match of a string **x** with a string **y**. In some cases, performing the matching sequentially may not be the best idea, since early decisions may completely impair the whole process. In order to see this, let us again consider matching the prototype shape to shapes (b) and (d) in Figure 6.18. The perfect matching of the first two segments of the prototype with shape (d) results in a better matching score than with shape (b) for a not too high substitution cost. The situation may worsen when there are many primitives, and complex relations among them. In such situations, a parallel approach that iteratively adjusts the matching at several points using local constraints may produce better results.

Relaxation labelling is a class of iterative algorithms that works in a parallel way, dealing with several constraints at the same time. In what follows we will describe the two main methods of performing relaxation, *probabilistic* and *discrete*, and we will also present a neural net approach implementing the relaxation.

Let us assume that there are n objects A_i that we want to label with m labels l_k. Suppose also that the label assignments of the objects are interdependent, i.e., the assignments $A_i \rightarrow l_j$ and $A_h \rightarrow l_k$ have some measure of compatibility $c(i{:}j; h{:}k)$ that varies in the interval [-1, 1], with 1 meaning full compatibility, -1 full incompatibility and 0 a "don't care" situation. Our goal is to obtain a compatible assignment of labels to objects, measured by a probability estimate, P_{ij}, of assigning l_j to A_i. For this purpose, we have to consider how we can iteratively update our probability estimates in order to obtain a final assignment, starting from an initial situation where the probability of the assignment $A_i \rightarrow l_j$ is $P_{ij}^{(0)}$.

The *probabilistic relaxation* method updates the probabilities of the assignment $A_i \rightarrow l_j$ by noticing first that, given the assignment $A_h \rightarrow l_k$, one would like to increment P_{ij} with $c(i{:}j; h{:}k)P_{hk}$ since one wants to increase P_{ij} proportionally to P_{hk} if the compatibility is high and, in the same way, decrease it if the compatibility is low. One way to combine, at each iteration r, the increments for all objects A_h and labels l_k, is to add up the increments for all possible labels as:

$$\sum_{k=1}^{m} c(i:j;h:k)P_{hk}^{(r)}, \tag{6-24a}$$

and average these increments for all objects $\mathbf{x}_h \neq \mathbf{x}_i$:

$$q_{ij}^{(r)} = \frac{1}{n-1} \sum_{\substack{h=1 \\ h \neq i}}^{n} \sum_{k=1}^{m} c(i:j; h:k) P_{hk}^{(r)} . \tag{6-24b}$$

The quantities q_{ij} are in $[-1, 1]$ and can be used to update the P_{ij}, satisfying the constraints that they are nonnegative and add up to one for each object, in the following way:

$$P_{ij}^{(r+1)} = \frac{P_{ij}^{(r)}\left(1+q_{ij}^{(r)}\right)}{\sum_{j=1}^{m} P_{ij}^{(r)}\left(1+q_{ij}^{(r)}\right)}. \tag{6-25}$$

The most important decisions one must make when applying probabilistic relaxation relate to the choice of compatibility measures and the estimation of the $P_{ij}^{(0)}$.

Let us consider the so-called image registration problem. This is a pattern recognition problem, where we want to establish a correspondence between two different patterns (images) A and B using two sets of points, called control points. The control points correspond to n points of A and m points of B, respectively, which share k common points, with k unknown. They are chosen so that they reflect clearly identifiable segments of the images. In an application to satellite images registration (Ton and Jain, 1989), the control points are centroids of clearly identifiable regions and have attributes that are the type and the size of the respective region. A matrix of $n \times m$ probabilities P_{ij} can then be established to represent the probability of matching each pair of points. The initial estimates are:

$$P_{ij}^{(0)} = \begin{cases} \min\left(\dfrac{size(A_i)}{size(B_j)}, \dfrac{size(B_j)}{size(A_i)}\right) & \text{if } A_i \text{ and } B_j \text{ are the same type,} \\ 0, & \text{otherwise.} \end{cases} \tag{6-26}$$

The compatibility factors use both the probability estimates and the relative distances among the points:

$$c^{(r)}(i:j; h:k) = P_{hk}^{(r)} . \min\left(\frac{d_{ih}}{d_{jk}}, \frac{d_{jk}}{d_{ih}}\right). \tag{6-27}$$

From these compatibility factors, one can compute the support that the other points lend to the assignment (A_i, B_j), at iteration r, as:

$$q_{ij}^{(r)} = \frac{1}{m-1} \sum_{\substack{h=1 \\ h \neq i}}^{n} \left[\max_{\substack{1 \leq k \leq m \\ k \neq j}} c^{(r)}(i:j; h:k) \right]. \tag{6-28}$$

The probabilities are then updated, as:

$$P_{ij}^{(r+1)} = q_{ij}^{(r)} P_{ij}^{(r)}. \tag{6-29}$$

As a result of this updating process, it is expected that the probabilities corresponding to a match will be close to one, while the other values will be close to zero. In practice, one may stop the iterative process when a sufficient discrimination of values above or below 0.5 is reached.

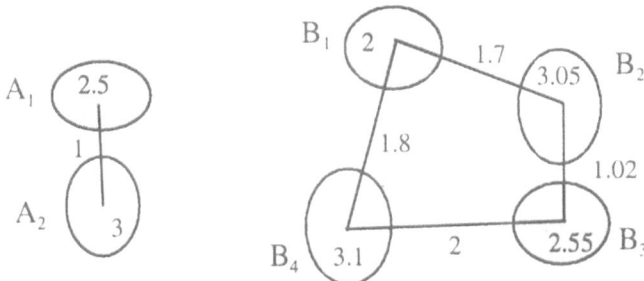

Figure 6.21. An image registration example, where the goal is to establish a correspondence of centroids of A regions with centroids of B regions.

We exemplify this method using the regions shown in Figure 6.21, where there are two types of regions (white and grey) with areas and distances among the centroids as indicated. Table 6.4 shows the probability matrix from the initial phase up to the second iteration. Initially, the probabilities depend only on the region size, and in this particular case, all non-zero values are initially close to one. In the following iterations, the compatibility factors play their role so that in the second iteration it is already clear that there is only one valid match: (A_1, B_3), (A_2, B_2).

Table 6.4. Estimates of centroid matching probabilities for the image registration example.

	$P^{(0)}$			$P^{(1)}$			$P^{(2)}$	
	A_1	A_2		A_1	A_2		A_1	A_2
B_1	0.8	0	B_1	0.463	0	B_1	0.257	0
B_2	0	0.984	B_2	0	0.945	B_2	0	0.876
B_3	0.980	0	B_3	0.945	0	B_3	0.876	0
B_4	0	0.968	B_4	0	0.474	B_4	0	0.224

In this case, the updating of the probabilities is quite easily done by hand. For instance, the first updating of P_{11} depends only on the compatibilities of (A_2, B_2) and of (A_2, B_4), with:

$$c(1{:}1; 2{:}2) = P_{22} (1/1.7) = 0.5788;$$
$$c(1{:}1; 2{:}4) = P_{24} (1/1.8) = 0.5378.$$

The maximum value of these compatibilities for A_2, updates $P_{11} = 0.8$ to $P_{11} = 0.8 \times 0.5788 = 0.463$.

This basic probabilistic relaxation scheme can also be applied to other pattern recognition tasks, including object classification, as exemplified in Exercise 6.22.

6.4.3 Discrete Relaxation Matching

In some situations it is not adequate to assign probabilities to the object labelling, since the only decision is whether the label is possible or not, i.e., P_{ij} is either 1 or 0. Usually, in these situations the compatibilities are also qualitative in nature: the $A_i \rightarrow l_j$ assignment is either compatible ($c=1$) or not ($c=0$). An example of such a situation is in graph matching, where correspondence between nodes is either possible or impossible.

There is a variant of the basic relaxation algorithm, called *discrete relaxation*, appropriate for these kinds of situations. In discrete relaxation, for every A_h relevant to A_i, there must be at least one label k, such that $c(i{:}j; h{:}k)=1$ with $P_{hk}=1$; otherwise the assignment $A_i \rightarrow l_j$ is impossible. Initially, the $P_{ij}^{(0)}$ are all set to one. At subsequent iterations, P_{ij} remains 1 if for every relevant A_h there is an assignment such that $c(i{:}j; h{:}k)P_{hk}=1$; otherwise P_{ij} becomes 0. This is equivalent to the following formula:

$$P_{ij}^{(r+1)} = \min_h \left[\max_{k=1}^{m} c(i{:}j; h{:}k)P_{hk}^{(r)} \right]. \tag{6-30}$$

i:j	11	13	22	24	31	33
h:k	22	-	11	-	-	22
			33			

i:j	11	13	22	31	33
h:k	22	-	11	-	-

a   b

Figure 6.22. Discrete relaxation applied to two simples examples of compatible (a) and incompatible (b) shapes.

Formula (6-30) estimates possible assignments for A_i by checking that each assignment is compatible with the surviving assignments of A_i's neighbours.

Let us apply discrete relaxation to the matching of the prototype shape of Figure 6.18 with shapes (b) and (d).

In this example we only distinguish whether the lines are horizontal or vertical, and consider that an assignment $i:j$ is compatible if they are of the same type. Further, $i:j$ is compatible with $h:k$ if h is an immediate neighbour of i, such that it is possible to find a translation $i:j$ that superimposes h over k. With these compatibility rules, we can list the compatible assignments as shown in Figure 6.22 for each pair $i:j$. For instance, for the matching (a), the assignment 1:1 is compatible with 2:2; for the assignment 1:3, one does not find any compatible primitives, since the neighbour segment 2 of the first shape is not compatible with the neighbour segment 4 of the second shape.

Starting with a matrix $[P_{ij}]$ filled in with ones, we can now apply the compatibility rules to arrive at the final matrix shown in Table 6.5 for the matching situation of Figure 6.22a. It is clear that a total match is reached (1:1, 2:2, 3:3). For the shape matching situation of Figure 6.22b, only the partial match (1:1, 2:2) is obtained.

Notice that for complex shapes, the computation of the compatibilities can be cumbersome. We will see in the next section a method to expedite their computation.

Table 6.5. Probability matrix for the matching situation of Figure 6.22a.

	$\mathbf{P}^{(0)}$					$\mathbf{P}^{(1)}$					$\mathbf{P}^{(2)}$			
	1	2	3	4		1	2	3	4		1	2	3	4
1	1	1	1	1	1	1	0	1	0	1	1	0	0	0
2	1	1	1	1	2	0	1	0	1	2	0	1	0	0
3	1	1	1	1	3	1	0	1	0	3	0	0	1	0

6.4.4 Relaxation Using Hopfield Networks

Relaxation methods can be implemented using neural networks. In particular, a modified version of the Hopfield network has been found useful in several applications of relaxation methods, namely in line drawing matching (Kuner and Ueberreiter, 1988) and in hierarchical recognition of three-dimensional objects such as machine parts (Lin *et al.*, 1991).

We will now describe how this approach is applied using the line drawings example. Imagine that we have two line drawings X and Y, constituted by line segments x_i $(i = 1,..., n)$ and y_j $(j = 1,..., m)$. The line drawing X is considered the prototype drawing that we want to match with a subset of the line drawing of Y.

For this purpose, we start by defining a function $t(x_i, x_h)$ that reflects the transformation that must be applied to x_i in order to obtain x_h. For some applications, function $t(x_i, x_h)$ just computes a matching score resembling the transforming function used in (6-22c).

Next, we compute the compatibility coefficients for the assignments $x_i \rightarrow y_j$ and $x_h \rightarrow y_k$ as follows:

$$c(i:j;h:k)=1 \quad \text{if} \quad t(x_i,x_h)=t(y_j,y_k); \tag{6-31a}$$

$$c(i:j;h:k)<1 \quad \text{if} \quad t(x_i,x_h)\neq t(y_j,y_k); \tag{6-31b}$$

$$c(h:k,i:j)=c(i:j;h:k). \tag{6-31c}$$

Therefore, full compatibility only exists if the matching between candidate segments in the prototype drawing is the same as between candidate segments in the unknown drawing.

Let us use a Boolean matrix $\mathbf{M}$ with n lines and m columns for the representation of the possible assignments of line segments of X to line segments of Y. Possible assignments are represented by $m_{ij}=1$, impossible assignments by $m_{ij}=0$. A matching of X with a subset of Y corresponds to a $n \times m$ matrix $\mathbf{X}$, generated from $\mathbf{M}$, such that:

$$x_{ij} =1 \quad \Rightarrow \quad x_{il} =0 \quad \text{if} \quad l \neq j, \tag{6-32}$$

since in any matching, a segment of X can only be assigned to one segment of Y. The optimal assignment corresponds to:

$$\max\left(\sum_{i=1}^{n}\sum_{h=1}^{n}\sum_{j=1}^{m}\sum_{k=1}^{m} x_{ij}\, c(i:j,h:k)x_{hk} \right), \tag{6-33a}$$

with $\displaystyle\sum_{j=1}^{m}x_{ij} = 1$ and $\displaystyle\sum_{i=1}^{n}x_{ij} \leq 1$. $\tag{6-33b}$

This is a quadratic assignment problem that can be solved using a probabilistic relaxation method (see Kuner and Ueberreiter, 1988). Initially, a probability matrix is initialised with a constant value, e.g. $1/n$. Next, the basic relaxation algorithm expressed by formulas (6-24) and (6-25) is applied until there is no significant difference between the probability matrices $\mathbf{P}$ in successive iterations. Matrix $\mathbf{P}$ represents then the probabilities of the assignments, with the higher values P_{ij} representing the best assignments $x_i \rightarrow y_j$. One then proceeds to solve the much simpler linear assignment problem:

$$\max\left(\sum_{i=1}^{n}\sum_{j=1}^{m} P_{ij}x_{ij} \right) \text{ with the constraints (6-33b).} \tag{6-34}$$

This relaxation assignment can be solved with a modified Hopfield net in the following way:

1. Set a two-dimensional Hopfield network with the rows representing the segments (objects) of X and the columns the segments (objects) of Y. Each node of the net, now denoted x_{ij}, represents an assignment $x_i \rightarrow y_j$;
2. Compute the connection weights of the net as $w_{ijhk} = c(i{:}j, h{:}k)$, which correspond to the weight that links neuron x_{ij} with x_{hk};
3. Initialise the inputs with a matrix **M** of possible assignments, $m_{ij} = 1/n$, and set a total compatibility factor $q=0$;
4. Perform the output updating of the network in a full parallel way:

$$P_{ij} = \text{sgn}\left(\sum_{h=1}^{n} \sum_{k=1}^{m} c(i:j, h:k) m_{hk} \right); \tag{6-35}$$

5. With the probability matrix obtained, solve the linear assignment problem (6-34) and evaluate the new value of q, q', using the objective function of (6-33a).
6. If $q' < q$ set **P** = **M** and stop, otherwise set **M** = **P**, $q = q'$ and go to step 4.

The *Hopfield* program (Appendix B) allows one to perform experiments of a Hopfield net in the particular case of discrete relaxation. Let us consider the simple example shown in Figure 6.22a. In order to derive the optimal assignment, we start by setting a network of 3x4 neurons. Next, since we are using the values {1, -1}, instead of {1, 0} for the discrete Hopfield net, we set all the weights to -1 (corresponding to incompatibility) except for the compatible assignments, where we set the corresponding weight to the value $n \times m = 12$, therefore insuring a positive result if at least one of the products $c(i:j, h:k)m_{hk}$ is positive. We initialise the net with a grid filled in with ones and get the final solution shown in Table 6.5, where the final assignment is easily derived.

Let us now consider a less trivial example of having to find the compatible assignment between the line drawings shown in Figure 6.23. We start by defining the function that reflects the transformation that must be applied to segment x_i in order to obtain segment x_h. For this purpose, we may choose the following vectorial function:

$$t(x_i, x_k) = [d_{\min} \quad r_l \quad \alpha]', \quad \text{with} \tag{6-36}$$

$d_{\min}$: minimum distance between segments;
r_l : ratio of the segments lengths;
α : angle between segments, in [0, 180°].

With this function it is easy to see, for instance, that the pair (x_2, x_3) is compatible with (y_4, y_6) but not with (y_5, y_6). When applying the comparisons

(6-31a) and (6-31b), it is convenient to set some tolerance for all components of $\mathbf{t}(x_i, x_k)$.

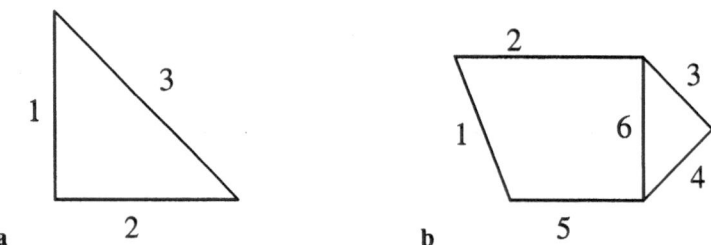

Figure 6.23. Line drawings for illustration of discrete matching with a Hopfield network: (a) prototype; (b) "unknown" drawing.

The compatibility matrix corresponding to the Hopfield net weights is a sparse matrix, since it is filled with -1 (incompatible assignment) for all elements w_{ijhk} such that $h=i$ or $k=j$ (shaded cells in Table 6.6). Also, since it is a symmetric matrix, one only has to fill in half of the matrix values. Table 6.6 shows part of the compatibility matrix using the binary set $\{1, 0\}$. The Hopfield weight matrix will be filled with -1 instead of 0, and $n \times m = 18$ instead of 1. For instance, since $(\mathbf{x}_2, \mathbf{x}_3)$ is compatible with $(\mathbf{y}_4, \mathbf{y}_6)$, the weight w_{2436} will be filled in with 18.

Table 6.6. Compatibility matrix for the example of Figure 6.23. Parts of the matrix not shown are filled in with zeros.

	21	22	23	24	25	26	31	32	33	34	35	36
11	0	0	0	0	0	0	0	0	0	0	0	0
12	0	0	0	0	0	0	0	0	0	0	0	0
13	0	0	0	1	0	0	0	0	0	0	0	1
14	0	0	1	0	0	0	0	0	0	0	0	1
15	0	0	0	0	0	1	0	0	0	0	0	0
16	0	0	0	0	1	0	0	0	0	0	0	0

	21	22	23	24	25	26	31	32	33	34	35	36
21	0	0	0	0	0	0	0	0	0	0	0	0
22		0	0	0	0	0	0	0	0	0	0	0
23			0	0	0	0	0	0	0	0	0	1
24				0	0	0	0	0	0	0	0	1
25					0	0	0	0	0	0	0	0
26						0	0	0	0	0	0	0

With the Hopfield network inputs set initially with ones, the net will iterate to the outputs shown in Figure 6.24a, which give a picture of all feasible assignments. We now solve the linear assignment problem (6-34), also using the Hopfield net. Since $\mathbf{x}_3 \rightarrow \mathbf{y}_6$ is the only feasible assignment for $\mathbf{x}_3$, we investigate other assignments satisfying (6-33b). One such assignment is shown in Figure 6.23b and has a final state shown in Figure 6.23c, with $q=2$, which corresponds to the partial assignment $\{x_3 \rightarrow y_6, x_2 \rightarrow y_5\}$. The maximum value of $q=3$ is only obtained with the full compatible assignments $\{x_3 \rightarrow y_6, x_2 \rightarrow y_3, x_1 \rightarrow y_4\}$ or $\{x_3 \rightarrow y_6, x_2 \rightarrow y_4, x_1 \rightarrow y_3\}$.

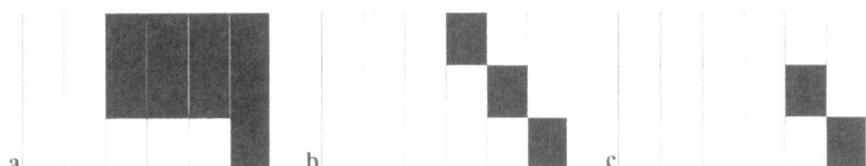

a   b   c

Figure 6.24. Hopfield net illustrating the probabilities associated with the assignments corresponding to the example shown in Figure 6.23. (a) Feasible assignments as solutions to the quadratic problem; (b) A candidate assignment; (c) final assignment corresponding to the previous situation ($q=2$).

The basic ideas that have just been described, concerning the application of a discrete Hopfield network for discrete relaxation matching, can be generalized for more complex probabilistic relaxation tasks, using a modified version of the continuous Hopfield network. In the work of Lin *et al.* (1991), the hierarchical recognition of machine parts using such modified Hopfield networks is described. The hierarchical process uses: at the first stage, a Hopfield network whose weights correspond to surface matching scores, picking up possible candidates from a database of machine parts; at the second stage, a Hopfield network performs vertex matching in order to achieve a finer selection.

6.4.5 Graph and Tree Matching

Consider two graphs (or trees) $G_1=\{N_1, R_1\}$ and $G_2=\{N_2, R_2\}$, describing the structural relations of two patterns. A *homomorphism* from G_1 to G_2 is any function f establishing a correspondence between the nodes of N_1 and the nodes of N_2 such that any pair of adjacent nodes in G_1 corresponds, through f, to adjacent nodes in N_2. Let (a, b) represent two adjacent nodes of N_1. Then a homomorphism f satisfies:

$$(a,b) \in R_1 \Rightarrow (f(a), f(b)) \in R_2. \qquad (6\text{-}37)$$

Consider the two digraphs represented in Figure 6.25. When assessing node adjacency, we have to take into consideration the direction of the arc connecting the nodes. There are two easily found homomorphisms between both digraphs.

Two similar patterns will have a homomorphic relation in at least a large part of their graph or tree representations. The two patterns will be structurally equivalent if an *isomorphism* exists:

$$(a,b) \in R_1 \Leftrightarrow (f(a),f(b)) \in R_2. \tag{6-38}$$

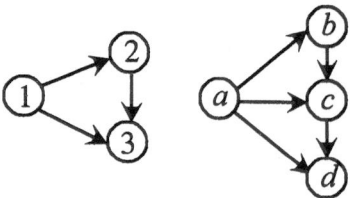

Figure 6.25. Two digraphs with two homomorphisms: (a) $f(1)=a$, $f(2)=b$, $f(3)=c$; (b) $f(1)=a$, $f(2)=c$, $f(3)=d$.

The structural descriptions are then the same except for a node re-labelling operation.

An algorithm for finding homomorphisms in two graphs $G_1=\{N_1, R_1\}$ and $G_2=\{N_2, R_2\}$ is based on the idea of first building the so-called *match graph*. This is a graph where each node represents an assignment from one of the N_1 nodes to one of the N_2 nodes. Let (n_1, n_2) and (n_1', n_2') be two such assignments, representing two distinct nodes in the match graph. An arc exists between these two nodes if the assignments are compatible or, equivalently, if the relation for the node pair (n_1, n_1') is the same as for the node pair (n_2, n_2').

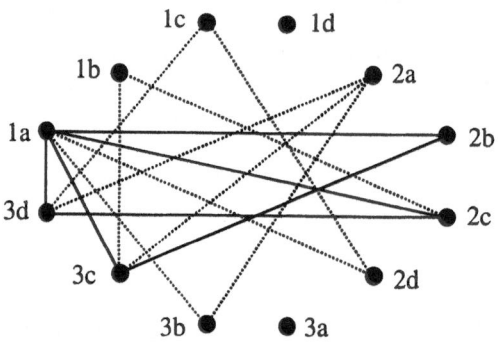

Figure 6.26. Match graph for the two graphs shown in Figure 6.25. The homomorphisms are shown with solid line.

Once the match graph is built, as shown in Figure 6.26 for the two graphs of Figure 6.25, one proceeds to determine its *cliques*. A clique is a totally connected sub-graph between any two different nodes, where totally connected means that there is a path linking any given pair of nodes. In our case, we are interested in maximal cliques involving different nodes of the source graphs. These are shown with solid line in Figure 6.26, representing the two known homomorphisms.

As seen in this example, finding isomorphisms or homomorphisms between graphs or trees can be a hard task in non-trivial situations, since it demands searching for compatible node adjacencies in the space of all possible node correspondences. This usually amounts to a long time-consuming task, for anything except a very small number of nodes. Existing algorithms that perform this search require a time that is approximately factorial-bound with the maximum number of nodes for the target correspondence. No polynomial-bound algorithms are known. The situation worsens when one has to assess not only node adjacency, but also attribute compatibility. For instance, if instead of the digraphs of Figure 6.25 we consider the digraphs of Figure 6.4, no homomorphism exists. However, an evident homomorphism exists between the digraphs of "F" and "E".

Practical applications of pattern recognition, with patterns described by trees or graphs, resort to faster methods of assessing the structural dissimilarity, namely to the idea of edit cost as explained in section 6.4.1 or to discrete relaxation as explained in section 6.4.3.

Tree matching based on edit operations is conceptually similar to the string matching method described in section 6.4.1. The following five edit operations are used:

1. Insertion of a node
2. Deletion of a node
3. Substitution of a node label
4. Splitting a node
5. Merging two nodes

Algorithms that assess tree dissimilarity using these edit operations are described in Sanfeliu (1990). These algorithms have a time complexity of the order of nm^2, where n and m are the number of nodes of the trees to be matched.

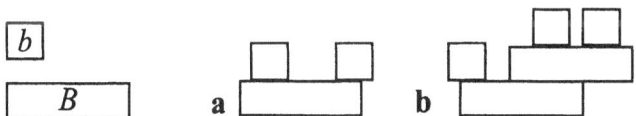

Figure 6.27. Two scene situations in a "block world", with primitives small block, b, and large block, B.

Relaxation techniques are quite attractive for assessing tree or graph dissimilarity, since they can be executed quickly and easily incorporate any constraints, namely those derived from the attributes. In some situations of tree or graph matching it is sufficient to perform discrete relaxation, much in the same way as we did in the previous sections. Consider for instance the scene situations shown in Figure 6.27. These can be represented by the trees of Figure 6.28, where a descendent node means "above". We can now perform discrete relaxation using the compatibilities of the neighbour nodes also shown in Figure 6.28. The probability matrix of the assignments evolves as shown in Table 6.7. A homomorphism of scene (a) relative to scene (b) is detected.

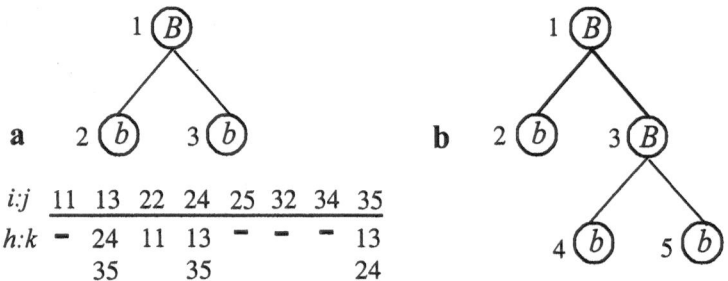

Figure 6.28. Trees describing the scene situations of Figure 6.27, with the compatibility table.

Table 6.7. Probability matrix of the tree matching problem shown in Figure 6.28.

$\mathbf{P}^{(0)}$						$\mathbf{P}^{(1)}$						$\mathbf{P}^{(2)}$				
	1	2	3	4	5		1	2	3	4	5		1	2	3	4	5
1	1	1	1	1	1	1	1	0	1	0	0	1	0	0	1	0	0
2	1	1	1	1	1	2	0	1	0	1	1	2	0	0	0	1	0
3	1	1	1	1	1	3	0	1	0	1	1	3	0	0	0	0	1

The Hopfield network approach can also be used for determining the graph homomorphisms, in the same way as explained in the previous section (see Exercise 6.24).

For attributed relational graphs such as those exemplified in Figure 6.4, one would have to compute similarities for the node properties (v, h, u, d, c, b) and for the relational properties (a, e, l, t). These would influence, through appropriate weighting, the compatibilities among the graph nodes. Work along these lines for generalized attributed relational graphs has been developed by Li (1992). In his work, a relaxation matching algorithm invariant to translations, rotations and scale changes is presented.

Special types of recurrent neural networks have also been developed for acyclic graph matching. Their application to automatic inference in syntactic and structural pattern recognition is described by Sperduti *et al.* (1996).

Bibliography

Biland HP, Wahl FM (1988) Hough-Space Decomposition for Polyhedral Scene Analysis. In: Ferraté G, Pavlidis T, Sanfeliu A, Bunke H (eds) Syntactic and Structural Pattern Recognition. Springer-Verlag.

Bunke H (1990a) String Grammars for Syntactic Pattern Recognition In: Bunke H, Sanfeliu A (eds) Syntactic and Structural Pattern Recognition. Theory and Applications. World Scientific Pub. Co., Singapore.

Bunke H (1990b) String Matching for Structural Pattern Recognition. In: Bunke H, Sanfeliu A (eds) Syntactic and Structural Pattern Recognition. Theory and Applications. World Scientific Pub. Co., Singapore.

Bunke H (1990c) Hybrid Pattern Recognition Methods. In: Bunke H, Sanfeliu A (eds) Syntactic and Structural Pattern Recognition. Theory and Applications. World Scientific Pub. Co., Singapore.

Chen JW, Lee SY (1996) A Hierarchical Representation for the Reference Database of On-line Chinese Character Recognition. In: Perner P, Wang P, Rosenfeld A (eds) Advances in Structural and Syntactical Pattern Recognition, Springer Verlag, pp. 351-360.

Davis LS (1979) Shape Matching Using Relaxation Techniques. IEEE Tr Patt An Mach Intell, 1:60-72.

DeMori R (1977) Syntactic Recognition of Speech Signals. In: Fu KS (ed) Syntactic Pattern Recognition Applications. Springer-Verlag.

Di Baja GS (1996) Representing Shape by Line Patterns. In: Perner P, Wang P, Rosenfeld A (eds) Advances in Structural and Syntactical Pattern Recognition, Springer Verlag, pp. 230-239.

Duda RO, Hart PE (1973) Pattern Classification and Scene Analysis. Wiley, New York.

Fu KS (1977) Introduction to Syntactic Pattern Recognition. In: Fu KS (ed) Syntactic Pattern Recognition Applications. Springer-Verlag.

Gdalyahu Y, Weinshall D (1999) Flexible Syntactic Matching of Curves and its Application to Automatic Hierarchical Classification of Silhouettes. IEEE Tr Patt An Mach Intell, 21:1312-1328.

Gold S, Rangarajan A (1996) A Graduated Assignment Algorithm for Graph Matching. IEEE Tr Patt An Mach Intell, 18:377-388.

Horowitz SL (1977) Peak Recognition in Waveforms. In: Fu KS (ed) Syntactic Pattern Recognition Applications. Springer-Verlag.

Hummel RA, Zucker SW (1983) On the Foundations of Relaxation Labeling Processes. IEEE Tr Patt An Mach Intell, 5:267-285.

Kuner P, Ueberreiter B (1988) Pattern Recognition by Graph Matching. Combinatorial Versus Continuous Optimization. Int. J. Patt. Rec. Artif. Intell., 2: 527-542.

Lapresté JT, Cartoux JY, Richetin M (1988) Face Recognition from Range Data by Structural Analysis. In: Ferraté G, Pavlidis T, Sanfeliu A, Bunke H (eds) Syntactic and Structural Pattern Recognition. Springer-Verlag.

Lee KH, Eom KB, Kashyap RL (1992) Character Recognition based on Attribute-Dependent Programmed Grammar. IEEE Tr. Patt. An. Mach. Intell., 14:1122-1128.

Li SZ (1992) Matching: Invariant to Translations, Rotations and Scale Changes. Pattern Recognition, 25:583-594.

Lin WC, Liao FY, Tsao CK, Lingutla T (1991) A Hierarchical Multiple-View Approach to Three-Dimensional Object Recognition. IEEE Tr Neural Networks, 2:84-92.

Mehrotra R, Grosky WI (1988) Smith: An Efficient Model-Based Two Dimensional Shape Matching Technique. In: Ferraté G, Pavlidis T, Sanfeliu A, Bunke H (eds) Syntactic and Structural Pattern Recognition. Springer-Verlag, pp. 233-248.

Miclet L (1990) Grammatical Inference. In: Bunke H, Sanfeliu A (eds) Syntactic and Structural Pattern Recognition. Theory and Applications. World Scientific Pub. Co., Singapore.

Miclet L, Quinqueton J (1988) Learning from Examples in Sequences and Grammatical Inference. In: Ferraté G, Pavlidis T, Sanfeliu A, Bunke H (eds) Syntactic and Structural Pattern Recognition. Springer-Verlag.

Moayer B, Fu KS (1977) Fingerprint Classification. In: Fu KS (ed) Syntactic Pattern Recognition Applications. Springer-Verlag.

Nishida H (1996) A Structural Analysis of Curve Deformation by Discontinuous Transformations. In: Perner P, Wang P, Rosenfeld A (eds) Advances in Structural and Syntactical Pattern Recognition, Springer Verlag, pp. 269-278.

Pao DCW, Li HF (1992) Shapes Recognition Using the Straight Line Hough Transform: Theory and Generalization. IEEE Tr Patt An Mach Intell, 14:1076-1128.

Pavlidis T (1973) Waveform Segmentation Through Functional Approximation. IEEE Tr Computers, 22:689-697.

Rosenfeld A, Kak A (1982) Digital Picture Processing, vol. 2. Academic Press Inc., Orlando, Florida.

Rosenfeld A (1990) Array, Tree and Graph Grammars. In: Bunke H and Sanfeliu A (eds) Syntactic and Structural Pattern Recognition. Theory and Applications. World Scientific Pub. Co., Singapore.

Sanfeliu A (1990) Matching Tree Structures. In: Bunke H, Sanfeliu A (eds) Syntactic and Structural Pattern Recognition. Theory and Applications. World Scientific Pub. Co., Singapore.

Schalkoff R (1992) Pattern Recognition. Statistical, Structural and Neural Approaches..John Wiley & Sons, Inc.

Shapiro L (1988) Ordered Structural Matching. In: Ferraté G, Pavlidis T, Sanfeliu A, Bunke H (eds) Syntactic and Structural Pattern Recognition. Springer-Verlag.

Shapiro LG, Haralick RM (1990) Matching Relational Structures Using Discrete Relaxation. In: Bunke H, Sanfeliu A (eds) Syntactic and Structural Pattern Recognition. Theory and Applications. World Scientific Pub. Co., Singapore.

Skordalakis E (1990) ECG Analysis. In: Bunke H, Sanfeliu A (eds) Syntactic and Structural Pattern Recognition. Theory and Applications. World Scientific Pub. Co., Singapore.

Sperduti A, Majidi D, Starita A (1996) Extended Cascade-Correlation for Syntactic and Structural Pattern Recognition. In: Perner P, Wang P, Rosenfeld A (eds) Advances in Structural and Syntactical Pattern Recognition, Springer Verlag, pp. 90-99.

Stenstrom JR (1988) Training and Model Generation for a Syntactic Curve Network Parser. In: Ferraté G, Pavlidis T, Sanfeliu A, Bunke H (eds) Syntactic and Structural Pattern Recognition. Springer-Verlag, pp. 249-267.

Tai JW, Liu YJ (1990) Chinese Character Recognition. In: Bunke H, Sanfeliu A (eds) Syntactic and Structural Pattern Recognition. Theory and Applications. World Scientific Pub. Co., Singapore.

Thomason GT (1990) Introduction and Overview. In: Bunke H, Sanfeliu A (eds) Syntactic and Structural Pattern Recognition. Theory and Applications. World Scientific Pub. Co., Singapore.

Ton J, Jain AK (1989) Registering Landsat Images by Point Matching. IEEE Tr Geosci and Rem Sensing, 27:642-651.

Tsai WH (1990) Combining Statistical and Structural Methods. In: Bunke H, Sanfeliu A (eds) Syntactic and Structural Pattern Recognition. Theory and Applications. World Scientific Pub. Co., Singapore.

Vámos T (1977) Industrial Objects and Machine Parts Recognition. In: Fu KS (ed) Syntactic Pattern Recognition Applications. Springer-Verlag.

Wong AKC, Constant J, You ML (1990) Random Graphs. In: Bunke H and Sanfeliu A (eds) Syntactic and Structural Pattern Recognition. Theory and Applications. World Scientific Pub. Co., Singapore.

You KC, Fu KS (1979) A Syntactic Approach to Shape Recognition Using Attributed Grammars. IEEE Tr Systems, Man and Cybernetics, 9:334-345.

Exercises

6.1 Consider the grammar presented in (6-7d).
   a) What type of grammar is it?
   b) Two grammars $G1$, $G2$ are considered equivalent if $L(G1)= L(G2)$. Is there a regular grammar equivalent to (6-7d)? Why?

6.2 A grammar for waveform description has the following production rules:

$$uP^+ \mapsto u(h \mid u)(P^+ \mid \lambda)d \; ;$$
$$hP^+ \mapsto hu(P^+ \mid \lambda)d \; .$$

   a) Interpret the production rules. What type of grammar is it?
   b) Which of the following sequences is parsed by the grammar: *hhud*; *huuhdd* ?

6.3 Modify the production rules (6-12a) so that the corresponding grammar will recognize positive and negative spikes formed by an arbitrary number of D and U primitives, with at most an h primitive between.

6.4 Consider the symbol set $T = \{h, p\}$ used to describe signals, where h represents a horizontal segment and p is a positive peak. Build a regular grammar capable of recognizing sequences terminated by *hph*, i.e., by isolated peaks. Draw the state diagram of the finite-state automaton that recognizes such sequences.

6.5 Improve the set of primitives and relations indicated in section 6.2.2 (Figure 6.4) in order to describe all capital letters by digraphs.

6.6 In section 6.3.2 two different PDL descriptions were given for the pattern "R", according to the traversing direction of the description. Develop a general rule that will generate a PDL description based on the description of the inverse traversing direction.

6.7 Consider "standard" prototype drawings of the decimal digits.
   a) Develop a PDL grammar that will generate the prototypes for each digit class.
   b) Perform string matching experiments (use *StrMatch.xls*) in order to determine which digit class an unknown PDL sequence can be assigned to. Also set a threshold for the matching score in order to establish a reject class.

6.8 An FHR spike (see Figure 6.11) has amplitude that is approximately half (negative spike) or double (positive spike) of its onset value.
   a) Determine the attributed grammar that will detect FHR spikes.
   b) Perform experiments with this grammar using the *FHR Signals* dataset, adjusting the appropriate attribute rules.

6.9 An upward FHR wave is considered an acceleration if it lasts for more than 15 s, reaching an amplitude of at least 15 bpm. Write the appropriate rules for the attributed grammar describing FHR accelerations (see rules (6-14)).

6.10 A downward FHR wave is considered a deceleration if it lasts for more than 15 s, reaching an amplitude of at least 10 bpm.
   a) Draw the state diagram describing decelerations, analogous to the one describing accelerations shown in Figure 6.12.
   b) Write the appropriate rules for the attribute vectors of this grammar, studying its behaviour by experimenting with the *FHR Signals* dataset.

6.11 Develop the grammar rules that will recognize the P, Q, R, S and T waves of ECG signals (see description in A.4). Use the *ECG Signals* dataset to carry out experiments with these rules.

6.12 A human expert has assigned the waves described by the following strings of $T=\{h, u, d\}$ to a certain class:

hudh
huudh
huhuhddh
huhudh
huhuuddh

Use the successor method in order to determine the state diagram that will recognize these strings.

6.13 Repeat the tank classification experiments, described in section 6.4.1, using other views of tanks available in the *Tanks* dataset. Determine whether an improvement of matching scores can be obtained by using scale and angular normalizations derived from alignment of segment references. Use as segment reference the upper edge of the tank cannon.

6.14 Use an attributed string matching approach for the detection of P waves in ECG signals, selecting one of the waves as prototype. Perform experiments using the column G signal of *ECG Signals.xls*, characterised by the presence of multiple P waves.

6.15 An impulsive signal sometimes appears buried in noise. The signal impulses can be described by:

$$S \xmapsto{0.3} hS; \quad S \xmapsto{0.7} uP; \quad P \xmapsto{0.3} dF; \quad P \xmapsto{0.7} uP;$$

$$F \xmapsto{0.2} dF; \quad F \xmapsto{0.4} hS; \quad F \xmapsto{0.4} uP.$$

a) Draw the state diagram corresponding to these rules.
b) What is the probability of the sequence *uudud* appearing, and what are the sequences most favoured by the transition probabilities?
c) The presence of noise enhances the occurrence rate of saw-tooth sequences of the *udud* type. Modify the transition probabilities so that such sequences have always a probability of occurring below 0.05.

6.16 Consider the chain code description of object contours, presented in section 6.1.2.

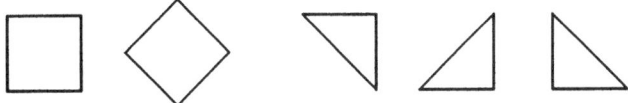

a) Write the string descriptions of the shapes above, assuming that the description starts with the upper left point.
b) Assuming that all sides are equal, as for the square, what is the correspondence rule between descriptions of the same object rotated by multiples of 45°?
c) Taking into consideration the descriptions of the triangles, how should one modify the previous rule in order to obtain the same chain code descriptions of any object rotated by multiples of 45°?
d) How must one modify the algorithm that computes the Levenshtein distance of such chain code strings, so that the matching score obtained is invariant to object rotations by multiples of 45°?

6.17 Consider the tree description of cupboards, as exemplified in Figure 6.6. Discard the body primitive and the *o*, *i* relations. Assume that the cupboards are built in a modular way, with modules constituted by at most two pieces (e.g., a module can have two shelves, another can have a drawer either on the top or on the bottom, etc.). Furthermore, there are equivalent modules; for instance, a module with a top shelf is considered equivalent to another one with a bottom shelf. Develop a discrete relaxation scheme that will be able to determine whether a cupboard includes a given assembly of modules or not.

6.18 Consider the tree description of cupboards as in the previous Exercise.

a) Show that the cupboards can also be described by a string grammar using the symbols of the primitives, plus:

Symbol operators: $\leftarrow$ (left of) ; $\uparrow$ (top of)
Parentheses indicating the precedence order of the operations: ( )

b) Interpret: $(s \uparrow d) \leftarrow (l \uparrow l)$; $((s \uparrow s) \leftarrow e) \uparrow ((d \uparrow d) \leftarrow (l \uparrow r))$.

c) The string grammar description of cupboards can discard the parentheses by using a *reverse Polish notation*, where the string is scanned from right to left, and whenever an operator is encountered, the corresponding operation is performed upon the previous operands. An example of this notation is $\leftarrow \uparrow s \, d \uparrow l \, l$ for the first string of b). Using this notation, what string corresponds to the second string of b)?

d) Perform string matching experiments using strings in reverse Polish notation to describe cupboards.

6.19 Develop a probabilistic relaxation scheme for the classification of profile silhouettes of tanks, using the line segment description presented in section 6.4.1 and available in the *Tanks* dataset.

6.20 A common operation performed on ECG signals consists of temporal alignment of the respective QRS wave sequences (see description in A.4) in order to obtain averaged waves. Consider the string descriptions of QRS wave sequences, using h, u, d, U and D primitives, obtained by the *SigParse* program for the ECGs of the *ECG Signals* dataset. Perform temporal alignment experiments of QRS waves using:

a) String matching.

b) Probabilistic relaxation.

6.21 Recompute the probability matrix **P** of Table 6.4, assuming that the distance between the centroids of A_1, A_2 (Figure 6.21) is 2.2.

6.22 Consider the aerial images of tanks, included in the *Tanks* dataset, with two prototype images TU4 and TU5.

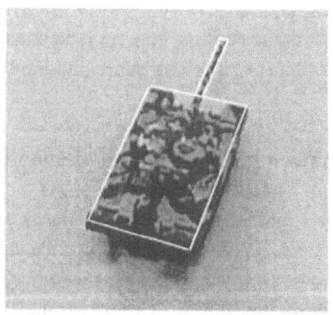

Use probabilistic relaxation in order to classify an "unknown" image as one of these prototypes. For this purpose, consider each tank described by two rectangular regions, as shown in the Figure above, and use the image registration approach described in section 6.4.2. As an alternative to the area of each region use the ratio l/w, where l and w are respectively the length and width of a rectangular region.

6.23 Consider the prototype drawing of Figure 6.23. Use the *Hopfield* program in order to determine the compatible assignments with the line drawings in the Figure below.

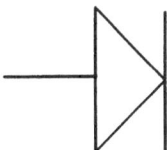 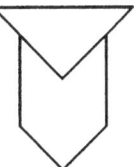

6.24 Use the *Hopfield* program in order to determine the homomorphisms for the graphs shown in Figure 6.28. Compare the results obtained with those of Table 6.7.

Appendix A – CD Datasets

CD datasets are presented in the form of *Microsoft Excel* files and other types of data files with examples of signals and images. All dataset Excel files have a description worksheet.

A.1 Breast Tissue

The *Breast Tissue.xls* file contains 106 electrical impedance measurements performed on samples of freshly excised tissue from the breast. Six classes of tissue were studied:

car - carcinoma (21 cases)
fad - fibro-adenoma (15 cases)
mas - mastopathy (18 cases)
gla - glandular (16 cases)
con - connective (14 cases)
adi - adipose (22 cases)

Impedance measurements were taken at seven frequencies and plotted in the (real, - imaginary) plane, constituting the impedance spectrum from which the features below were computed:

I0   impedivity (ohm) at zero frequency
PA500   phase angle at 500 KHz
HFS   high-frequency slope of phase angle
DA   impedance distance between spectral ends
AREA   area under spectrum
A/DA   area normalized by DA
MAX IP   maximum of the spectrum
DR   distance between I0 and real part of the max. frequency point
P   length of the spectral curve

Source: J Jossinet, INSERM U.281, Lyon, France.
Reference: JE Silva, JP Marques de Sá, J Jossinet (2000) Classification of Breast Tissue by Electrical Impedance Spectroscopy. Med & Bio Eng & Computing, 38:26-30.

A.2 Clusters

The *Clusters.xls* file contains four sets with two-dimensional (A, B) sets of points with different cluster shape:

"Glob" :   globular clusters data
"Filam" :   filamentary clusters data
"+Cross":   + shaped Cross data
"xCross" :   x shaped Cross data

Author: JP Marques de Sá, Engineering Faculty, Oporto University.

A.3 Cork Stoppers

The *Cork Stoppers.xls* file contains measurements performed automatically by an image processing system on 150 cork stoppers belonging to three classes. Each image was digitised with an adequate threshold in order to enhance the defects as shown in Figure A.1.

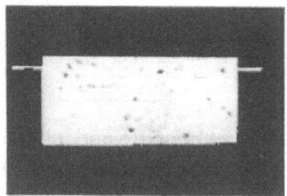 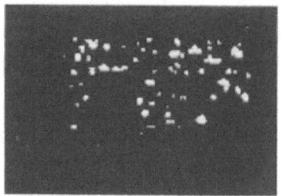

Figure A.1. Example of a cork stopper image at the left and the corresponding binary image of the defects at the right.

The first column of the *Cork Stoppers.xls* spreadsheet contains the class labels assigned by human experts:

ω_1 - Quality Super   (n_1=50 cork stoppers)
ω_2 - Quality Normal   (n_2=50 cork stoppers)
ω_3 - Quality Poor   (n_3=50 cork stoppers)

The following columns contain the measurements performed automatically:

N   :   Total number of defects
PRT :   Total perimeter of the defects (in pixels)
ART :   Total area of the defects (in pixels)

PRM :   Average perimeter of the defects (in pixels)=PRT/N
ARM :   Average area of the defects (in pixels)=ART/N
NG   :   Number of big defects (area bigger than an adequate threshold)
PRTG: Total perimeter of big defects (in pixels)
ARTG: Total area of big defects (in pixels)
RAAR: Area ratio of the defects = ARTG/ART
RAN :   Ratio of the number of defects = NG/N

Source: A Campilho, Engineering Faculty, Oporto University.
Reference: A Campilho (1985), Ph.D. Thesis, Engineering Faculty/DEEC, Oporto
University.

A.4 Crimes

The *Crimes.xls* file contains the number of crimes per thousand inhabitants in
Portuguese districts during 1988, categorized as:

CAPeople - Crimes against people
CAProperty - Crimes against property

Source: "Diário de Notícias" collection, 1989.

A.5 Cardiotocographic Data

The *CTG.xls* file contains measurements and classification results of
cardiotocographic (CTG) examinations of 2126 foetuses. The examinations were
performed at S. João Hospital, Oporto. Cardiotocography is a popular diagnostic
method in Obstetrics, consisting of the analysis and interpretation of the following
signals: foetal heart rate; uterine contractions; foetal movements.

The measurements included in the *CTG.xls* file correspond only to foetal heart
rate features (e.g., basal value, accelerative/decelerative events), computed by an
automatic system. The classification corresponds to a diagnostic category assigned
by expert obstetricians independent of the CTG.

The following cardiotocographic features are available in the *CTG.xls* file:

LBE	baseline value (medical expert)	LB	baseline value (system)
AC	accelerations	FM	foetal movement
UC	uterine contractions		
ASTV	percentage of time with abnormal short term (beat-to-beat) variability		
MSTV	mean value of short term variability		
ALTV	percentage of time with abnormal long term (one minute) variability		
MLTV	mean value of long term variability		
DL	light decelerations	DS	severe decelerations

DP	prolonged decelerations	DR	repetitive decelerations
WIDTH	histogram width (histogram of foetal heart rate values)		
MIN	low freq. of the histogram	MAX	high freq. of the histogram
NMAX	number of histogram peaks	NZER	number of histogram zeros
MODE	histogram mode	MEAN	histogram mean
MEDIAN	histogram median	VAR	histogram variance
TEND	histogram tendency: -1=left assym.; 0=symm.; 1=right assym.		

The data is classified into ten classes:

A   calm sleep
B   rapid eye movement sleep
C   calm vigilance
D   active vigilance
SH   shift pattern (A or SUSP with shifts)
AD   accelerative/decelerative pattern (stress situation)
DE   decelerative pattern (vagal stimulation)
LD   largely decelerative pattern
FS   flat-sinusoidal pattern (pathological state)
SUSP suspect pattern

A column containing the codes of Normal (1), Suspect (2) and Pathologic (3) classification is also included.

Source: J Bernardes, Faculty of Medicine, Oporto University.
Reference: D Ayres de Campos *et al.* (2000) SisPorto 2.0 A Program for Automated Analysis of Cardiotocograms. J Matern Fetal Med 5:311-318.

A.6 Electrocardiograms

The *ECG Signals.xls* file contains seven electrocardiographic signals (ECG) acquired at S. João Hospital, Oporto. An ECG records the electrical activity of the heart. Its amplitude is measured in microvolts and is represented along a column of the Microsoft Excel file, sampled at f_s=250Hz (250 signal rows represent 1 second).

All seven ECG tracings have 5 second durations and basically consist of the repetition of wave packets in correspondence with the atrial and ventricular activities as mentioned in section 1.3 (Figure 1.9):

– P wave: reflects the atrial activity. P waves can be unipolar, positive or negative, or bipolar (positive followed by negative or vice-versa).
– Q, R, S waves: a sequence of high slope negative, positive, negative waves, reflecting the ventricular polarisation. Some of these waves can be absent: an ECG can contain only QR, QS, RS, R or Q sequences.

− T wave: reflects the ventricular depolarisation and can be unipolar, positive or negative, or bipolar (positive followed by negative or vice-versa).

The *ECG Signals.xls* file contains examples illustrating several wave morphologies appropriate for testing structural description methods.

Text files obtained from *ECG Signals.xls* are also included, containing signals processed by the *SigParse* program and illustrated in chapter 6.

Source: C Abreu Lima, JP Marques de Sá, Medicine Faculty, Engineering Faculty, Oporto University.

Reference: C Abreu Lima, JP Marques de Sá (1990) Interpretation of Short ECGs with a Personal Computer: The Porto Program. Methods of Information in Medicine, Schattauer, 29:410-412.

A.7 Foetal Heart Rate Signals

The *FHR Signals.xls* file contains nine foetal heart rate (FHR) signals representing three classes: A - calm sleep; B - rapid eye movement sleep; FS - Flat-sinusoidal (pathologic).

Each FHR signal records the instantaneous frequency of the heart in beats per minute. The signals were acquired at S. João Hospital, Oporto by an automatic system (*SisPorto*). They are appropriate for training structural description of FHR signals, namely the detection of spikes, accelerations and decelerations.

A text file obtained from *FHR Signals.xls* is also included, containing the signal processed by the *SigParse* program and illustrated in chapter 6 (Figure 6.11).

Source: J Bernardes, Faculty of Medicine, Oporto University.

Reference: D Ayres de Campos *et al.* (2000) SisPorto 2.0 A Program for Automated Analysis of Cardiotocograms. J Matern Fetal Med 5:311-318.

A.8 FHR-Apgar

The *FHR-Apgar.xls* file contains 227 measurements of foetal heart rate tracings, recorded just previous to birth, and the respective Apgar index, evaluated by obstetricians according to a standard clinical procedure, one minute and five minutes after birth. All data was collected in Portuguese Hospitals following a strict protocol. The Apgar index is a ranking index in the [0, 10] interval, assessing the well-being of the newborn babies. Low values (below 5) are considered bad prognosis. Normal newborns have an Apgar above 6.

The following measurements are available in the *FHR-Apgar.xls* file:

Apgar1	Apgar measured at 1 minute after birth
Apgar5	Apgar measured at 5 minutes after birth

Duration	Duration in minutes of the FHR tracing
Baseline	Basal value of the FHR in beat/min
Acelnum	Number of FHR accelerations
Acelrate	Number of FHR accelerations per minute
AbSTV	Percentage of time with abnormal short term variability
AverSTV	Average duration of abnormal short term variability
AbLTV	Percentage of time with abnormal long term variability
AverLTV	Average duration of abnormal long term variability

Source: D Ayres de Campos, Faculty of Medicine, Oporto University.
Reference: SisPorto Multicentre Study, http://sisporto.med.up.pt/.

A.9 Firms

The *Firms.xls* file contains values of the following economic indicators relative to 838 Portuguese firms, during the year 1995:

Branch	1=Services; 2=Commerce; 3=Industry; 4=Construction
GI	Gross Income (millions of Portuguese Escudos)
Cap	Invested Capital (millions of Portuguese Escudos)
CA	Capital+Assets
NI	Net Income (millions of Portuguese Escudos) = GI minus wages +taxes
NW	Number of Workers
P	Apparent Productivity=GI/NW
GIR	Gross Income Revenue=NI/GI
CapR	Capital Revenue=NI/Cap
A/C	Assets share =(CA-Cap)/Cap %
Depr	Depreciations + provisions

Source: "Jornal de Notícias" Supplement, November 1995.

A.10 Foetal Weight

The *Foetal Weight.xls* file contains echographic measurements obtained from 414 newborn babies, shortly before delivery, at four Portuguese Hospitals. Obstetricians use such measurements in order to predict the foetal weight at birth.

The following measurements, all obtained under a strict protocol, are available:

MW	Mother weight	MH	Mother height
GA	Gestation age in weeks	DBMB	Days between meas. and birth
BPD	Biparietal diameter	CP	Cephalic perimeter
AP	Abdominal perimeter	FL	Femur length

FTW   Foetal weight at birth
FTL   Foetal length at birth
CPB   Cephalic perimeter at birth

Source: A Matos, S. João Hospital, Oporto.
Reference: F Sereno *et al.* (2000) The Application of Radial Basis Functions and Support Vector Machines to the Foetal Weight Prediction. Intell Eng Syst Through Artif Neural Networks, 10: 801-806.

A.11 Food

The *Food.xls* file contains a table with the following contents for 36 food products:

CAL   Calories per g
P   Phosphor (mg per g)
Ca   Calcium (mg per g)
Fe   Iron (mg per g)
PROT   Proteic substances (mg per g)
B1B2   Vitamins B1 and B2 (mg per g)

Source: Portuguese pharmacy flyer, 1990.

A.12 Fruits

The *Fruits* dataset contains colour image files of apples (22), oranges (15) and peaches (36). The fruit images shown in chapter 1 (Figures 1.1 and 1.2) are also included. All images are in 256 colours, obtained with a low-resolution digital camera.

Source: JP Marques de Sá, Engineering Faculty, Oporto University.

A.13 Impulses on Noise

The *Signal Noise.xls* file contains 100 samples of noise with a chi-square distribution, to which were added impulses with arrival times following a Poisson distribution. The amplitudes of the impulses were also generated with a chi-square distribution.

    A threshold value can be specified in order to detect the signal impulses. Changing the value of the threshold will change the number of true and false impulse detections.

The computed sensibility and specificity are shown at the bottom of the data worksheet.

Author: JP Marques de Sá, Engineering Faculty, Oporto University.

A.14 MLP Sets

The *MLPSets.xls* file contains 26 pairs of points (X1, X2) and 2-class classification columns, exemplifying the following situations:

C1   linearly separable classes with one perceptron
C2   XOR-like classes, separable with a two-layer MLP
C3   Separable with a three-layer MLP

Author: JP Marques de Sá, Faculty of Engineering, Oporto University.

A.15 Norm2c2d

The *Norm2c2d.xls* file contains two sets with $n=50$ points of 2-dimensional distributions with the same covariance matrix. The distributions were generated by linear transformation of $N(0,1)$, using the following transformation matrix:

$$\mathbf{A} = \begin{bmatrix} 1.5 & 0.5 \\ 0.5 & 1 \end{bmatrix}$$

The dataset is as follows:

Set 1: columns n11 and n12;   Mean=[1 1]'
Set 2: columns n21 and n22;   Mean=[3 4]'

$$\text{Covariance} = \begin{bmatrix} 2.5 & 1.25 \\ 1.25 & 1.25 \end{bmatrix}; \quad \text{Inverse Covariance} = \begin{bmatrix} 0.8 & -0.8 \\ -0.8 & 1.6 \end{bmatrix}$$

The distribution parameters can be easily changed, altering the values in the spreadsheet column m, C containing the means and the coefficients of matrix $\mathbf{A}$.

Author: JP Marques de Sá, Engineering Faculty, Oporto University.

A.16 Rocks

The *Rocks.xls* file contains a table of 134 Portuguese rocks with values of oxide composition in percentages (SiO_2, ..., TiO_2) and measurements obtained from physical-mechanical tests:

RMCS   Compression breaking load, norm DIN 52105/E226 (Kg/cm2)
RCSG   Compression breaking load, after freezing/thawing tests, norm DIN 52105/E226 (Kg/cm2)
RMFX   Bending strength, norm DIN 52112 (Kg/cm2)
MVAP   Volumetric weight, norm DIN 52102 (Kg/m3)
AAPN   Water absorption at NP conditions, norm DIN 52103 (%)
PAOA   Apparent porosity, norm LNEC E-216-1968 (%)
CDLT   Thermal linear expansion coefficient (x $10^{-6}/°C$)
RDES   Abrasion test, NP-309 (mm)
RCHQ   Impact test: minimum fall height (cm)

Source: Instituto Geológico Mineiro (IGM), Oporto, Portugal, collected by J. Góis, Engineering Faculty, Oporto University.
Reference: Rochas Ornamentais Portuguesas. Complementary Technical Files, IGM, Oporto, Portugal.

A.17 Stock Exchange

The *Stock Exchange.xls* file contains data from daily share values of Portuguese enterprises (Lisbon Stock Exchange Bourse), together with important economic indicators, during the period of June 1, 1999 through August 31, 2000:

Lisbor6M   Bank of Portugal Interest Rate for 6 months
Euribor6M   European Interest Rate for 6 months
BVL30   Lisbon Stock Exchange index ("Bolsa de Valores de Lisboa")
BCP   Banco Comercial Português
BESC   Banco Espírito Santo
BRISA   Road construction firm
CIMPOR   Cement firm
EDP   Electricity of Portugal
SONAE   Large trade firm
PTEL   Portuguese telephones
CHF   Swiss franc (exchange rate in Euros)
JPY   Japanese yen (exchange rate in Euros)
USD   US dollar (exchange rate in Euros)

Source: Bulletins of Portuguese banks.

A.18 Tanks

The *Tanks* dataset contains:

- Grey-level image files (12) of tank models. They comprise profile views of three prototype tanks (T1, T2 and T3) and three views of each prototype (numbered T_{ij}, where i refers to the prototype and j to the view), taken at variable distance and perspective.
- Processed images of the tank models, with piecewise linear contours superimposed. The contours were determined using an active contour technique, with adjusted number of segments.
- Excel file with two columns for each tank containing the length and the angular orientation of each contour segment, in clockwise traversing order, starting at the lower corner of the cannon mouth.

Source: JP Marques de Sá, Jorge Barbosa, Engineering Faculty, Oporto University.

A.19 Weather

The *Weather.xls* file contains the measurements made at 12H00 for the period of January 1, 1999 through August 23, 2000 of the following variables:

T   Temperature (°C)
H   Humidity (%)
WS   Wind speed (m/s)
WD   Wind direction (anticlockwise, relative to North)
NS   Projection of WD in the North-South direction
EW   Projection of WD in the East-West direction

Source: "Estação Meteorológica da FEUP", Weather Station (WEB Service), authored by J Góis, Engineering Faculty, Oporto University.

Appendix B – CD Tools

CD tools include both didactical *Microsoft Excel* files and installable programs for assisting in PR design.

B.1 Adaptive Filtering

The *ECG 50Hz.xls* file allows one to perform adaptive filtering of a 50Hz noise signal added to an electrocardiographic signal (ECG), using an LMS linear discriminant (two-input linear neural network). The user can change the learning rate and other parameters of the filter in order to get insight into the learning properties of the gradient descent method.
   Variables:

T	Time in seconds	ECG	Original ECG signal
sin	50 Hz sinusoidal noise	nG	Noise gain
t	Target signal: ECG + noise	eta	Learning factor
n1, n2	Discriminant inputs	r	Discriminant output
w1, w2	Weights	e	Error signal
phi	Phase angle of discriminant inputs		
g	Amplitude factor of discriminant inputs		

Author: JP Marques de Sá, Engineering Faculty, Oporto University.

B.2 Density Estimation

The *Parzen.xls* file allows one to perform experiments of density estimation on data with *log norm* distribution, using the Parzen window method. The user can see the effect of changing the window width and the number of training samples. A worksheet containing the values of feature ARM for the first two classes of the *Cork Stoppers* dataset allows one to perform a Bayesian classification based on Parzen window estimation of the distributions.

Author: JP Marques de Sá, Engineering Faculty, Oporto University.

B.3 Design Set Size

The *PR Size* program is intended to provide some guidance to the PR designer on the choice of the appropriate system complexity, given the design set size. It has the following modules:

SC Size (Statistical Classifier Design)

Displays a picture box containing graphics of the following variables, for a two-class linear classifier with specified Battacharrya distance and for several values of the dimensionality ratio, n/d:

Bayes error;
Expected design set error (resubstitution method);
Expected test set error (holdout method).

Both classes are assumed to be represented by the same number of patterns per class, n.

The user only has to specify the dimension d and the square of the Battacharrya distance (computable by several statistical software products).

For any chosen value of n/d, the program also displays the standard deviations of the error estimates when the mouse is clicked over a selected point of the picture box.

The expected design and test set errors are computed using the formulas presented in the work of Foley (1972) mentioned in the bibliography of Chapter 4. The formula for the expected test set error is an approximation formula, which can produce slightly erroneous values, below the Bayes error, for certain n/d ratios.

NN Size (Neural Network Design)

Displays tables of the following values, for a two-class two-layer MLP and for a user-specified interval of the number of hidden nodes, h:

– Number of neurons.
– Number of weights (including biases).
– Lower bound of the Vapnik-Chervonenkis dimension (formula 5-52).
– Upper bound of the Vapnik-Chervonenkis dimension (formula 5-56).
– Lower bound of learning set size needed for generalization (formula 5-53).
– Upper bound of learning set size sufficient for generalization (formula 5-56a).

The user has to specify the dimension, d, corresponding to the number of MLP inputs, the training set error and the confidence level of the training set error.

Author: JP Marques de Sá, Engineering Faculty, Oporto University.

B.4 Error Energy

The *Error Energy.xls* file allows the inspection of error energy surfaces corresponding to several LMS discriminants, including the possibility of inspecting the progress of a gradient descent process for one of the examples (iterations performed along the columns).

The following worksheets, exemplifying different LMS situations, are included:

minglob
   Error energy surface for an LMS discriminant with 2 target values (-1, 1), with only a global minimum. There are two variable weights, one with values along the rows of column A, the other with values along columns B1 to B11.

minglob2
   Similar to minglob for an error energy surface with two global minima, corresponding to 3 target points (1, 0, 1).

minloc
   Similar to minglob2 with the possibility of positioning the "3rd point" in order to generate error energy surfaces with local minima (see section 5.2, Figure 5.9).

minloc(zoom), minloc(zoom1)
   Zoomed areas of minloc for precise minima determination.

perceptron
   Similar to minglob using the perceptron learning rule.

ellipt-error
   Ellipsoidal error surface ($a^2+pb^2-2a-qb+1$), including the possibility for the user to inspect the progress of gradient descent, by performing iterations along the columns, namely by specifying the initial values for the weights and the learning rate.
   The worksheet columns are labelled as:

eta	Learning rate
a(new), b(new)	New weight values
dE/da, dE/db	Error derivatives
da db	Weight increments

Author: JP Marques de Sá, Engineering Faculty, Oporto University.

B.5 Genetic Neural Networks

The *Neuro-Genetic* program allows the user to perform classification of patterns using multilayer perceptrons (up to three layers) trained with the back-propagation or with a genetic algorithm. It is therefore possible to compare both training methods.

In order to use *Neuro-Genetic*, an MLP classification project must first be defined (go to menu *Project* and select *New Project* or click the appropriate button in the toolbar), specifying the following items:

1. Data file. This is a text file with the information organized by rows and columns, separated by tabs. Each column corresponds to a network input or output and each row corresponds to a different pattern.
2. Training set and test set. To specify the training set input values, the initial and final columns and the initial and final rows in the data file should be indicated. For the output values, only the initial and final columns are needed (the rows are the same). The same procedure must be followed for the test set.
3. Training procedure (genetic algorithm or back-propagation).
4. Neural network architecture. It is possible to specify a network with 1 or 2 hidden layers . One linear output layer (with the purpose of scaling the output value) can also be specified. If the check box corresponding to the linear output layer is checked, the number of neurons for the first hidden and second hidden layers must be indicated.
5. Initial weights. The complete path for the initial weight file must also be filled in, or else a file with random weights must be generated (by clicking the appropriate button). This file includes all the weights and bias values for the defined neural network. It is a text file, with extension *.wgt*, containing the weight values in individual rows, ordered as:

$w_{n-i/j}$, where

n varies from 1 to the number of layers (includes output layer);
i varies from 1 to the number of neurons in that layer;
j varies from 0 (bias value) to the number of inputs or neurons in the previous layer (if $n>1$).

Once a project has been defined, it can be saved for later re-use with the menu option *Save Project*. Network training can be started (or stopped) using the respective buttons. No validation set is used during training, therefore the user must decide when to stop the training, otherwise training stops when the specified error goal or the maximum number of iterations is reached.

Once the training is complete the user can inspect the weights and the predicted values and errors in the training set and test set. It is also possible to visualize the error evolution during the training procedure by selecting the *Errors Chart* option.

The following parameters must be indicated independently of the training technique:

- Error goal;
- Maximum number of iterations;
- Number of iterations between chart updates.

When back-propagation training is chosen, the following values must be indicated:

- Learning rate;
- Learning rate increase;
- Learning rate decrease;
- Momentum factor;
- Maximum error ratio.

When genetic algorithm training is chosen, the following values must be indicated:

- Initial population;
- Mutation rate;
- Crossover rate;
- Crossover type.

The following crossover types can be specified:

- 1 point crossover: change 1 point value between 2 population elements, using the crossover rate as probability.
- 2 points crossover: change 2 point values between 2 population elements, using the crossover rate as probability.
- Uniform crossover: perform a uniform change of point values between 2 population elements, using the crossover rate as probability.
- NN 1 point crossover: change the values corresponding to the weights and bias of 1 neuron between 2 population elements, using the crossover rate as probability.
- NN 2 points crossover: change the values corresponding to the weights and bias of 2 neurons between 2 population elements, using the crossover rate as probability.
- NN uniform crossover: perform a uniform change of the values corresponding to the neurons' weights and bias between 2 population elements, using the crossover rate as probability.
- Elitism: the population element with lowest error will always be transferred without any change to the next generation.

The following training results appear in the training results frame and are continuously updated during the learning process:

- Training set error;

- Iteration number;
- Average time for each iteration (epoch);
- Total learning time;
- Test set error;
- Learning rate value (only for back-propagation).

Neuro-Genetic also affords the possibility of creating macros for sequences of projects to be executed sequentially. The next project in the sequence will be started after the execution of the previous one is finished. By double-clicking over the line of a column project a selection box appears for easy insertion of the project file name (with extension *.prj*). The macro can be saved in a file with extension *.mcr*.

This macro possibility can be particularly useful when a network is first trained during some epochs with a genetic algorithm (attempting to escape local minima), followed by back-propagation training for a quicker and finer adjustment.

An examples folder is included, containing the project files for an XOR-like dataset and for the cork stoppers dataset used in the experiment described in section 5.8.

Author: A Garrido, Engineering Faculty, Oporto University.

B.6 Hopfield network

The *Hopfield* program implements a discrete Hopfield network appropriate for CAM experiments with binary patterns, and for discrete relaxation matching. In this case, the binary patterns represent object assignments.

The binary patterns are specified in a rectangular grid whose dimensions, *mxn*, are specified by the user at the beginning of each experiment. When the patterns are read in from a file, with the button "Load", the dimensions are set to the values specified in the file. A binary pattern can also be saved in a file with the button "Save".

Files with binary patterns are text files with the extension *.HNF*. The first line of the text file has the information regarding the grid dimensions. Example:

```
[9X6]
0 0 0 0 0 0
0 0 1 1 1 0
0 1 0 0 0 1
0 1 0 0 0 1
0 1 0 0 0 1
0 1 0 0 0 1
0 1 0 0 0 1
0 1 0 0 0 1
0 1 0 0 0 1
```

The user can specify the desired pattern directly on the grid, either by clicking each grid cell or by dragging the mouse over grid cells, then inverting the previous values of those cells. "Clear Window" clears the whole grid.

In order to use the network as a CAM device, proceed as follows:

1. The prototype patterns must either be loaded or specified in the grid, and then memorized using the "Store" button. When loading from a file, they are immediately stored if the "Load and Store" option is set. Using the scroll bar, each of the stored prototypes can be inspected.
2. Choose "Random serial" in the combo box for asynchronous updating of the weights. In "Full serial", mode the neurons are updated in sequence from (1,1) to (m, n).
3. Draw or load in the grid the unknown binary pattern to be classified. Random noise with uniform distribution can be added to this pattern by clicking on the button "Add Noise". When needed, use the "Clear Window" button to wipe out the pattern from the grid.
4. Use "Recall" to train the net until the best matching prototype is retrieved. Use "Step" to inspect the successive states until the final state. The "Used as a Classifier" option should be selected before "Recall" to impose the final selection of the best matching prototype; otherwise the final state is displayed. The weight matrix can be inspected with the "Get Weight" button.

A new experiment with other dimensions must be preceded by "Clean", wiping out all the stored prototype patterns.

In order to use the network for discrete relaxation matching, proceed as follows:

1. Dimension the grid with the set cardinalities of the two sets to be matched.
2. Fill in the weight matrix using the "New Weight" button. The weights can be edited either directly or loaded in from a file with the same format as above with extension .HNW. Only one half of the matrix has to be specified if the "Matrix is Symmetric" option is selected. In this case, when editing cell (i,j), the cell (j,i) gets the same value.
3. When filling in the weight matrix, it is convenient to start by clicking the "Weights Initialisation" button, which initializes all matrix values with the one specified in the text box. See section 6.4.4 for the choice of weight values.
4. Choose the "Full parallel" mode in the combo box, imposing a synchronous updating of all neurons.
5. Click "Step" to update the assignment probabilities.

When performing several experiments with the same weight matrix, it is usually convenient to define it only once and save it using the "Save" button. The weight matrix can also be cleared using the "Clear Weight" button.

Author: Paulo Sousa, Engineering Faculty, Oporto University.

B.7 k-NN Bounds

The *k-NN Bounds.xls* file allows the computation of error bounds for a k-NN classifier. Bounds for a number of neighbours k=1, 3, 9 and 21 are already computed and presented (p denotes the Bayes error). Bounds for other values of k are easily computed by filling in the $C(k, i)$ column.

Author: JP Marques de Sá, Engineering Faculty, Oporto University.

B.8 k-NN Classification

The *KNN* program allows k-NN classification to be performed on a two-class dataset using either a partition or an edition approach.
    Data is read from a text file with the following format:

n	number of patterns.
n_1	number of patterns of the first class.
d	dimension.
...	n lines with d values, first n_1 lines for the first class, followed by n-n_1 lines for the second class.

The first line of the text file is the total number of patterns, n (n $\leq$ 500); n_1 is the number of patterns belonging to class ω_1; d is the number of features ($d \leq 6$). Succeeding lines represent the feature vectors, with d feature values separated by commas. The first n_1 lines must contain the feature values relative to class ω_1 patterns.
    In the "Specifications" frame the user must fill in the file name, the value of k (number of neighbours) and choose either the partition or the edit method. If the partition method is chosen, the number of partitions must also be specified.
    Classification of the data is obtained by clicking the "Compute" button. The program then shows the classification matrix with the class and overall test set errors, in percentage values. For the partition method, the standard deviation of the errors across the partitions is also presented.
    Suppose that the distributed *N-PRT10.txt* file is used. This file contains the N, *PRT10* feature values corresponding to the first two classes of the cork stoppers data, with a total of 100 patterns, the first 50 from class ω_1.
    Performing a k-NN classification with one neighbour and 2 partitions, one obtains an overall error of 21% with 9.9% standard deviation. If the "Stepwise" box is checked, the classification matrices for the individual partitions can be observed. For the first step, patterns 1 through 25 and 51 though 75 are used for test, the others for training. An overall error of 28% is obtained. For the second step, the set roles are reversed and an overall error of 14% is obtained. The individual test set errors are distributed around the 21% average value with 9.9% standard deviation.

Performing a K-NN classification with one neighbour and the "edit" approach, the data is partitioned into two halves. A resubstitution classification method is applied to the first half, which is classified with 10% error. Edition is then performed by "discarding" the wrongly classified patterns. Finally, the second half is classified using the edited first half. An overall test set error of 18% is obtained.

Author: JP Marques de Sá, Engineering Faculty, Oporto University.

B.9 Perceptron

The *Perceptron* program has didactical purposes, showing how the training of a linear discriminant using the perceptron learning rule progresses in a pattern-by-pattern learning fashion for the case of separable and non-separable pattern clusters.

The patterns are handwritten *u*'s and *v*'s drawn in an 8x7 grid. Two features computed from these grids are used (see section 5.3). The user can choose either a set of linearly separable patterns (set 1) or not (set 2).

Placing the cursor on each point displays the corresponding *u* or *v*.

Learning progresses by clicking the button "Step" or "Enter", in this case allowing fast repetition.

Authors: JP Marques de Sá, F Sousa, Engineering Faculty, Oporto University.

B.10 Syntactic Analysis

The *SigParse* program allows syntactic analysis experiments of signals to be performed and has the following main functionalities:

- Linear piecewise approximation of a signal.
- Signal labelling.
- String parsing using a finite-state automaton.

Usually, operation with *SigParse* proceeds as follows:

1. Read in a signal from a text file, where each line is a signal value, up to a maximum of 2000 signal samples. The signal is displayed in a picture box with scroll, 4x zoom and sample increment ("step") facilities. The signal values are also shown in a list box.
2. Derive a linear piecewise approximation of the signal, using the algorithm described in section 6.1.1. The user specifies the approximation norm and a deviation tolerance for the line segments. Good results are usually obtained using the Chebychev norm. The piecewise linear approximation is displayed in the picture box with black colour, superimposed on the original signal displayed

with grey colour. The program also shows the number of line segments obtained and lists the length (number of samples), accumulated length and slope of each line segment in a "results" list box.

3. Perform signal labelling by specifying two slope thresholds, s_1 and s_2. Line segments with absolute slope values below s_1 are labelled h (horizontal) and displayed green. Above s_1 are labelled u (up) or d (down), according to the slope sign (positive or negative) and are displayed with red or cyan colour, respectively. Above s_2 are labelled U (large up) or D (large down), according to the slope sign (positive or negative) and are displayed with magenta or blue colour, respectively. The labels are shown in the "results" list box.

4. Specify a state transition table of a finite-state automaton, either by directly filling in the table or by reading in the table from a text file (the "Table" option must be checked then), where each line corresponds to a table row with the symbols separated by commas. The table has a maximum of 50 rows. The letter "F" must be used to designate final states.

5. Parse the signal. Line segments corresponding to final states are shown in black colour. State symbols resulting from the parse operation are shown in the "results" list box.

The contents of the "results" list box can be saved in a text file. The user can perform parsing experiments for the same string by modifying the state transition table.

The program also allows the user to parse any string read in with the "String" option checked. The corresponding text file must have a string symbol (character) per line.

Author: JP Marques de Sá, Engineering Faculty, Oporto University.

Appendix C - Orthonormal Transformation

Suppose that we are presented with feature vectors $\mathbf{y}$ that have correlated features and covariance matrix $\mathbf{C}$. The aim is to determine a linear transformation that will yield a new space with uncorrelated features. Following the explanation in section 2.3, assume that we knew the linear transformation matrix $\mathbf{A}$ that generated the vectors, $\mathbf{y} = \mathbf{A}\mathbf{x}$, with $\mathbf{x}$ representing feature vectors that have unit covariance matrix $\mathbf{I}$ as illustrated in Figure 2.9.

Given $\mathbf{A}$, it is a simple matter to determine the matrix $\mathbf{Z}$ of its unit length eigenvectors:

$$\mathbf{Z} = \begin{bmatrix} \mathbf{z}_1 & \mathbf{z}_2 & \dots & \mathbf{z}_d \end{bmatrix}, \tag{B-1}$$

with $\mathbf{z}_i'\mathbf{z}_j = 0$ and $\mathbf{Z}'\mathbf{Z} = \mathbf{I}$ (i.e., $\mathbf{Z}$ is an *orthonormal matrix*). $\tag{B-1a}$

Let us now apply to the feature vectors $\mathbf{y}$ a linear transformation with the transpose of $\mathbf{Z}$, obtaining new feature vectors $\mathbf{u}$:

$$\mathbf{u} = \mathbf{Z}'\mathbf{y}. \tag{B-2}$$

Notice that from the definition of eigenvectors, $\mathbf{A}\mathbf{z}_i = \lambda_i \mathbf{z}_i$, one has:

$$\mathbf{A}\mathbf{Z} = \Lambda\mathbf{Z}, \tag{B-3}$$

where Λ is the diagonal matrix of the eigenvalues:

$$\Lambda = \begin{bmatrix} \lambda_1 & 0 & \dots & 0 \\ 0 & \lambda_2 & \dots & 0 \\ \dots & \dots & \dots & \dots \\ 0 & 0 & \dots & \lambda_d \end{bmatrix}. \tag{B-4}$$

Using (B-3) and well-known matrix properties, one can compute the new covariance matrix $\mathbf{K}$ of the feature vectors $\mathbf{u}$, as:

$$\mathbf{K} \overset{(2-18b)}{=} \mathbf{Z}'\mathbf{C}\mathbf{Z} = \mathbf{Z}'\mathbf{A}\mathbf{I}\mathbf{A}'\mathbf{Z} = \mathbf{Z}'\mathbf{A}\mathbf{A}'\mathbf{Z} \overset{(\text{A is symmetric})}{=} \mathbf{Z}'\mathbf{A}'\mathbf{A}\mathbf{Z} =$$
$$= (\mathbf{A}\mathbf{Z})'\mathbf{A}\mathbf{Z} \overset{(B-3)}{=} (\Lambda\mathbf{Z})'\Lambda\mathbf{Z} = \mathbf{Z}'\Lambda^2\mathbf{Z} = \Lambda^2\mathbf{Z}'\mathbf{Z} \overset{(B-1a)}{=} \Lambda^2. \tag{B-5}$$

Conclusions:

- The linear and orthonormal transformation with matrix $\mathbf{Z'}$ does indeed transform correlated features into uncorrelated ones.
- The squares of the eigenvalues of $\mathbf{A}$ are the variances in the new system of coordinates.

It can also be shown that:

- The orthonormal transformation preserves the Mahalanobis distances, the matrix Λ of the eigenvalues and the determinant of the covariance matrix.
  Notice that the determinant of the covariance matrix has a physical interpretation as the volume of the pattern cluster.
- The orthonormal transformation can also be performed with the transpose matrix of the eigenvectors of $\mathbf{C}$. This is precisely what is usually done, since in a real problem we seldom know the matrix $\mathbf{A}$. The only difference is that now the eigenvalues themselves are the new variances.
  For the example of section 2.3 (Figure 2.15), the new variances would be $\lambda_1 = 6.854$ and $\lambda_2 = 0.1458$.

We present two other interesting results:

Positive definiteness

Consider the quadratic form of a real and symmetric matrix $\mathbf{C}$ with all eigenvalues positive:

$$d^2 = \mathbf{y'Cy}. \tag{B-6}$$

Without loss of generality, we can assume the vectors $\mathbf{y}$ originated from an orthonormal transformation of the vectors $\mathbf{x}$: $\mathbf{y} = \mathbf{Zx}$. Thus:

$$d^2 = \mathbf{y'Cy} = (\mathbf{Zx})'\mathbf{C}(\mathbf{Zx}) = \mathbf{x'Z'CZx} = \mathbf{x'}\Lambda\mathbf{x} = \sum_{i=1}^{d} \lambda_i x_i^2 \ . \tag{B-7}$$

This proves that d^2 is positive for all non-null $\mathbf{x}$.

Since covariance (and correlation) matrices are real symmetrical matrices with positive eigenvalues (representing variances after the orthonormal transformation), they are also *positive definite*.

Whitening transformation

Suppose that after applying the orthonormal transformation to the vectors $\mathbf{y}$, as expressed in (B-2), we apply another linear transformation using the matrix Λ^{-1}. The new covariance is:

$$K = \Lambda^{-1} \Lambda^2 \Lambda^{-1} = I. \tag{B-8}$$

Therefore, this transformation yields uncorrelated and equal variance (whitened) features.

The use of uncorrelated features is often desirable. Unfortunately, the whitening transformation is not orthonormal and, therefore, does not preserve the Euclidian distances.

Through a process similar to the whitening transformation it is also possible to perform the simultaneous diagonalisation of two distributions, therefore obtaining uncorrelated features in two-class classification problems. Details on this method can be obtained from (Fukunaga, 1990).

Index